Drug-Induced
Ocular Side Effects
and Drug Interactions

Drug-Induced Ocular Side Effects and Drug Interactions

F. T. FRAUNFELDER, M.D.

Professor and Chairman
Department of Ophthalmology
University of Arkansas Medical Center
Little Rock Veterans Administration
Arkansas Children's Hospital
Little Rock, Arkansas

Lea & Febiger

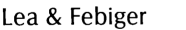

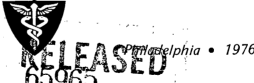

Philadelphia • 1976

Library of Congress Cataloging in Publication Data

Fraunfelder, F   T
   Drug-induced ocular side effects and drug interactions.

   Includes bibliographical references and index.
   1. Ocular pharmacology. 2. Drugs—Side effects.
3. Drug interactions. I. Title. [DNLM: 1. Drug
therapy—Adverse effects.   2.   Drug interactions.
3. Eye—Drug effects. 4. Iatrogenic disease.
WW100 F845d]   -   -
RE994.F7   615'.78   76-12572
ISBN   0-8121-0551-6

Published in Great Britain by Henry Kimpton Publishers, London
Printed in the United States of America

To
Yvonne, Yvette, Helene Jean,
Nina, Ricky, and Nicholas

FOREWORD

This reference work will be a fitting companion for the clinical ophthalmologist in both office and hospital. With startling clarity, the author impresses the ophthalmologist with the importance of asking each patient: "What medicines are you taking?" Whatever the reply, the ophthalmologist can determine its significance by consulting this thoughtfully prepared book.

As Sir William Osler said: "To study the phenomena of disease without books is to sail an uncharted sea, while to study books without patients is not to go to sea at all." Dr. Fraunfelder's book is a worthy follower of the Oslerian tradition, using the master word of Osler: "Work." The author has surveyed the literature extensively and has compiled huge amounts of data about the clinical significance of drugs, their side effects, and their cross reactions. This information is especially useful when a patient is taking drugs with which the ophthalmologist is not familiar.

However, I wish that the list could include, between the letter O and the letter Q, the word Physician. I believe that treating the patient with oneself, the physician, is the most important remedy that doctors have had or ever will have.

Robert P. Burns, M.D.
Professor
Department of Ophthalmology
University of Oregon Medical School

PREFACE

The clinician is overwhelmed by the volume of ocular toxicology in the medical literature and is in need of a reference book that "boils it down." It is for the busy practitioner that this book is designed. The subject of our work is the *probable* medication-induced ocular side effects and the *possible* interactions of drugs prescribed by the ophthalmologist with those the patient is already taking. These areas are of increasing importance to the clinician, and possibly only in presentations of this type can he efficiently make use of the volume of data available. If a patient receiving medication has ocular signs or symptoms, these are not necessarily drug-related. It is the physician's experience, his knowledge, and previous reports on the effects of a particular drug that will lead him to suspect a drug relationship. In a controlled experimental environment it is often difficult to prove that a sign or symptom is drug related; in clinical practice, with multiple variables, it may in many instances be impossible. The clinician, however, needs to remember that there is no active drug known which is without undesirable side actions. It is the intent of this book to compile and organize "previous reports" into a format useful to the physician. No animal data have been included, since ocular toxicologic studies, except in primates, have had limited clinical correlation. Owing to the nature of this book and the volume of material covered, errors, omissions, and misemphasis are inevitable. In the hope of improving future editions, I welcome suggestions or corrections.

Data in this book have been accumulated by innumerable physicians and scientists who have suspected adverse reactions secondary to drug therapy. My sincere thanks to Sir Duke-Elder and Dr. Calvin Hanna for their helpful comments and constructive suggestions, and to Professor Barrie Jones, Institute of Ophthalmology and Moorfields Eye Hospital, London, England, in whose department this book was completed. The enormous amount of library research and organization has been most ably done by Mrs. Martha Meyer and her assistant, Miss Robin Ross, without whom this text would not have been possible. Also, many thanks to Mrs. Lee Hallmark and Mrs. Margaret Casinger for hours of secretarial work expertly performed.

Little Rock, Arkansas   F. T. Fraunfelder, M.D.

INSTRUCTIONS TO USERS

The basic format used in each chapter for each drug or group of drugs in this book includes

Class: The general category of the primary action of the drug is given.

Generic Name: The United States national formulary name of each drug is listed. A name in parenthesis following the national formulary name is the international generic name if it differs from the one used in the United States.

Proprietary Name: The more common trade names are given. In a group of drugs, the number before a generic name corresponds to the number preceding the proprietary drug. This is true for both the systemic and ophthalmic forms of the drug. If a proprietary name differs from that of the United States, the country is given in parentheses after that particular proprietary name. Combination drugs are seldom included.

Primary Use: The type of drug and its current use in the management of various conditions are listed.

Ocular Side Effects:
   A. Systemic Administration — Ocular side effects as reported from oral, intravenous, intramuscular, or intrathecal administration.
   B. Local Ophthalmic Use or Exposure — Ocular side effects as reported from topical ocular application or subconjunctival, retrobulbar, or intracameral injection.
   C. Inadvertent Ocular Exposure — Ocular side effects as reported due to accidental ocular exposure from any form of the drug.
   The ocular side effects are listed in probable order of importance. The determination of importance is based on incidence of significance of the side effect. Side effects of inadequate documentation or current debate are followed by (?). The name of a drug in parenthesis adjacent to an adverse reaction indicates that this is the only agent in the group reported to have caused this side effect.

Clinical Significance: A concise overview of the general importance is given to the clinician of the ocular side effects produced.

Interactions with Other Drugs:
   A. Effect of This Drug on Activity of Other Drugs
   B. Effect of Other Drugs on Activity of This Drug
   C. Synergistic Activity
   D. Cross Sensitivity
   E. Contraindications — specific

The amount of data in this area is voluminous. To make its use practical, only drugs which ophthalmologists might commonly prescribe are listed. If no interactions are listed, then none of major significance to the ophthalmologist have been reported. The symbol (↑) means enhanced or increased effect on the activity of a drug while (↓) means decreased effect on the activity of a drug. When (↑↓) is used, this means a variable response, in some cases increased, in others decreased.

References: References have been limited to either the best articles, the most current, or to those with the most complete bibliography. Since references for drug interactions are even more extensive, to save space they have not been included; however, a majority of the references are cited in Martin, E. W. (Ed.): *Hazards of Medication.* Philadelphia, J. B. Lippincott Co., 1971; Hansten, P. D.: *Drug Interactions.* 3rd Ed., Philadelphia, Lea & Febiger, 1975; and Garb, S.: *Clinical Guide to Undesirable Drug Interactions and Interferences.* New York, Springer Publishing Co., Inc., 1971.

Index of Side Effects: The lists of adverse ocular side effects due to drugs are intended in part to be indexes in themselves. The adverse ocular reactions are not separated in this index as to route of administration; however, this can be obtained by going to the text.

Index: The index includes both the drugs' generic and proprietary names. No indexing of drug interactions has been done, but this can be obtained by looking up the specific drug. The index is the primary source of entry into this book. This is a necessity since many drugs are in groups and would otherwise be missed.

In the following section, the services of the National Registry of Drug-Induced Ocular Side Effects are outlined. The intent of this registry is to make available data of possible drug-induced ocular side effects and to provide a central area where possible adverse ocular drug reactions can be reported.

* *

NATIONAL REGISTRY OF DRUG-INDUCED OCULAR SIDE EFFECTS

Rationale:

Collecting clinical data of drug-induced side effects for any organ system is still in its infancy. Reporting systems, registries, and surveys are currently being used along with costly prospective studies; however, none of these are being extensively used in ophthalmology. In a specialized area such as ophthalmology, seldom does a practitioner or even a group of practitioners see the patient volume necessary to make a correlation between possible cause and effect of drug-related or drug-induced ocular disease. A national registry to correlate this type of data may be of value, since this task would be difficult to carry out by any other method. If a number of these "possible" associations are found with a particular drug, then definitive controlled studies could be undertaken to obtain valid data. It is hoped that future editions of this book will present data with greater scientific significance, in part due to the reports of possible drug-induced ocular side effects which physicians will send to the registry.

Objectives:

To establish a national center where possible drug-induced ocular side effects can be accumulated.

To review possible drug-induced ocular side effect data collected through the FDA Forum 1639 and the FDA total community studies.

To compile the data in the world literature on reports of possible drug-induced ocular side effects.

To make available this data to physicians who feel they have a possible drug-induced ocular side effect.

Format:

The cases of primary interest are those adverse ocular reactions not previously recognized and those that are rare, severe, serious, or unusual. Data, to be of value, should be complete and follow the basic format as shown below.

Age:

Sex:

Suspected drug — trade name:

Suspected reaction — date of onset:

Route, dose and when drug started:

Improvement after suspected drug stopped — if restarted, did adverse reaction recur:

Other drugs taken at time of suspected adverse reaction:

Comments — optional: (Your opinion if drug-induced, probably related, possibly related, or unrelated.)

Your name and address — optional:

We would welcome, however, your impressions even without specific cases. To ensure confidentiality, no names of patients or physicians are used in any files or reports. This will protect you and the registry from legal interference.

Send to:

Ms. Martha Meyer, Associate Director
National Registry of Drug-Induced Ocular Side Effects
University of Arkansas for Medical Sciences
4301 W. Markham Street
Little Rock, Arkansas 72201

Phone: (501) 661-6011

Abbreviations

($\uparrow$) — Increase
($\downarrow$) — Decrease
($\uparrow\downarrow$) — Variable response — increased or decreased
Arg. — Argentina
Austral. — Australia
Aust. — Austria
Belg. — Belgium
Braz. — Brazil
Canad. — Canada
Cz. — Czechoslovakia
Denm. — Denmark
Fr. — France
G.B. — Great Britain
Germ. — Germany
Ind. — India
Isr. — Israel
Ital. — Italy
Jap. — Japan
Neth. — Netherlands
Norw. — Norway
Pol. — Poland
Scand. — Scandinavian
Span. — Spanish
Swed. — Sweden
Switz. — Switzerland
U.S.S.R. — Union of Soviet Socialist Republics

CONTENTS

I. Anti-infectives

Class: Amebicides

Generic Name: 1. Amodiaquine; 2. Chloroquine; 3. Hydroxychloroquine. See under *Class: Antimalarial Agents.*

* * * * * * * * * * * *

Generic Name: 1. Diiodohydroxyquin (Diiodohydroxyquinoline); 2. Iodochlorhydroxyquin

Proprietary Name: 1. Diodoquin, Embequin (G.B.), Floroquin, Vaam-DHQ (Austral.), Yodoxin; 2. Enteroquin (Austral.), Entero-Vioform

Primary Use: These amebicidal agents are effective against *Entamoeba histolytica.*

Ocular Side Effects

A. Systemic Administration
1. Decreased vision
2. Optic atrophy
3. Optic neuritis — subacute myelo-opticoneuropathy
4. Nystagmus
5. Blindness
6. Macular edema
7. Macular degeneration
8. Diplopia
9. Absence of foveal reflex
10. Problems with color vision
    a. Dyschromatopsia
    b. Purple spots on white background
11. Corneal opacities (?)

Clinical Significance: Major toxic ocular effects may occur with long-term oral administration of these amebicidal agents. Since they are given orally for *Entamoeba histolytica*, most reports are from the Far East. Data suggest that these amebicides may cause subacute myelo-opticoneuropathy (SMON). This neurologic disease has a 19 percent incidence of decreased vision and a 2.5 percent incidence of blindness. Possibly diiodohydroxyquin causes fewer side effects since less is absorbed through the gastrointestinal tract than with iodochlorhydroxyquin.

1

References

Behrens, M. M.: Optic atrophy in children after diiodohydroxyquin therapy. JAMA *228*:693, 1974.

Berggren, L. and Hansson, O.: Treating acrodermatitis enteropathica. Lancet *1*:52, 1966.

Etheridge, J. E., Jr., and Stewart, G. T.: Treating acrodermatitis enteropathica. Lancet *1*:261, 1966.

Nakae, K., Yamamoto, S., and Igata, A.: Subacute myelo-optico-neuropathy (SMON) in Japan. Lancet *2*:510, 1971.

Van Balen, A. T. M.: Toxic damage to the optic nerve caused by iodochlorhydroxyquinoline (Enteovioform). Ophthalmologica *163*:8, 1971.

Warshawsky, R. S., et al.: Acrodermatitis enteropathica. Corneal involvement with histochemical and electron micrographic studies. Arch. Ophthalmol. *93*:194, 1975.

* * * * * * * * * * * * *

Generic Name: Emetine

Proprietary Name: Emetine

Primary Use: This alkaloid is effective in the treatment of acute amebic dysentery, amebic hepatitis, and amebic abscesses.

Ocular Side Effects

A. Systemic Administration
　　1. Nonspecific ocular irritation
　　　　a. Lacrimation
　　　　b. Hyperemia
　　　　c. Photophobia
　　2. Pupils
　　　　a. Mydriasis
　　　　b. Absence of reaction to light
　　3. Paralysis of accommodation
　　4. Decreased vision
　　5. Blindness
　　6. Visual fields
　　　　a. Scotomas — central
　　　　b. Constriction
B. Inadvertent Ocular Exposure
　　1. Irritation
　　　　a. Lacrimation
　　　　b. Hyperemia
　　　　c. Photophobia
　　2. Eyelids or conjunctiva
　　　　a. Allergic reactions
　　　　b. Conjunctivitis — nonspecific
　　　　c. Edema
　　　　d. Blepharospasm
　　3. Keratitis
　　4. Corneal ulceration
　　5. Iritis
　　6. Corneal opacities

Clinical Significance: Systemic emetine occasionally causes adverse ocular effects; however, discontinuation of the drug returns the eyes to normal within a few days to weeks. Topical ocular exposure may cause a severe irritative response lasting from 24 to 48 hours. Typically, this ocular discomfort does not occur until 4 to 10 hours after the initial contact. Only one case of permanent blindness secondary to corneal opacities has been reported from inadvertent ocular exposure of emetine.

References

Blacow, N. W. (Ed.): Martindale: The Extra Pharmacopoeia. 26th Ed., London, Pharmaceutical Press, 1972, pp. 101–102.
Blue, J. B.: Emetin: A warning. (Correspondence). JAMA *65*:1297, 1915.
Duke-Elder, S.: Systems of Ophthalmology. St. Louis, C. V. Mosby, Vol. XIV, Part 2, 1972, p. 1187.
Grant, W. M.: Toxicology of the Eye. 2nd Ed., Springfield, Charles C Thomas, 1974, pp. 445–446.
Jacovides: Troubles visuels a la suite d'injections fortes d'emetine. Arch. Ophtalmol. (Paris) *40*:657, 1923.
Lasky, M. A.: Corneal response to emetine hydrochloride. Arch. Ophthalmol. *44*:47, 1950.
Porges, N.: Tragedy in compounding. (Letter). J. Am. Pharm. Assoc. Pract. Pharm. *9*:593, 1948.
Torres Estrada, A.: Ocular lesions caused by emetine. Bol. Hosp. Oftal. NS Luz. (Mex.) *2*:145, 1944 (Am. J. Ophthalmol. *28*:1060, 1945).

* * * * * * * * * * * *

Class: Antibiotics

Generic Name: 1. Ampicillin; 2. Carbenicillin; 3. Cloxacillin; 4. Dicloxacillin; 5. Hetacillin; 6. Methicillin; 7. Nafcillin; 8. Oxacillin

Proprietary Name: 1. Alpen, Amcill, Ampicin (Canad.), Austrapen (Austral.), Doktacillin (Swed.), Omnipen, Pen A or A/N, Penbriten, Penicline (Fr.), Pensyn, Polycillin, Principen, QIDamp, Supen, Totacillin; 2. Geocillin, Geopen, Pyopen; 3. Austrastaph (Austral.), Ekvacillin (Swed.), Orbenin, Tegopen; 4. Dynapen, Pathocil, Veracillin; 5. Penplenum, Versapen; 6. Belfacillin (Swed.), Celbenin, Lucopenin (Denm.), Metin (Austral.), Penistaph (Fr.), Staphcillin, Synticillin (Denm.); 7. Unipen; 8. Bactocill, Bristopen (G.B., Fr.), Prostaphlin

Primary Use: Semisynthetic penicillins are primarily effective against staphylococci, streptococci, pneumococci, and various other gram-positive and gram-negative bacteria.

Ocular Side Effects

A. Systemic Administration
    1. Eyelids or conjunctiva
        a. Allergic reactions
        b. Conjunctivitis — nonspecific
        c. Angioneurotic edema
        d. Stevens-Johnson syndrome
        e. Exfoliative dermatitis
        f. Lyell's syndrome
    2. Subconjunctival or retinal hemorrhages secondary to drug-induced anemia
    3. Diplopia (?)
B. Local Ophthalmic Use or Exposure — Topical Application or Subconjunctival Injection
    1. Irritation — primarily with subconjunctival injection
        a. Hyperemia
        b. Ocular pain
        c. Edema
    2. Eyelids or conjunctiva
        a. Allergic reactions
        b. Angioneurotic edema
    3. Overgrowth of nonsusceptible organisms
    4. Corneal opacities (cloxacillin) — primarily with subconjunctival injection
C. Local Ophthalmic Use or Exposure — Intracameral Injection
    1. Uveitis (methicillin)
    2. Corneal edema (methicillin)
    3. Lens damage (methicillin)

Clinical Significance: Surprisingly few ocular side effects other than dermatologically or hematologically related conditions have been reported with the semisynthetic penicillins. The incidence of allergic skin reactions due to ampicillin, however, is quite high.

Interactions with Other Drugs

A. Effect of Other Drugs on Activity of Semisynthetic Penicillins
    1. Salicylates ↑
    2. Sulfonamides ↑
    3. Antibiotics ↓
        (Chloramphenicol, Erythromycin, Tetracyclines)
B. Cross Sensitivity
    1. Other penicillins

References

AMA Drug Evaluations. 2nd Ed., Acton, Mass., Publishing Sciences Group, 1973, pp. 514–521, 702–703, 707.

Davidson, S. I.: Reports of ocular adverse reactions. Trans. Ophthalmol. Soc. U. K. *93*: 495–510, 1973.

Ellis, P. P., and Smith, D. L.: Handbook of Ocular Therapeutics and Pharmacology. 4th Ed., St. Louis, C. V. Mosby, 1973, pp. 113–120.
Goodman, L. S., and Gilman, A. (Eds.): The Pharmacological Basis of Therapeutics. 4th Ed., New York, Macmillan, 1970, pp. 1219–1229.
Physicians' Desk Reference. 28th Ed., Oradell, N. J., Medical Economics Co., 1974, pp. 601, 603, 635, 1081.

* * * * * * * * * * * *

Generic Name: Bacitracin

Proprietary Name: Baciguent (*Systemic* and *Ophthalmic*)

Primary Use: This polypeptide bactericidal agent is primarily effective against gram positive cocci, *Neisseria*, and organisms causing gas gangrene.

Ocular Side Effects

A. Systemic Administration
   1. Myasthenic neuromuscular blocking effect
      a. Paralysis of extraocular muscles
      b. Ptosis
   2. Decreased vision
   3. Diplopia
   4. Eyelids or conjunctiva
      a. Allergic reactions
      b. Angioneurotic edema
B. Local Ophthalmic Use or Exposure — Topical Application or Subconjunctival Injection
   1. Irritation
   2. Eyelids or conjunctiva — allergic reactions
   3. Overgrowth of nonsusceptible organisms
C. Local Ophthalmic Use or Exposure — Intracameral Injection
   1. Uveitis
   2. Corneal edema
   3. Lens damage

Clinical Significance: Ocular side effects from either systemic or ocular administration of bacitracin are rare. The myasthenic neuromuscular blocking effect is more commonly seen if bacitracin is used in combination with neomycin, kanamycin, polymyxin, or colistin. Severe ocular or periocular allergic reactions, while rare, have been seen due to topical ophthalmic bacitracin application.

References

Blacow, N. W. (Ed.): Martindale: The Extra Pharmacopoeia. 26th Ed., London, Pharmaceutical Press, 1972, pp. 1310–1312.
Goodman, L. S., and Gilman, A. (Eds.): The Pharmacological Basis of Therapeutics. 4th Ed., New York, Macmillan, 1970, pp. 1293–1294.
McQuillen, M. P., Cantor, H. E., and O'Rourke, J. R.: Myasthenic syndrome associated with antibiotics. Arch. Neurol. *18*:402, 1968.

Small, G. A.: Respiratory paralysis after a large dose of intraperitoneal polymyxin B and bacitracin. Anesth. Analg. *43*:137,1964.

Walsh, F. B., and Hoyt, W. F.: Clinical Neuro-Ophthalmology. 3rd Ed., Baltimore, Williams & Wilkins, Vol. III, 1969, p. 2680.

* * * * * * * * * * * *

Generic Name: 1. Benzathine Penicillin G; 2. Hydrabamine Phenoxymethyl Penicillin; 3. Phenoxymethyl Penicillin, Potassium Penicillin V, Potassium Phenoxymethyl Penicillin; 4. Potassium Penicillin G; 5. Potassium Phenethicillin; 6. Procaine Penicillin G

Proprietary Name: 1. Bicillin, LPG (Austral.), Penidural (G.B.), Permapen; 2. Abbocillin-V (Austral.), Compocillin-V; 3. Abbocillin VK (Austral.), Acocillin (Scand.), Apsin VK (G.B.), Betapen-VK, Calciopen (Scand.), Calcipen (Scand.), Caps-Pen V (Austral.), Cillaphen (Austral.), Co-Caps Penicillin V-K (G.B.), Compocillin-VK, Crystapen V (G.B.), CVK (G.B.), Distaquàine V or V-K (G.B.), Econocil-VK (G.B.), Econopen V (G.B.), Falcopen V or VK (Austral.), Fenoxcillin (Scand.), Fenoxypen (Scand.), GPV (G.B.), la-pen (G.B.), Icipen (G.B.), Kesso-Pen-VK, Ledercillin VK, LPV (Austral.), Norcillin (G.B.), Oracilline (Fr.), Oratren (Germ.), Orvepen (Neth.), Ospeneff (G.B.), Pancillen (Austral.), Penapar VK, Penicals (G.B.), Peni-Vee (K) (Austral.), Penoxyl VK (G.B.), Pen-Vee K, Pfipen V (Austral.), Pfizerpen VK, Propen-VK (Austral.), PVK (Austral.), PVO (Austral.), QIDpen VK, Robicillin VK, Roscopenin (Scand.), Rosilin (Scand.), SK-Penicillin VK, Stabillin V-K (G.B.), Suspen V (Austral.), Uticillin VK, V-Cil-K (G.B.), V-Cillin K, Veecillin (Austral.), Veetids, Viacillin (Scand.), Vicin (Austral.), Viraxacillin-V (Austral.), VPV (Austral.), Weifapenin (Scand.); 4. Crystapen (G.B.), Eskacillin 100 (G.B.), Falapen (G.B.), Hyasorb, Kesso-Pen, Penevan (Austral.), Peniset (Austral.), Pensol (Austral.), Pentids, Pfizerpen G, Purapen G (G.B.), QIDpen G, Solupen (G.B.), Tabillin (G.B.); 5. Bendralan (Norw.), Broxil (G.B.), Darcil, Dramicillin, Maxipen, Pensig (Austral.), Ro-Cillin, Syncillin, Synthecilline (Fr.); 6. Aquacaine G (Austral.), Aquacillin (Austral.), Crysticillin AS, Depo-Penicillin, Distaquaine (G.B.), Diurnal-Penicillin, Duracillin AS, Eskacillin 200 (G.B.), Evacilin (Austral.), Flocilline (Fr.), Hydracillin (Swed.), Lentopen, Leopenicillin Retard (Swed.), Megapen (Austral.), Pentids-P, Pfizerpan-AS, Procillin (Austral.), Pro-Stabillin AS (G.B.), Suspenin (Swed.), Viraxacillin (Austral.), Wycillin

Primary Use: These bactericidal penicillins are effective against streptococci, *S. aureus*, gonococci, meningococci, pneumococci, *T. pallidium, Clostridium, B. anthracis, C. diphtheriae,* and several species of *Actinomyces.*

Ocular Side Effects

A. Systemic Administration
  1. Mydriasis
  2. Decreased accommodation
  3. Diplopia

      4. Papilledema
      5. Blindness
      6. Visual hallucinations
      7. Visual agnosia
      8. Eyelids or conjunctiva
         a. Allergic reactions
         b. Blepharitis
         c. Angioneurotic edema
         d. Stevens-Johnson syndrome
         e. Lyell's syndrome
      9. Subconjunctival or retinal hemorrhages secondary to drug-induced anemia

B. Local Ophthalmic Use or Exposure -- Topical Application or Subconjunctival Injection
      1. Irritation
      2. Eyelids or conjunctiva — allergic reactions
      3. Overgrowth of nonsusceptible organisms

C. Local Ophthalmic Use or Exposure — Intracameral Injection
      1. Uveitis
      2. Corneal edema
      3. Lens damage

Clinical Significance: Systemic administration of penicillin only rarely causes ocular side effects; however, topical ocular administration results in a high incidence of allergic reactions. The incidence of allergic reactions is greater in patients with Sjögren's syndrome or rheumatoid arthritis than in other individuals. The most serious adverse ocular reaction is papilledema secondary to elevated intracranial pressure. Most other ocular side effects due to penicillin are transient and reversible.

Interactions with Other Drugs

A. Effect of Other Drugs on Activity of Penicillin
      1. Analgesics ↑
      2. Bacitracin ↑
      3. Salicylates ↑
      4. Antacids ↓
      5. Antibiotics ↓
         (Chloramphenicol, Erythromycin, Kanamycin, Neomycin, Streptomycin, Tetracyclines)

B. Synergistic Activity
      1. Cephalosporins
      2. Erythromycin
      3. Kanamycin
      4. Other penicillins
      5. Streptomycin
      6. Sulfonamides (occasionally indifferent or inhibitory)

C. Cross Sensitivity
      1. Cephalosporins

References

Bjornberg, A.: Hallucinatory reactions in association with oral administration of Probenecid Penicillin. Acta Med. Scand. *165*:207, 1959.
Bjornberg, A., and Selstam, J.: Acute psychotic reaction after injection of Procaine Penicilline. Acta Dermatovener. *37*:50, 1957.
New, P. S., and Wells, C. E.: Cerebral toxicity associated with massive intravenous penicillin therapy. Neurology *15*:1053, 1965.
Utley, P. M., Lucas, J. B., and Billings, T. E.: Acute psychotic reactions to aqueous Procaine Penicillin (G). Southern Med. J. *59*:1271, 1966.

* * * * * * * * * * * * *

Generic Name: 1. Cefazolin; 2. Cephalexin; 3. Cephaloglycin; 4. Cephaloridine; 5. Cephalothin

Proprietary Name: 1. Ancef, Kefzol; 2. Ceporex (G.B.), Keflex; 3. Kafocin; 4. Ceporin (G.B.), Loridine; 5. Keflin

Primary Use: Cephalosporins are effective against streptococci, staphylococci, pneumococci, and strains of *E. coli, P. mirabilis*, and *Klebsiella*.

Ocular Side Effects

A. Systemic Administration
    1. Nystagmus
    2. Eyelids or conjunctiva
        a. Allergic reactions
        b. Angioneurotic edema
        c. Urticaria
    3. Subconjunctival or retinal hemorrhages secondary to drug-induced anemia
    4. Visual hallucinations
    5. Diplopia (cephaloridine)
    6. Decreased vision (?)
    7. Papilledema (?) (cephaloridine)
    8. Retinal pigmentary changes (?) (cephaloridine)
B. Local Ophthalmic Use or Exposure — Topical Application or Subconjunctival Injection
    1. Irritation
        a. Hyperemia
        b. Ocular pain
        c. Edema
    2. Eyelids or conjunctiva
        a. Allergic reactions
        b. Angioneurotic edema
        c. Urticaria
    3. Overgrowth of nonsusceptible organisms

Clinical Significance: Few significant ocular side effects have been reported with these antibiotics. All reported adverse ocular reactions are transitory when use of these drugs is discontinued. Only with cephaloridine has one possible instance of toxic papilledema or retinal change been suspected.

Interactions with Other Drugs
A. Cross Sensitivity
   1. Penicillins

References

AMA Drug Evaluations. 2nd Ed., Acton, Mass., Publishing Sciences Group, 1973, pp. 523–527, 703–704.

Ballingall, D. L. K., and Trupie, A. G. G.: Cephaloridine toxicity (Letter to editor). Lancet 2:835, 1967.

Crosbie, R. B.: Cephaloridine toxicity. Lancet 1:422, 1968.

Goodman, L. S., and Gilman, A. (Eds.): The Pharmacological Basis of Therapeutics. 4th Ed., New York, Macmillan, 1970, pp. 1277–1282.

Grant, W. M.: Toxicology of the Eye. 2nd Ed., Springfield, Charles C Thomas, 1974, p. 249.

* * * * * * * * * * * * *

Generic Name: Chloramphenicol

Proprietary Name: *Systemic:* Amphicol, Austracol (Austral.), Bipimycetin (Ind.), Chlomin (Austral.), Chloramphycin (Ind.), Chloromycetin, Clorcetin (G.B.), Enicol (Canad.), Eusynthomycin (U.S.S.R.), Kemicetine (G.B.), Leukomycin (Germ.), Mycinol (Canad.), Paraxin (Germ.), Tifomycine (Fr.) *Ophthalmic:* AntiBiOpto, Chloromycetin, Chloroptic, Kemicetine (G.B.), Ophthochlor, Opulets (G.B.)

Primary Use: This bacteriostatic dichloracetic acid derivative is particularly effective against *Salmonella typhi, H. influenzae meningitis,* rickettsia, the lymphogranuloma-psittacosis group, and is useful in the management of cystic fibrosis.

Ocular Side Effects
A. Systemic Administration
   1. Decreased vision
   2. Visual fields
      a. Scotomas
      b. Constriction
   3. Retrobulbar neuritis
   4. Optic atrophy
   5. Blindness
   6. Problems with color vision
      a. Dyschromatopsia
      b. Objects have yellow tinge
   7. Eyelids or conjunctiva
      a. Allergic reactions
      b. Angioneurotic edema
   8. Paralysis of accommodation

        9. Pupils
           a. Mydriasis
           b. Absence of reaction to light
      10. Retinal pigmentary changes
      11. Retinal edema
      12. Subconjunctival or retinal hemorrhages secondary to drug-induced anemia
  B. Local Ophthalmic Use or Exposure — Topical Application or Subconjunctival Injection
      1. Irritation
      2. Eyelids or conjunctiva — allergic reactions
      3. Overgrowth of nonsusceptible organisms
  C. Local Ophthalmic Use or Exposure — Intracameral Injection
      1. Uveitis
      2. Corneal edema
      3. Lens damage

Clinical Significance: Ocular side effects from systemic chloramphenicol administration are uncommon in adults, but occur often in children, especially if the total dose exceeds 100 grams or if therapy lasts over 6 weeks. Topical ophthalmic application causes infrequent ocular side effects. Although chloramphenicol has fewer allergic reactions than neomycin, those due to chloramphenicol are often the more severe. Like other antibiotics, this agent may cause latent hypersensitivity which lasts for many years. Three instances of significant adverse changes in the hemopoietic system secondary to topical ocular chloramphenicol administration have been reported. Topical ocular chloramphenicol probably has fewer toxic effects on the corneal epithelium than any other antibiotic.

Interactions with Other Drugs

  A. Effect of Chloramphenicol on Activity of Other Drugs
      1. Analgesics ↑
      2. Barbiturates ↑
      3. Cephalosporins ↓
      4. Penicillins ↓
  B. Effect of Other Drugs on Activity of Chloramphenicol
      1. Barbiturates ↓
  C. Synergistic Activity
      1. Erythromycin
      2. Sulfonamides

References

Cocke, J. G., Brown, R. E., and Geppert, L. J.: Optic neuritis with prolonged use of chloramphenicol. J. Pediatr. 68:27, 1966.

Cole, J. G., Cole, H. G., and Janoff, L. A.: A toxic ocular manifestation of chloramphenicol therapy. Am. J. Ophthalmol. 44:18, 1957.

Davidson, S. I.: Systemic effects of eye drops. Trans. Ophthalmol. Soc. U. K. 94:487, 1974.

Joy, R. J. T., Scalettar, R., and Sodee, D. B.: Optic and peripheral neuritis. Probable effect of prolonged chloramphenicol therapy. JAMA 173:1731, 1960.

Lamda, P. A., Sood, N. N., and Moorthy, S. S.: Retinopathy due to chloramphenicol. Scot. Med. J. *13*:166, 1968.

Rosenthal, R. L., and Blackman, A.: Bone marrow hypoplasia following use of chloramphenicol eyedrops. JAMA *191*:136, 1965.

* * * * * * * * * * * * *

Generic Name: 1. Chlortetracycline; 2. Demeclocycline; 3. Doxycycline; 4. Methacycline; 5. Minocycline; 6. Oxytetracycline; 7. Tetracycline

Proprietary Name: *Systemic:* 1. Aureomycin, Chlortet (Austral.), Chlortetrin (G.B.); 2. Declomycin, Ledermycin (G.B.); 3. Doxy-II, Vibramycin; 4. Adriamicina (Ital.), Roliteracycline, Rondomycin; 5. Minocin, Vectrin; 6. Abbocin (G.B.), Adamycin (Austral.), Anprox (G.B.), Berkmycen (G.B.), Bobbamycin (Austral.), Clinimycin (G.B.), Galenomycin (G.B.), Ia-Ioxin (G.B.), Imperacin (G.B.), Oxatets (G.B.), Oxycycline (Austral.), Oxydon (G.B.), Oxy-Kesso-Tetra, Oxymycin (G.B.), Oxytetrin (G.B.); Stecsolin (G.B.), Terramycin, Unimycin (G.B.), Uri-Tet, Vendarcin (G.B.); 7. Achromycin, Anpocine (G.B.), Austramycin (Austral.), Bristacycline, Clinitetrin (G.B.), Co-Caps Tetracycline (G.B.), Cyclopar, Democracin (G.B.), Economycin (G.B.), Hostacycline (Germ.), Kesso-Tetra, Oppacyn (G.B.), Panmycin, Polycycline, QIDtet, Quadracycline (Austral.), Retet, Rexamycin, Robitet, SK-Tetracycline, Steclin, Sumycin, T-125/250, Telotrex (G.B.), Tetrabid (G.B.), Tetrachel (G.B.), Tetracin, Tetracyn, Tetrex, Totmycin (G.B.) *Ophthalmic:* 1. Aureomycin; 7. Achromycin

Primary Use: These bacteriostatic derivatives of polycyclic naphthacene carboxamide are effective against a wide range of gram-negative and gram-positive organisms, mycoplasm, and members of the lymphogranuloma-psittacosis group.

Ocular Side Effects

- A. Systemic Administration
    1. Myopia
    2. Papilledema secondary to pseudotumor cerebri
    3. Decreased vision
    4. Photophobia
    5. Problems with color vision (chlortetracycline)
        a. Dyschromatopsia
        b. Objects have yellow tinge
    6. Eyelids or conjunctiva
        a. Erythema
        b. Photosensitivity
        c. Angioneurotic edema
        d. Erythema multiforme
        e. Stevens-Johnson syndrome
    7. Myasthenic neuromuscular blocking effect
        a. Paralysis of extraocular muscles
        b. Ptosis

       8. Subconjunctival or retinal hemorrhages secondary to drug-induced anemia
       9. Enlarged blind spot
     10. Visual hallucinations
     11. Congenital cataracts (?)
  B. Local Ophthalmic Use or Exposure — Topical Application or Subconjunctival Injection
      1. Irritation
      2. Eyelids or conjunctiva — allergic reactions
      3. Overgrowth of nonsusceptible organisms
  C. Local Ophthalmic Use or Exposure — Intracameral Injection
      1. Uveitis
      2. Corneal edema
      3. Lens damage

Clinical Significance: Systemic or ocular use of the tetracyclines rarely causes ocular side effects. While a large variety of drug-induced ocular side effects has been attributed to tetracyclines, most are reversible. Transient color defects have been reported only with chlortetracycline. The lowest reported incidence of contact dermatitis due to commonly used antibiotics is with chlortetracycline.

Interactions with Other Drugs

  A. Effect of Tetracyclines on Activity of Other Drugs
      1. Penicillins ↓
  B. Effect of Other Drugs on Activity of Tetracyclines
      1. Alcohol ↑
      2. Antacids ↓
      3. Riboflavin ↓
  C. Synergistic Activity
      1. Streptomycin

References

Edwards, T. S.: Transient myopia due to tetracycline. JAMA 186:69, 1963.
Furey, W. W., and Tan, C.: Anaphylactic shock due to oral dimethylchlortetracycline. Ann. Intern. Med. 70:357, 1969.
Gewin, H. M., and Friou, G. J.: Manifestation of vitamin deficiency during aureomycin and chloramphenicol therapy of endocarditis due to Staphylococcus aureus. Yale J. Biol. Med. 23:332, 1951.
Giles, C. L., and Soble, A. R.: Intracranial hypertension and tetracycline therapy. Am. J. Ophthalmol. 72:981, 1971.
Minkin, W., Cohen, H. J., and Frank, S. B.: Fixed-drug eruption due to tetracycline. Arch. Derm. 100:749, 1969.

* * * * * * * * * * * * *

Generic Name: 1. Clindamycin; 2. Erythromycin; 3. Lincomycin; 4. Vancomycin

Proprietary Name: *Systemic:* 1. Cleocin, Dalacin C (G.B.); 2. Bristamycin, EMU-V (Austral.), E-Mycin, Eromycin (Austral.), Erostin (Austral.), Erycen (G.B.), Erycinum (Germ.), Erypar, Erythrocin, Erythromid (G.B.), Erythrop-red (G.B.), Ethril, Ethryn (Austral.), Ilosone, Ilotycin, Kesso-Mycin, Pediamy-cin, Pfizer-E, QIDmycin, Retcin (G.B.), Robimycin, R-P Mycin, SK-Erythro-mycin; 3. Lincocin, Mycivin (G.B.); 4. Vancocin *Ophthalmic:* 2. Ilotycin; 3. Lincocin

Primary Use: These bactericidal antibiotics are effective against gram-positive or gram-negative organisms.

Ocular Side Effects

A. Systemic Administration
   1. Problems with color vision (erythromycin)
      a. Dyschromatopsia
      b. Achromatopsia, blue-yellow defect
   2. Eyelids or conjunctiva
      a. Allergic reactions
      b. Hyperemia
      c. Photosensitivity
      d. Angioneurotic edema
      e. Stevens-Johnson syndrome
      f. Exfoliative dermatitis
   3. Subconjunctival or retinal hemorrhages secondary to drug-induced anemia
B. Local Ophthalmic Use or Exposure — Topical Application or Subcon-junctival Injection
   1. Irritation
      a. Hyperemia
      b. Ocular pain
      c. Edema
   2. Eyelids or conjunctiva
      a. Allergic reactions
      b. Angioneurotic edema
   3. Overgrowth of nonsusceptible organisms
   4. Subconjunctival hemorrhages (lincomycin)
C. Local Ophthalmic Use or Exposure — Intracameral Injection
   1. Uveitis (erythromycin)
   2. Corneal edema (erythromycin)
   3. Lens damage (erythromycin)

Clinical Significance: Few adverse ocular reactions due to either systemic or ophthalmic use of these antibiotics are seen. Nearly all ocular side effects are transitory and reversible after the drug is discontinued. Most adverse ocular reactions are secondary to dermatologic or hematologic conditions.

Interactions with Other Drugs

A. Effect of These Antibiotics on Activity of Other Drugs
  1. Clindamycin ↓
  2. Erythromycin ↓
  3. Lincomycin ↓
  4. Penicillins ↓
B. Effect of Other Drugs on Activity of These Antibiotics
  1. Clindamycin ↓
  2. Erythromycin ↓
  3. Lincomycin ↓

References

AMA Drug Evaluations. 2nd Ed., Acton, Mass., Publishing Sciences Group, 1973, pp. 529–535, 578, 705–706, 710.

Goodman, L. S., and Gilman, A. (Eds.): The Pharmacological Basis of Therapeutics. 4th Ed., New York, Macmillan, 1970, pp. 1274–1277, 1292–1293, 1296–1297.

Kastrup, E. K., and Schwach, G. H. (Eds.): Facts and Comparisons. St. Louis, Facts and Comparisons, Inc., 1974, p. 423.

Physicians' Desk Reference. 28th Ed., Oradell, N. J., Medical Economics Co., 1974, pp. 508, 715, 912, 937, 1487, 1498.

* * * * * * * * * * * *

Generic Name: 1. Colistimethate; 2. Colistin

Proprietary Name: *Systemic:* 1. Colomycin Injection (G.B.), Coly-Mycin M; 2. Colomycin (G.B.), Coly-Mycin S *Ophthalmic:* 2. Coly-Mycin S

Primary Use: These bactericidal polypeptides are effective against *Aerobacter, E. coli, K. pneumoniae, Ps. aeruginosa, Shigella,* and *Salmonella.*

Ocular Side Effects

A. Systemic Administration
  1. Nystagmus
  2. Myasthenic neuromuscular blocking effect
    a. Paralysis of extraocular muscles
    b. Ptosis
  3. Diplopia
  4. Mydriasis
B. Local Ophthalmic Use or Exposure − Topical Application or Subconjunctival Injection
  1. Irritation
  2. Eyelids or conjunctiva − allergic reactions
  3. Overgrowth of nonsusceptible organisms
C. Local Ophthalmic Use or Exposure − Intracameral Injection
  1. Uveitis
  2. Corneal edema
  3. Lens damage

Clinical Significance: Only a few cases of ocular side effects from systemic or ocular colistimethate or colistin therapy have been reported. These adverse ocular reactions are usually transitory, reversible, and of little clinical importance. In resistant cases with overgrowth of nonsusceptible organisms, *Proteus* has been the most common bacterial organism found. Unfortunately, Colimycin is also the name given to an antibiotic of the neomycin group available in the U.S.S.R.

Interactions with Other Drugs

A. Effect of Colistimethate or Colistin on Activity of Other Drugs
   1. Antibiotics (apnea) ↑
      (Kanamycin, Neomycin, Polymyxin, Streptomycin)
   2. Anticholinesterases (apnea) ↑
   3. General anesthetics (apnea) ↑
B. Synergistic Activity
   1. Sulfonamides
C. Cross Sensitivity
   1. Gentamicin
   2. Kanamycin
   3. Polymyxin B
   4. Streptomycin

References

Gold, G. N., and Richardson, A. P.: An unusual case of neuromuscular blockade seen with therapeutic blood levels of colistin methanesulfonate. (Coly-Mycin). Am. J. Med. *41*:316, 1966.
Lund, M. H.: Colistin sulfate ophthalmic in the treatment of ocular infections. Arch. Ophthalmol. *81*:4, 1969.
McQuillen, M. P., Cantor, H. E., and O'Rourke, J. R.: Myasthenic syndrome associated with antibiotics. Arch. Neurol. *18*:402, 1968.
Wolinsky, E., and Hines, J. D.: Neurotoxic and nephrotoxic effects of colistin in patients with renal disease. N. Engl. J. Med. *266*:759, 1962.

* * * * * * * * * * * * *

Generic Name: Cycloserine. See under *Class: Antitubercular Agents.*

* * * * * * * * * * * * *

Generic Name: 1. Framycetin; 2. Neomycin

Proprietary Name: *Systemic:* 1. Enterfram (G.B.); 2. Mycifradin, Myciguent, Neobiotic, Neolate (G.B.), Neomate (Austral.), Neomin (G.B.), Neopt (Austral.), Neosulf (Austral.), Nivemycin (G.B.), Siguent (Austral.) *Ophthalmic:* 1. Framygen (G.B.), Soframycin (G.B.); 2. Myciguent, Nivemycin (G.B.)

Primary Use: These bactericidal aminoglycosidic agents are effective against *Ps. aeruginosa, Aerobacter, K. pneumoniae, P. vulgaris, E. coli, Salmonella, Shigella*, and most strains of *S. aureus*.

Ocular Side Effects
  A. Systemic Administration — Neomycin
    1. Myasthenic neuromuscular blocking effect
       a. Paralysis of extraocular muscles
       b. Ptosis
    2. Decreased or absent pupillary reaction to light
  B. Local Ophthalmic Use or Exposure — Topical Application or Subconjunctival Injection
    1. Irritation
    2. Eyelids or conjunctiva
       a. Allergic reactions
       b. Conjunctivitis — follicular
    3. Punctate keratitis
    4. Overgrowth of nonsusceptible organisms
  C. Local Ophthalmic Use or Exposure — Intracameral Injection
    1. Uveitis (neomycin)
    2. Corneal edema (neomycin)
    3. Lens damage (neomycin)

Clinical Significance: It is rare for nontopical ophthalmic application to cause ocular side effects; however, there are well-documented reports of decreased or absent pupillary reactions due to application of neomycin to the pleural or peritoneal cavities during a thoracic or abdominal operation. Topical ocular application of neomycin has been reported to cause allergic conjunctival or lid reactions in 4 percent of patients using this drug. In a recent series, neomycin was found to be one of the three more common drugs causing periocular allergic contact dermatitis. In addition, some feel that, of the more commonly used antibiotics, topical neomycin has the greatest toxicity to the corneal epithelium. After long-term ocular exposure to framycetin or neomycin, fungi superinfections have been reported. Nystagmus has been reported in a nine-year-old child following topical treatment of the skin with 1 percent neomycin in 11 percent dimethyl sulfoxide ointment.

Interactions with Other Drugs
  A. Effect of Framycetin or Neomycin on Activity of Other Drugs
    1. EDTA (apnea) ↑
    2. General anesthetics (apnea) ↑
    3. Other antibiotics (apnea) ↑
       (Bacitracin, Colistin, Gentamicin, Kanamycin, Polymyxin B, Streptomycin)
    4. Oral penicillins ↓
    5. Oral vitamin B_{12} ↓
  B. Effect of Other Drugs on Activity of Framycetin or Neomycin
    1. EDTA ↑
    2. Anticholinesterases ↓
  C. Synergistic Activity
    1. Bacitracin

D. Cross Sensitivity
    1. Gentamicin
    2. Kanamycin
    3. Streptomycin

References

Ferrara, B. E., and Phillips, R. D.: Respiratory arrest following administration of intraperitoneal neomycin. Am. Surg. 23:710, 1957.

Gordon, D. M.: Gentamicin sulfate in external eye infections. Am. J. Ophthalmol. 69:300, 1970.

Herd, J. K., et al.: Ototoxicity of topical neomycin augmented by dimethyl sulfoxide. Pediatrics 40:905, 1967.

McCorkle, R. G.: Neomycin toxicity. A case report. Arch. Pediat. 75:439, 1958.

McQuillen, M. P., Cantor, H. E., and O'Rourke, J. R.: Myasthenic syndrome associated with antibiotics. Arch. Neurol. 18:402, 1968.

Stechishin, O., Voloshin, P. C., and Allard, C. A.: Neuromuscular paralysis and respiratory arrest caused by intrapleural neomycin. Can. Med. Assoc. J. 81:32, 1959.

* * * * * * * * * * * * *

Generic Name: Gentamicin

Proprietary Name: *Systemic:* Cidomycin (G.B.), Garamycin, Genticin (G.B.), Refobacin (Germ.) *Ophthalmic:* Garamycin

Primary Use: This aminoglycoside is effective against *Ps. aeruginosa, Aerobacter, E. coli, K. pneumoniae,* and *Proteus.*

Ocular Side Effects

A. Systemic Administration
    1. Decreased vision
    2. Papilledema secondary to pseudotumor cerebri
    3. Loss of eyelashes or eyebrows
    4. Subconjunctival or retinal hemorrhages secondary to drug-induced anemia
    5. Blindness (?)
B. Local Ophthalmic Use or Exposure — Topical Application or Subconjunctival Injection
    1. Irritation
    2. Eyelids or conjunctiva
        a. Allergic reactions
        b. Conjunctivitis — follicular
    3. Overgrowth of nonsusceptible organisms

Clinical Significance: Surprisingly few drug-induced ocular side effects from either systemic or topical ocular administration have been reported with gentamicin. However, pseudotumor cerebri with secondary papilledema and visual loss has been well documented. Other adverse ocular effects are reversible and transitory after discontinued use of the drug.

Interactions with Other Drugs

A. Effect of Gentamicin on Activity of Other Drugs
   1. General anesthetics (apnea) ↑
B. Effect of Other Drugs on Activity of Gentamicin
   1. Penicillins ↓
C. Cross Sensitivity
   1. Kanamycin
   2. Neomycin
   3. Streptomycin

References

AMA Drug Evaluations. 2nd Ed., Acton, Mass., Publishing Sciences Group, 1973, pp. 569–570, 706.

Boe, R., and Conner, C. S.: Pseudotumor cerebri. JAMA 226:567, 1973.

Gordon, D. M.: Gentamicin sulfate in external eye infections. Am. J. Ophthalmol. 69:300, 1970.

Kastrup, E. K., and Schwach, G. H. (Eds.): Facts and Comparisons. St. Louis, Facts and Comparisons, Inc., 1974, p. 347.

Meyler, L., and Herxheimer, A. (Eds.): Side Effects of Drugs. Amsterdam, Excerpta Medica, Vol. VII, 1972, pp. 374–376.

* * * * * * * * * * * *

Generic Name: Kanamycin

Proprietary Name: Kamycine (Fr.), Kanasig (Austral.), Kannasyn (G.B.), Kantrex, Kantrox (Swed.)

Primary Use: This aminoglycoside is effective against gram-negative organisms and in drug-resistant staphylococcus.

Ocular Side Effects

A. Systemic Administration
   1. Decreased vision
   2. Myasthenic neuromuscular blocking effect
      a. Paralysis of extraocular muscles
      b. Ptosis
   3. Eyelids or conjunctiva
      a. Allergic reactions
      b. Lyell's syndrome
   4. Optic neuritis (?)
B. Local Ophthalmic Use or Exposure — Subconjunctival Injection
   1. Irritation
   2. Eyelids or conjunctiva — allergic reactions
   3. Overgrowth of nonsusceptible organisms

Clinical Significance: Systemic and ocular side effects due to kanamycin are quite rare, partially due to its poor gastrointestinal absorption. Myasthenic neuromuscular blocking effect occurs more frequently if kanamycin is given in combination with other antibiotics such as neomycin, gentamicin, polymyxin B, colistin, or streptomycin. Adverse ocular reactions to this agent are reversible, transitory, and seldom have residual complications.

Interactions with Other Drugs

A. Effect of Kanamycin on Activity of Other Drugs
    1. General anesthetics (apnea) ↑
    2. Other antibiotics (apnea) ↑
B. Effect of Other Drugs on Activity of Kanamycin
    1. EDTA (apnea) ↑
    2. Anticholinesterases (apnea) ↓
C. Synergistic Activity
    1. Cephalosporins
    2. Penicillins
D. Cross Sensitivity
    1. Gentamicin
    2. Neomycin
    3. Streptomycin

References

Finegold, S. M.: Kanamycin. Arch. Intern. Med. *104*:15, 1959.

Finegold, S. M.: Toxicity of kanamycin in adults. Ann. N. Y. Acad. Sci. *132*:942, 1966.

Freemon, F. R., Parker, R. L., Jr., and Greer, M.: Unusual neurotoxicity of kanamycin. JAMA *200*:410, 1967.

McQuillen, M. P., Cantor, H. E., and O'Rourke, J. R.: Myasthenic syndrome associated with antibiotics. Arch. Neurol. *18*:402, 1968.

Walsh, F. B., and Hoyt, W. F.: Clinical Neuro-Ophthalmology. 3rd Ed., Baltimore, Williams & Wilkins, Vol. III, 1969, pp. 2655, 2680.

* * * * * * * * * * * * *

Generic Name: Nalidixic Acid

Proprietary Name: NegGram, Negram (G.B.)

Primary Use: This bactericidal naphthyridine derivative is effective against *E. coli, Aerobacter,* and *Klebsiella;* however, its primary clinical use is against *Proteus.*

Ocular Side Effects

A. Systemic Administration
    1. Visual sensations
        a. Glare phenomenon
        b. Flashing lights — white or colored
        c. Scintillating scotomas — may be colored
    2. Problems with color vision
        a. Dyschromatopsia
        b. Objects have yellow, blue, or purple tinge

3. Photophobia
4. Paresis of extraocular muscles
5. Papilledema
6. Decreased vision
7. Decreased accommodation
8. Diplopia
9. Mydriasis
10. Eyelids or conjunctiva
    a. Photosensitivity
    b. Angioneurotic edema
    c. Urticaria
11. Blindness
12. Subconjunctival or retinal hemorrhages secondary to drug-induced anemia
13. Congenital ptosis (?)

Clinical Significance: Numerous ocular side effects due to nalidixic acid have been reported. In fact, in the annual report of adverse ocular reactions of the United Kingdom, almost one-third of all report cases were due to this drug. The most common adverse ocular reaction is a curious visual disturbance which includes as the main feature brightly colored appearances of objects. This often appears soon after the drug is taken. Temporary visual loss also occurs and lasts from half an hour to 72 hours. Probably the most serious ocular reaction is papilledema secondary to elevated intracranial pressure. This side effect is more frequent in the younger age groups. Most adverse ocular reactions due to nalidixic acid are transitory and reversible after use of the drug is discontinued.

Interactions with Other Drugs

A. Effect of Nalidixic Acid on Activity of Other Drugs
   1. Alcohol ↑
B. Effect of Other Drugs on Activity of Nalidixic Acid
   1. EDTA ↑
   2. Antacids ↓

References

AMA Drug Evaluations. 2nd Ed., Acton, Mass., Publishing Sciences Group, 1973, p. 576.
Boreus, L. O., and Sundstrom, B.: Intracranial hypertension in a child during treatment with nalidixic acid. Br. Med. Jr. 2:744, 1967.
Davidson, S. I.: Reports of ocular adverse reactions. Trans. Ophthalmol. Soc. U. K. 93:495, 1973.
Marshall, B. Y.: Visual side effects of nalidixic acid. Practitioner 199:222, 1967.
VanDyk, H. J. L., and Swan, K. C.: Drug-induced pseudotumor cerebri. In Leopold, I. H. (Ed.): Symposium on Ocular Therapy. St. Louis, C. V. Mosby, Vol. IV, 1969, pp. 71–77.
Walker, S. H., Salanio, I., and Standiford, W. E.: Nalidixic acid in childhood urinary tract infection; clinical and laboratory experience with 50 patients. Clin. Pediat. 5:718, 1966.

* * * * * * * * * * * *

Generic Name: Nitrofurantoin

Proprietary Name: Berkfurin (G.B.), Ceduran (G.B.), Co-Caps Nitrofurantoin (G.B.), Cyantin, Furadantin, Furadoine (Fr.), Furan (G.B.), Macrodantin, Nifosept (Pol.), Nitoin (G.B.), Trantoin

Primary Use: This bactericidal furan derivative is effective against specific organisms which cause urinary tract infections, especially *E. coli*, enterococci, and *S. aureus*.

Ocular Side Effects

A. Systemic Administration
  1. Nonspecific ocular irritation
     a. Lacrimation
     b. Burning sensation
  2. Vertical diplopia
  3. Nystagmus
  4. Decreased vision
  5. Paralysis of extraocular muscles
  6. Eyelids or conjunctiva
     a. Allergic reactions
     b. Angioneurotic edema
     c. Lyell's syndrome
  7. Subconjunctival or retinal hemorrhages secondary to drug-induced anemia
  8. Problems with color vision (?)
     a. Dyschromatopsia
     b. Objects have yellow tinge

Clinical Significance: The most aggravating ocular side effects due to nitrofurantoin are the severe itching, burning, and tearing which may persist long after use of the drug is stopped in some patients. All adverse ocular reactions due to this drug have been transitory and reversible if use was discontinued. Only a few cases of paralysis of extraocular muscles have been reported.

Interactions with Other Drugs

A. Effect of Other Drugs on Activity of Nitrofurantoin
  1. Antacids ↓
  2. Barbiturates ↓
  3. Carbonic anhydrase inhibitors ↓

References

Kastrup, E. K., and Schwach, G. H. (Eds.): Facts and Comparisons. St. Louis, Facts and Comparisons, Inc. 1974, pp. 382a–382b.

Peritt, R. A.: Eye complications resulting from systemic medication. Ill. Med. J. *117*:423, 1960.

Physicians' Desk Reference. 28th Ed., Oradell, N. J., Medical Economics Co., 1974, pp. 743, 844, 963.

Toole, J. F., et al.: Neural effects of nitrofurantoin. Arch. Neurol. *18*:680, 1968.

Walsh, F. B., and Hoyt, W. F.: Clinical Neuro-Ophthalmology. 3rd Ed., Baltimore, Williams & Wilkins, Vol. III, 1969, p. 2653.

* * * * * * * * * * * * *

Generic Name: Polymyxin B

Proprietary Name: *Systemic:* Aerosporin, Polmix (Austral.) *Ophthalmic:* Aerosporin

Primary Use: This bactericidal polypeptide is effective against gram-negative bacilli, especially *Ps. aeruginosa.*

Ocular Side Effects

A. Systemic Administration
  1. Myasthenic neuromuscular blocking effect
      a. Paralysis of extraocular muscles
      b. Ptosis
  2. Decreased vision
  3. Diplopia
B. Local Ophthalmic Use or Exposure — Topical Application or Subconjunctival Injection
  1. Irritation — ocular pain
  2. Eyelids or conjunctiva — allergic reactions
  3. Overgrowth of nonsusceptible organisms
C. Local Ophthalmic Use or Exposure — Intracameral Injection
  1. Uveitis
  2. Corneal edema
  3. Lens damage

Clinical Significance: Although ocular side effects due to polymyxin B are well documented, they are quite rare and seldom of major clinical importance. The most significant side effects are secondary to intracameral injections where permanent changes to the cornea and lens have occurred.

Interactions with Other Drugs

A. Effect of Polymyxin B on Activity of Other Drugs
  1. General anesthetics (apnea) ↑
B. Effect of Other Drugs on Activity of Polymyxin B
  1. Other antibiotics (apnea) ↑
      (Colistin, Gentamicin, Kanamycin, Neomycin, Streptomycin)
  2. Anticholinesterases (apnea) ↑↓
C. Cross Sensitivity
  1. Colistin

References

Goodman, L. S., and Gilman, A. (Eds.): The Pharmacological Basis of Therapeutics. 4th Ed., New York, Macmillan, 1970, pp. 1287–1290.

McQuillen, M. P., Cantor, H. E., and O'Rourke, J. R.: Myasthenic syndrome associated with antibiotics. Arch. Neurol. *18*:402, 1968.

Pohlmann, G.: Respiratory arrest associated with intravenous administration of polymyxin B sulfate. JAMA *196*:181, 1966.

Small, G. A.: Respiratory paralysis after a large dose of intraperitoneal polymyxin B and bacitracin. Anesth. Analg. *43*:137, 1964.

* * * * * * * * * * * * *

Generic Name: Streptomycin

Proprietary Name: Strepolin 33 (G.B.), Streptaquaine (G.B.), Streptevan (Austral.)

Primary Use: This bactericidal aminoglycosidic agent is effective against *Brucella*, *Pasteurella*, *Mycobacterium*, and *Shigella.*

Ocular Side Effects

A. Systemic or Intrathecal Administration
  1. Nystagmus
  2. Decreased vision
  3. Blindness
  4. Myasthenic neuromuscular blocking effect
    a. Paresis or paralysis of extraocular muscles
    b. Ptosis
  5. Visual sensations
    a. Visual disturbance during motion
    b. Continuance of image after ocular movement
  6. Photophobia
  7. Problems with color vision
    a. Dyschromatopsia
    b. Objects have yellow tinge
    c. Achromatopsia, blue or green defect
  8. Decreased accommodation
  9. Retrobulbar or optic neuritis
  10. Scotomas
  11. Optic atrophy
  12. Retinal vasospasm
  13. Eyelids or conjunctiva
    a. Allergic reactions
    b. Conjunctivitis — nonspecific
    c. Edema
    d. Angioneurotic edema
    e. Lupoid syndrome
  14. Subconjunctival or retinal hemorrhages secondary to drug-induced anemia
B. Local Ophthalmic Use or Exposure — Subconjunctival Injection
  1. Irritation
  2. Eyelids or conjunctiva — allergic reactions
  3. Overgrowth of nonsusceptible organisms
C. Local Ophthalmic Use or Exposure — Intracameral Injection
  1. Uveitis
  2. Corneal edema
  3. Lens damage
  4. Retinal damage (?)

Clinical Significance: Since more effective aminoglycosidic antibiotics exist, the clinical use of streptomycin is limited. Toxic visual effects are rare, usually transitory, and reversible with systemic administration; however, permanent blindness and optic atrophy have been reported with intrathecal injection. Nystagmus due to streptomycin can be produced without vestibular damage. Skin sensitization is common among medical personnel who handle this drug and may lead to dermatitis not infrequently associated with periorbital edema and conjunctivitis.

Interactions with Other Drugs

A. Effect of Streptomycin on Activity of Other Drugs
   1. Colistin (apnea) ↑
   2. EDTA (apnea) ↑
   3. General anesthetics (apnea) ↑
   4. Penicillins ↑
B. Effect of Other Drugs on Activity of Streptomycin
   1. Oxygen ↑
   2. Anticholinesterases (apnea) ↓
C. Synergistic Activity
   1. Cephalosporins
   2. Chloramphenicol
   3. Erythromycin
   4. Penicillins
   5. Sulfonamides
   6. Tetracycline
D. Cross Sensitivity
   1. Gentamicin
   2. Kanamycin
   3. Neomycin

References

AMA Drug Evaluations. 2nd Ed., Acton, Mass., Publishing Sciences Group, 1973, pp. 572–573, 588.
Blacow, N. W. (Ed.): Martindale: The Extra Pharmacopoeia. 26th Ed., London, Pharmaceutical Press, 1972, pp. 1424–1430.
Sannella, L. S.: An early symptom of streptomycin neurotoxicity. Arch. Ophthalmol. 50:331, 1953.
Sykowski, P.: Streptomycin causing retrobulbar optic neuritis. Am. J. Ophthalmol. 34:1446, 1951.
Thomas, E. B.: Scotomas in conjunction with streptomycin therapy. Report of 11 cases. Arch. Ophthalmol. 43:729, 1950.
Walker, G. F.: Blindness during streptomycin and chloramphenicol therapy. Br. J. Ophthalmol. 45:555, 1961.

* * * * * * * * * * * *

Generic Name: 1. Sulfacetamide; 2. Sulfachlorpyridazine; 3. Sulfadiazine; 4. Sulfadimethoxine; 5. Sulfamerazine; 6. Sulfameter; 7. Sulfamethizole; 8. Sulfamethoxazole;   9. Sulfamethoxypyridazine;   10. Sulfanilamide; 11. Sulfaphenazole; 12. Sulfisoxazole (Sulfafurazole)

Proprietary Name: *Systemic:* 1. Acetosulfamine (Jap.), Optamide (Austral.), Sulamyd, Sulphacetamide (G.B.); 2. Sonilyn; 3. Adiazine (Fr.), Coco-Diazine, Diazyl (Austral.), Sulphadiazine (G.B.); 4. Madribon, Madroxine (Pol.), Sulfoplan (Denm.), Sulphadimethoxine (G.B.); 5. Sulfamerazini (Switz.), Sulphamerazine (G.B.); 6. Bayrena (Scand.), Durenat (Germ.), Durenate (G.B.), Kirocid (Austral.), Kiron (Swed.), Sulla, Sulphamethoxydiazine (G.B.); 7. Famet (Austral.), Lucosil (Scand.), Methisul (G.B.), Microsul, Mizol (G.B.), Proklar-M, Sulfametin (Swed.), Sulfasol, Sulfstat, Sulfurine, Sulphamethizole (G.B.), Thiosulf, Urolex (Austral.), Urolin (Austral.), Uroz (Austral.), Urolucosil (G.B.), Utrasul; 8. Gantanol; 9. Kynex, Lederkyn (G.B.), Midicel, Midikel (Belg., Scand.), Sulfdurazin (Scand.), Sulphamethoxypyridazine (G.B.); 10. Sulphanilamide (G.B.); 11. Orisul (Switz.), Orisulf (G.B.), Sulfabid, Sulphaphenazole (G.B.); 12. Chemovag, Gantrisin, SK-Soxazole, Sosol, Soxomide, Sulfagan (Austral.), Sulfazole (Austral.), Sulfisin (Austral.), Sulphafurazole (G.B.), Urogan (Austral.) *Ophthalmic:* 1. Acetopt (Austral.) Albucid (G.B.), Bleph-10/30, Cetamide, Isopto Cetamide, Opulets Sulfacetamide (G.B.), Sodium Sulamyd, Sulf-10/30, Sulfacel-15; 7. Oculoguttae Sulfamethizoli (Scand.); 12. Gantrisin

Primary Use: The sulfonamides are bacteriostatic agents effective against most gram-positive and some gram-negative organisms. Sulfonamides are the agents of choice for treatment of nocardiosis, chancroid, and toxoplasmosis.

Ocular Side Effects

A. Systemic Administration
1. Decreased vision
2. Myopia — with or without astigmatism
3. Decreased depth perception — with or without decreased adduction at near
4. Nonspecific ocular irritation
   a. Lacrimation
   b. Photophobia
5. Keratitis
6. Problems with color vision
   a. Dyschromatopsia
   b. Objects have yellow or red tinge
7. Subconjunctival or retinal hemorrhages
8. Visual fields
   a. Scotomas
   b. Constriction
9. Optic neuritis
10. Myasthenic neuromuscular blocking effect
    a. Paralysis of extraocular muscles
    b. Ptosis
11. Periorbital edema
12. Visual hallucinations
13. Papilledema
14. Cortical blindness

15. Vivid light lavender colored retinal vascular tree
16. Decreased anterior chamber depth — may precipitate narrow-angle glaucoma
17. Eyelids or conjunctiva
    a. Allergic reactions
    b. Conjunctivitis — nonspecific
    c. Stevens-Johnson syndrome
    d. Exfoliative dermatitis
    e. Lyell's syndrome
    f. Pemphigoid lesion with or without symblepharon
18. Blindness (?)
19. Optic atrophy (?)
20. Hypermetropia (?)
B. Local Ophthalmic Use or Exposure — Topical Application
    1. Irritation
    2. Eyelids or conjunctiva
       a. Allergic reactions
       b. Conjunctivitis — follicular
    3. Overgrowth of nonsusceptible organisms
    4. Delayed healing of corneal wound
    5. Conjunctival concretions

Clinical Significance: While there are numerous reported ocular side effects from systemic sulfa medication, most are rare and reversible. Probably the most common ocular side effect seen in patients on systemic therapy is myopia. This is transient, with or without induced astigmatism, usually bilateral, and may exceed several diopters. This is most likely due to refractive changes within the lens. Since sulfa not infrequently causes dermatologic problems, associated conjunctivitis, keratitis, and lid problems may be seen. Optic neuritis has been reported even in low dosages and is usually reversible with complete recovery of vision. Optic nerve and retinal disorders have been seen, but are quite rare.

Interactions with Other Drugs

A. Effect of Sulfonamides on Activity of Other Drugs
    1. Penicillins ↑
    2. Pyrimethamine ↑
    3. Ascorbic acid ↓
B. Effect of Other Drugs on Activity of Sulfonamides
    1. Analgesics ↑
    2. Ascorbic acid ↑
    3. Phenothiazines ↑
    4. Salicylates ↑
    5. Antacids ↓
    6. Local anesthetics ↓
    7. Mineral oil ↓
C. Synergistic Activity
    1. Colistin

2. Erythromycin
3. Penicillin (occasionally indifferent or inhibitory)
D. Cross Sensitivity
 1. Carbonic anhydrase inhibitors
 2. Other sulfonamides
E. Contraindications
 1. Ophthalmic solutions containing silver or aminobenzoic acid

References

Boettner, E. A., Fralick, F. B., and Wolter, J. R.: Conjunctival concretions of sulfadiazine. Arch. Ophthalmol. 92:446, 1974.
Bucy, P. C.: Toxic optic neuritis resulting from sulfanilamide. JAMA 109:1007, 1937.
Haviland, J. W., and Long, P. H.: Skin and ocular reactions in sulfathiazole therapy. Bull. Johns Hopkins Hosp. 66:263, 1940.
Hornbogen, D. P.: Transient myopia during sulfanilamide therapy. Am. J. Ophthalmol. 24:323, 1941.
Newell, F. W., and Greetham, J. S.: Pemphigus conjunctivae. Am. J. Ophthalmol. 29:1426, 1946.
Taub, R. G., and Hollenhorst, R. W.: Sulfonamides as a cause of toxic amblyopia. Am. J. Ophthalmol. 40:486, 1955.

* * * * * * * * * * * *

Class: Antifungal Agents

Generic Name: Amphotericin B

Proprietary Name: Fungilin (G.B.), Fungizone

Primary Use: This polyene fungistatic agent is effective against *Blastomyces*, *Histoplasma*, *Cryptococcus*, *Coccidiomyces*, *Candida*, and *Aspergillus*.

Ocular Side Effects

A. Systemic Administration
 1. Decreased vision
 2. Paresis of extraocular muscles
 3. Retinal exudates
 4. Subconjunctival or retinal hemorrhages secondary to drug-induced anemia
 5. Diplopia
B. Local Ophthalmic Use or Exposure — Topical Application or Subconjunctival Injection
 1. Irritation
  a. Ocular pain
  b. Burning sensation
 2. Punctate keratitis

   3. Eyelids or conjunctiva
      a. Allergic reactions
      b. Ulceration
      c. Conjunctivitis — follicular
   4. Overgrowth of nonsusceptible organisms
   5. Iridocyclitis
C. Local Ophthalmic Use or Exposure — Intracameral Injection
   1. Uveitis
   2. Corneal edema
   3. Lens damage

Clinical Significance: Ocular complications due to amphotericin B are primarily seen with intrathecal injection; otherwise, few ocular side effects have been reported. With topical ocular application, however, local irritation and pruritus are not uncommon. A case of marked iridocyclitis with small hyphema has been seen each time after restarting application of topical ocular amphotericin B.

Interactions with Other Drugs

A. Effect of Amphotericin B on Activity of Other Drugs
   1. Corticosteroids ↓

References

AMA Drug Evaluations. 2nd Ed., Acton, Mass., Publishing Sciences Group, 1973, pp. 597–599, 711–712.
Burns, R. P.: Repeated iridocyclitis following topical ocular amphotericin B therapy. Personal communication, 1975.
Meyler, L., and Herxheimer, A. (Eds.): Side Effects of Drugs. Amsterdam, Excerpta Medica, Vol. VII, 1972, p. 405.
Spickard, A., et al.: The improved prognosis of cryptococcal meningitis with amphotericin B therapy. Ann. Intern. Med. 58:66, 1963.
Utz, J. P.: Current concepts in therapy. Chemotherapeutic agents for the systemic mycoses. N. Engl. J. Med. 268:938, 1963.

* * * * * * * * * * * *

Generic Name: Griseofulvin

Proprietary Name: Fulcin (G.B.), Fulvicin-U/F, Grifulvin V, Grisactin, Grisefuline (Fr.), Grisovin (G.B.), Gris Owen, Gris-Peg, Lamoryl Novum (Swed.)

Primary Use: This is the only commercially available oral antifungal agent effective against *Microsporum, Epidermophyton*, and *Trichophyton*.

Ocular Side Effects

A. Systemic Administration
   1. Decreased vision
   2. Problems with color vision — objects have green tinge
   3. Macular degeneration
   4. Macular edema

5. Visual hallucinations
6. Eyelids or conjunctiva
   a. Allergic reactions
   b. Edema
   c. Photosensitivity
   d. Angioneurotic edema
   e. Lupoid syndrome
   f. Exfoliative dermatitis
7. Papilledema secondary to pseudotumor cerebri
8. Congenital blindness
9. Subconjunctival or retinal hemorrhages secondary to drug-induced anemia
10. Paresis of extraocular muscles (?)

Clinical Significance: Griseofulvin rarely causes ophthalmic problems; however, it may cause severe allergic reactions with ocular involvement. Most of the preceding adverse ocular reactions are based on only a few cases.

Interactions with Other Drugs

A. Effect of Griseofulvin on Activity of Other Drugs
   1. Alcohol ↑
   2. Barbiturates ↑
B. Effect of Other Drugs on Activity of Griseofulvin
   1. Antihistamines ↓
   2. Phenylbutazone ↓
   3. Sedatives and hypnotics ↓
C. Cross Sensitivity
   1. Penicillins

References

AMA Drug Evaluations. 2nd Ed., Acton, Mass., Publishing Sciences Group, 1973, pp. 600–601.

Delman, M., and Leubuscher, K.: Transient macular edema due to griseofulvin. Am. J. Ophthalmol. 56:658, 1963.

Duverne, J., et al.: Accidents hallucinatoires repetes chez une enfant traitee par la grisefuline pour dermatophyties multiples. Lyon Med. 211:1773, 1964.

Goodman, L. S., and Gilman, A. (Eds.): The Pharmacological Basis of Therapeutics. 4th Ed., New York, Macmillan, 1970, pp. 1302–1304.

Meyler, L., and Herxheimer, A. (Eds.): Side Effects of Drugs. Amsterdam, Excerpta Medica, Vol. VII, 1972, pp. 404–405.

* * * * * * * * * * * * *

Generic Name: Nystatin

Proprietary Name: Mycostatin, Nilstat, Nitacin (G.B.), Nystan (G.B.)

Primary Use: This polyene fungistatic and fungicidal agent is effective against *Candida*.

Ocular Side Effects

   A. Systemic Administration
      1. Optic neuritis
      2. Decreased vision
   B. Local Ophthalmic Use or Exposure — Topical Application or Subconjunctival Injection
      1. Irritation
      2. Eyelids or conjunctiva — allergic reactions
      3. Overgrowth of nonsusceptible organisms

Clinical Significance: Ocular side effects from systemic or ocular nystatin administration are unusual. Most adverse ocular reactions due to it are reversible and transitory.

References

Physicians' Desk Reference. 28th Ed., Oradell, N. J., Medical Economics Co., 1974, pp. 864, 1411.

Saraux, H.: La nevrite optique par intoxication medicamenteuse. Communication Soc. Med. Milit. December 17, 1970.

Wasilewski, C.: Allergic contact dermatitis from nystatin. Arch. Derm. *102:*216, 1970.

* * * * * * * * * * * *

Generic Name: Thiabendazole. See under *Class: Anthelmintics.*

* * * * * * * * * * * *

Class: Antileprosy Agents

Generic Name: Amithiozone. See under *Class: Antitubercular Agents.*

* * * * * * * * * * * *

Generic Name: Ethionamide. See under *Class: Antitubercular Agents.*

* * * * * * * * * * * *

Class: Antimalarial Agents

Generic Name: 1. Amodiaquine; 2. Chloroquine; 3. Hydroxychloroquine

Proprietary Name: 1. Camoquin, Flavoquine (Fr.); 2. Aralen, Avloclor (G.B.), Bemaphate (G.B.), Bemasulf (G.B.), Chloroquin (Austral.), Imagon (Swed.), Nivaquaine (G.B.), Resochin (G.B.); 3. Ercoquin (Norw.), Plaquenil

Primary Use: These aminoquinolines are used in the treatment of malaria, extraintestinal amebiasis, rheumatoid arthritis, and lupus erythematosus.

Ocular Side Effects

A. Systemic Administration
1. Decreased vision
2. Corneal deposits
3. Macular or retinal degeneration — pigmentary retinopathy, bull's eye, doughnut
4. Visual fields
    a. Scotomas — annular, central, or paracentral
    b. Constriction
5. Problems with color vision
    a. Dyschromatopsia
    b. Objects have yellow tinge
    c. Achromatopsia, red-green or blue-yellow defect
    d. Colored haloes around lights
6. Retinal vasoconstriction
7. Blindness
8. Decreased accommodation
9. Photophobia
10. Corneal edema
11. Night blindness
12. Decreased corneal reflex
13. Visual hallucinations
14. Poliosis
15. Absence of foveal reflex
16. Diplopia
17. Flashing lights
18. Paralysis of extraocular muscles
19. Ptosis
20. Retinal edema
21. Subconjunctival or retinal hemorrhages secondary to drug-induced anemia
22. Optic atrophy
23. Eyelids or conjunctiva
    a. Allergic reactions
    b. Photosensitivity
    c. Erythema multiforme
    d. Stevens-Johnson syndrome
    e. Exfoliative dermatitis
24. Uveitis (?)
25. Lens opacities (?)
26. Decreased dark adaptation (?)

27. Loss of eyelashes or eyebrows (?)
28. Ocular teratogenic effects (?)
B. Inadvertent Ocular Exposure
   1. Corneal deposits

Clinical Significance: Significant ocular side effects are rarely found in patients taking 250 mg or less of aminoquinolines daily. However, if this dosage (250 mg) is maintained for over 6 months, significant ocular side effects are seen in some patients. Corneal deposits have no direct relationship to posterior segment disease and are reversible. Toxic maculopathy usually is reversible only in its earliest phases. If these drugs have caused skin, eyelid, or hair changes, this is an excellent indicator of possible drug-induced retinopathy. Since these agents are concentrated in pigmented tissue, macular changes may progress long after the drug therapy is stopped. The "bull's eye" macula is not diagnostic for aminoquinoline-induced disease since a number of other entities can cause this same clinical picture. Amodiaquine has not been as extensively used as chloroquine or hydroxychloroquine, and thus far, few ocular side effects have been reported for it.

Interactions with Other Drugs

A. Effect of Other Drugs on Activity of Aminoquinolines
   1. Antacids ↑
   2. Monoamine oxidase inhibitors ↑

References

Arden, G. B., and Kolb, H.: Antimalarial therapy and early retinal changes in patients with rheumatoid arthritis. Br. Med. J. 1:270, 1966.
Bernstein, H. N.: Chloroquine ocular toxicity. Surv. Ophthalmol. 12:415, 1967.
Blacow, N. W. (Ed.): Martindale: The Extra Pharmacopoeia. 26th Ed., London, Pharmaceutical Press, 1972, pp. 418–426, 428–430.
Burns, R. P.: Delayed onset of chloroquine retinopathy. N. Engl. J. Med. 275:693, 1966.
Lazar, M., Regenbogen, L., and Stein, R.: Anterior uveitis due to chloroquine. Ophthalmologica 146:411, 1963.
Percival, S. P. B., and Behrman, J.: Ophthalmological safety with chloroquine. Br. J. Ophthalmol. 53:101, 1969.

* * * * * * * * * * * *

Generic Name: Quinacrine (Mepacrine). See under *Class: Anthelmintics.*

* * * * * * * * * * * *

Generic Name: Quinine

Proprietary Name: Quinbisan (Austral.), Quinsan (Austral.)

Primary Use: This alkaloid is effective in the management of nocturnal leg cramps, myotonia congenita, and in resistant *P. falciparum.* It is also used in attempted abortions. Ophthalmologically, it is useful in the treatment of eyelid myokymia.

Ocular Side Effects

A. Systemic Administration
    1. Decreased vision
    2. Mydriasis
    3. Papilledema
    4. Visual fields
        a. Scotomas
        b. Constriction
    5. Optic atrophy
    6. Iris atrophy
    7. Blindness
    8. Retinal vasodilatation followed by marked constriction
    9. Photophobia
    10. Night blindness
    11. Problems with color vision
        a. Dyschromatopsia
        b. Objects have red or green tinge
        c. Achromatopsia, red-green or blue defect
    12. Visual hallucinations
    13. Vertical nystagmus
    14. Macular degeneration
    15. Subconjunctival or retinal hemorrhages secondary to drug-induced anemia
    16. Eyelids or conjunctiva
        a. Allergic reactions
        b. Angioneurotic edema
        c. Purpura
        d. Erythema multiforme
        e. Stevens-Johnson syndrome
    17. Congenital blindness
    18. Retinal or macular edema
    19. Absence of foveal reflex
    20. Retinal exudates
    21. Flashing lights
    22. Ocular teratogenic effects (?)

Clinical Significance: The most severe adverse ocular reactions with irreversible changes due to quinine are seen primarily in cases of attempted abortions. Quinine-induced blindness in offspring of mothers with unsuccessful abortions has also been seen. Ocular side effects, however, are quite rare at suggested dosage levels.

Interactions with Other Drugs

A. Effect of Quinine on Activity of Other Drugs
    1. Antibiotics (apnea) ↑
        (Kanamycin, Neomycin, Streptomycin)
    2. Anticholinergics ↑
    3. Anticholinesterases ↓

References

Bard, L. A., and Gills, J. P.: Quinine amblyopia. Arch. Ophthalmol. *72*:328, 1964.
Behrman, J., and Mushin, A.: Electrodiagnostic findings in quinine amblyopia. Br. J. Ophthalmol. *52*:925, 1968.
Braveman, B. L., Koransky, D. S., and Kulvin, M. M.: Quinine amaurosis. Am. J. Ophthalmol. *31*:731, 1948.
Francois, J., De Rouck, A., and Cambie, E.: Retinal and optic evaluation in quinine poisoning. Ann. Ophthalmol. *4*:177, 1972.
Knox, D. L., Palmer, C. A. L., and English, F.: Iris atrophy after quinine amblyopia. Arch. Ophthalmol. *76*:359, 1966.

* * * * * * * * * * * *

Class: Antiprotozoal Agents

Generic Name: Tryparsamide

Proprietary Name: Tryparsamide

Primary Use: This organic arsenical is used in the treatment of trypanosomiasis (African sleeping sickness).

Ocular Side Effects
- A. Systemic Administration
    1. Constriction of visual fields
    2. Decreased vision
    3. Visual sensations
        a. Smokeless fog
        b. Shimmering effect
    4. Optic neuritis
    5. Optic atrophy
    6. Blindness

Clinical Significance: The most serious and common adverse drug reactions due to tryparsamide involve the eye. Incidences of ocular side effects vary from 3 to 20 percent of cases, with constriction of visual fields followed by decreased vision as the characteristic sequence. Almost 10 percent of individuals taking tryparsamide experience visual changes consisting of "shimmering" or "dazzling" which may persist for days or even weeks. If the medication is not immediately discontinued following these visual changes, the pathologic condition of the optic nerve may become irreversible and progress to blindness.

References

AMA Drug Evaluations. 2nd Ed., Acton, Mass., Publishing Sciences Group, 1973, p. 626.
Blacow, N. W. (Ed.): Martindale: The Extra Pharmacopoeia. 26th Ed., London, Pharmaceutical Press, 1972, p. 1865.

Goodman, L. S., and Gilman, A. (Eds.): The Pharmacological Basis of Therapeutics. 4th Ed., New York, Macmillan, 1970, p. 1149.

Grant, W. M.: Toxicology of the Eye. 2nd Ed., Springfield, Charles C Thomas, 1974, pp. 1069–1070.

LeJeune, J. R.: Les oligo-elements et chelateurs. Bull. Soc. Belge Ophtalmol. *160*:241, 1972.

Walsh, F. B., and Hoyt, W. F.: Clinical Neuro-Ophthalmology. 3rd Ed., Baltimore, Williams & Wilkins, Vol. III, 1969, pp. 2594–2596.

* * * * * * * * * * * *

Class: Anthelmintics

Generic Name: 1. Antimony Lithium Thiomalate; 2. Antimony Potassium Tartrate; 3. Antimony Sodium Tartrate; 4. Antimony Sodium Thioglycollate; 5. Sodium Antimonylgluconate; 6. Stibocaptate; 7. Stibophen

Proprietary Name: 1. Anthiomaline (G.B.); 2. Antimonial Wine (G.B.); 3. Antimony Sodium Tartrate; 4. Antimonio E Sodio Tioglicolato (Ital.); 5. Triostam (G.B.); 6. Astiban; 7. Fuadin

Primary Use: These trivalent antimony compounds are used in the treatment of schistosomiasis and filariasis.

Ocular Side Effects

A. Systemic Administration
1. Eyelids or conjunctiva
   a. Edema
   b. Urticaria
2. Yellow discoloration of skin or sclera
3. Decreased vision
4. Pupils
   a. Mydriasis
   b. Absence of reaction to light
5. Papilledema
6. Optic atrophy
7. Blindness
8. Subconjunctival or retinal hemorrhages secondary to drug-induced anemia

Clinical Significance: Since antimonials are rarely used in developed countries, only limited data on their complete toxicologic effects are available. While the preceding adverse reactions have been reported, few are well documented. Serious adverse ocular reactions have been seen, although infrequently.

References

Blacow, N. W. (Ed.): Martindale: The Extra Pharmacopoeia. 26th Ed., London, Pharmaceutical Press, 1972, pp. 1610–1615.

D'Amino, D.: Considerazioni sopra un caso di cecita instantanea bilaterale da avvelenamento per tartaro stibiato nella cura del Kala-azar. Lett. Oftalmol. 8:474, 1931.

Goodman, L. S. and Gilman, A. (Eds.): The Pharmacological Basis of Therapeutics, 4th Ed., New York, Macmillan, 1970, pp. 965–967.

Grant, W. M.: Toxicology of the Eye. 2nd Ed., Springfield, Charles C Thomas, 1974, p. 150.

* * * * * * * * * * * * *

Generic Name: Diethylcarbamazine

Proprietary Name: Banocide, Hetrazan, Notezine

Primary Use: This antifilarial agent is particularly effective against *W. bancrofti*, *W. malayi*, *O. volvulus*, and *Loa loa*.

Ocular Side Effects

A. Systemic Administration
   1. Conjunctivitis — nonspecific
   2. Iridocyclitis
   3. Posterior uveitis
   4. Loss of eyelashes or eyebrows
   5. Blindness

Clinical Significance: Adverse ocular reactions to diethylcarbamazine may occur, but primarily only indirectly. After the filaria has been killed by the drug, an allergic reaction due to the release of foreign protein from the dead larvae or adult worms may occur. This reaction in the eye may be so marked that blindness follows.

References

AMA Drug Evaluations. 2nd Ed., Acton, Mass., Publishing Sciences Group, 1973, pp. 634, 713.

Dralands, L.: Les anthelminthiques. Bull. Soc. Belge Ophtalmol. 160:436, 1972.

Duke, B. O. L.: Medicine in the tropics. Onchocerciasis. Br. Med. J. 4:301, 1968.

Gray, H. H.: Alopecia totalis after diethylcarbamazine treatment of loiasis. Trans. R. Soc. Trop. Med. Hyg. 59:718, 1965.

Meyler, L., and Herxheimer, A. (Eds.): Side Effects of Drugs. Amsterdam, Excerpta Medica, Vol. VII, 1972, p. 433.

* * * * * * * * * * * *

Generic Name: Piperazine

Proprietary Name: Adipalit (Ital.), Antepar, Antivermine (Pol.), Entacyl, Entazin (Denm.), Eraverm (Germ.), Helmezine (G.B.), Lumbrioxyl (Fr.), Minox (G.B.), Multifuge, Parazine, Perin, Piperasol (Pol.), Piperate, Pipizan, Piprosan (Austral.), Pripsen (G.B.), Uvilon (Germ.), Vermicompren (Germ.), Vermidol, Vermizine, Vermolina (Austral.)

Primary Use: This anthelmintic agent is used in the treatment of ascariasis and enterobiasis.

Ocular Side Effects

A. Systemic Administration
1. Decreased vision
2. Problems with color vision — dyschromatopsia
3. Paralysis of accommodation
4. Miosis
5. Nystagmus
6. Visual hallucinations
7. Paralysis of extraocular muscles
8. Visual sensations
a. Flashing lights
b. Entopic light flashes
9. Eyelids or conjunctiva
a. Allergic reactions
b. Edema
c. Photosensitivity
d. Urticaria
e. Purpura
10. Cataracts (?)

Clinical Significance: While a number of ocular side effects have been attributed to piperazine, they are rare, reversible, and usually of little clinical importance. Adverse ocular reactions generally occur only in instances of overdose or impaired excretion. Only one well-documented case of extraocular muscle paralysis has been reported.

References

AMA Drug Evaluations. 2nd Ed., Acton, Mass., Publishing Sciences Group, 1973, pp. 635–636.

Brown, H. W., Chan, K. F., and Hussey, K. L.: Treatment of enterobiasis and ascariasis with piperazine. JAMA *161*:515, 1956.

Combes, B., Damon, A., and Gottfried, E.: Piperazine (Antepar) neurotoxicity. Report of a case probably due to renal insufficiency. N. Engl. J. Med. *254*:223, 1956.

Mezey, P.: The role of piperazine derivates in the pathogenesis of cataract. Klin. Monatsbl. Augenheilkd. *151*:885, 1967.

Walsh, F. B., and Hoyt, W. F.: Clinical Neuro-Ophthalmology. 3rd Ed., Baltimore, Williams & Wilkins, Vol. III, 1969, pp. 2637–2638.

* * * * * * * * * * * * *

Generic Name: Quinacrine (Mepacrine)

Proprietary Name: Atabrine, Atebrin

Primary Use: This methoxyacridine agent is effective in the treatment of tapeworm infestations and in the prophylaxis and treatment of malaria.

Ocular Side Effects

A. Systemic Administration
   1. Decreased vision
   2. Visual fields
      a. Scotomas
      b. Enlarged blind spot
   3. Optic neuritis
   4. Corneal edema
   5. Yellow, white, clear, brown, blue, or grey punctate deposits
      a. Conjunctiva
      b. Cornea
      c. Nasolacrimal system
   6. Problems with color vision
      a. Dyschromatopsia
      b. Objects have yellow, green, blue, or violet tinge
      c. Colored haloes around lights — mainly blue
   7. Subconjunctival or retinal hemorrhages secondary to drug-induced anemia
   8. Eyelids or conjunctiva
      a. Blue-black pigmentation
      b. Yellow discoloration
      c. Eczema
      d. Exfoliative dermatitis
   9. Ocular teratogenic effects (?)
B. Inadvertent Ocular Exposure
   1. Blue haloes around lights
   2. Eyelids, conjunctiva, or cornea
      a. Edema
      b. Yellow discoloration
   3. Irritation
      a. Lacrimation
      b. Ocular pain

Clinical Significance: Adverse ocular reactions due to quinacrine are common but seldom of clinical significance. Nearly all are reversible and fairly asymptomatic. Topical ocular application has been used for self-inflicted ocular damage; however, it has been apparently fairly devoid of any permanent ocular damage.

References

Abbey, E. A., and Lawrence, E. A.: The effect of Atabrine suppressive therapy on eyesight of pilots. JAMA *130*:786, 1946.
Chamberlain, W. P., and Boles, D. J.: Edema of the cornea precipitated by quinacrine (Atabrine). Arch. Ophthalmol. *35*:120, 1946.
Dame, L. R.: The effects of Atabrine on the human visual system. Am. J. Ophthalmol. *29*:1432, 1946.
Ferrara, A.: Optic neuritis from high doses of Atebrin. Rass. Ital. Ottalmol. *12*:123, 1943.
Mann, I.: "Blue haloes" in Atebrin workers. Br. J. Ophthalmol. *31*:40, 1947.

* * * * * * * * * * * * *

Generic Name: Thiabendazole

Proprietary Name: Mintezol

Primary Use: This benzimidazole compound is used in the treatment of enterobiasis, strongyloidiasis, ascariasis, uncinariasis, trichuriasis, and cutaneous larva migrans. It has been advocated as an antimycotic in corneal ulcers.

Ocular Side Effects

A. Systemic Administration
1. Decreased vision
2. Problems with color vision
a. Dyschromatopsia
b. Objects have yellow tinge
3. Abnormal visual sensations
4. Eyelids or conjunctiva
a. Allergic reactions
b. Hyperemia
c. Angioneurotic edema
d. Stevens-Johnson syndrome
e. Exfoliative dermatitis
5. Subconjunctival or retinal hemorrhages secondary to drug-induced anemia.

Clinical Significance: While thiabendazole is one of the more potent therapeutic agents known, it has surprisingly few reported ocular or systemic toxic side effects. Ocular side effects are transitory, reversible, and seldom of clinical importance.

References

AMA Drug Evaluations. 2nd Ed., Acton, Mass., Publishing Sciences Group, 1973, pp. 639, 713.
Goodman, L. S., and Gilman, A. (Eds.): The Pharmacological Basis of Therapeutics. 4th Ed., New York, Macmillan, 1970, pp. 1083–1085.
Meyler, L., and Herxheimer, A. (Eds.): Side Effects of Drugs, Amsterdam, Excerpta Medica, Vol. VII, 1972, p. 435.
Physicians' Desk Reference. 28th Ed., Oradell, N. J., Medical Economics Co., 1974, p. 1034.
Thiabendazole. Med. Lett. Drugs Ther. 11:28, 1969.

* * * * * * * * * * * * *

Class: Antitubercular Agents

Generic Name: Aminosalicylic Acid

Proprietary Name: Pamisyl, Para-Pas, Parasal, PAS-C, Pascorbic, Rezipas

Primary Use: Aminosalicylic acid is a bacteriostatic agent which is effective against *M. tuberculosis.*

Ocular Side Effects

A. Systemic Administration
1. Decreased accommodation (?)
2. Decreased vision (?)
3. Optic neuritis (?)
4. Scotomas (?)
5. Optic atrophy (?)
6. Eyelids or conjunctiva
   a. Allergic reactions (?)
   b. Blepharitis (?)
   c. Edema (?)
   d. Stevens-Johnson syndrome (?)
   e. Exfoliative dermatitis (?)
7. Subconjunctival or retinal hemorrhages secondary to drug-induced anemia (?)

Clinical Significance: Aminosalicylic acid is so seldom used by itself that many, if not most, of the preceding ocular side effects may be due to other drugs. Even so, the total number of reported cases of possible adverse ocular reactions is very small.

Interactions with Other Drugs

A. Effect of Aminosalicylic Acid on Activity of Other Drugs
1. Barbiturates ↑
2. Sulfonamides ↓
3. Vitamin B_{12} ↓
B. Effect of Other Drugs on Activity of Aminosalicylic Acid
1. Salicylates ↑
2. Streptomycin ↑

References

AMA Drug Evaluations. 2nd Ed., Acton, Mass., Publishing Sciences Group, 1973, pp. 582–583.

Meyler, L., and Herxheimer, A. (Eds.): Side Effects of Drugs. Amsterdam, Excerpta Medica, Vol. VII, 1972, pp. 423–426.

O'Hara, H.: Blepharitis squamosa occurred before dermatitis exfoliativa caused by PAS-Ca and streptomycin. J. Clin. Ophthalmol. (Tokyo) *10*:1421,`1956.

Pohjola, S., and Horsmanheimo, A.: Keratitis sicca after erythema exudativum multiforme caused by P.A.S. (Case report). Acta Ophthalmol. *44*:415, 1966.

Steiner, C.: Un cas d'intoxication par PAS et produits analogues. Bull. Soc. Ophtalmol. Fr., p. 527, April, 1951.

* * * * * * * * * * * *

Generic Name: Amithiozone

Proprietary Name: Couteben (Germ.), Panrone, Thiacetazone (G.B.), Thiopara-mizone (G.B.), Tibione

Primary Use: This tuberculostatic agent is effective against *M. tuberculosis* and *M. leprae.*

Ocular Side Effects

A. Systemic Administration
  1. Decreased vision
  2. Nonspecific ocular irritation
     a. Photophobia
     b. Ocular pain
     c. Burning sensation
  3. Eyelids or conjunctiva
     a. Allergic reactions
     b. Erythema multiforme
     c. Stevens-Johnson syndrome
     d. Exfoliative dermatitis
  4. Retinal edema
  5. Subconjunctival or retinal hemorrhages secondary to drug-induced anemia

Clinical Significance: Numerous adverse ocular reactions due to amithiozone have been seen. Skin manifestations have been the most frequent. Nearly all ocular side effects are reversible and of minor clinical significance. One instance of toxic amblyopia has been reported; however, the patient was also receiving aminosalicylic acid.

Interactions with Other Drugs

A. Effect of Other Drugs on Activity of Amithiozone
  1. Corticosteroids ↓

References

Blacow, N. W. (Ed.): Martindale: The Extra Pharmacopoeia. 26th Ed., London, Pharmaceutical Press, 1972, pp. 1884–1886.
Jopling, W. H., and Kirwan, E. W. O'G.: Toxic amblyopia caused by TB3: A case record. Trans. R. Soc. Trop. Med. Hyg. 46:656, 1952.
Steiner, C.: Un cas d'intoxication par P.A.S. et produits analogues. Bull. Soc. Ophtalmol. Fr. p. 527, April 1951.
von Oettingen, W. F.: Poisoning. 2nd Ed., Philadelphia, W. B. Saunders, 1958.

* * * * * * * * * * * *

Generic Name: Capreomycin

Proprietary Name: Capastat

Primary Use: This polypeptide tuberculostatic antibiotic is effective against *M. tuberculosis.* It is used when less toxic antitubercular agents have been ineffective.

Ocular Side Effects

    A. Systemic Administration
        1. Visual sensations
            a. Flickering vision
            b. Flashing lights
        2. Problems with color vision — objects have white tinge
        3. Eyelids or conjunctiva
            a. Angioneurotic edema
            b. Urticaria
        4. Blindness
        5. Visual hallucinations (?)

Clinical Significance: Adverse ocular reactions due to capreomycin are not common, and all ocular side effects are transitory and reversible. Blindness is usually of only short duration and reversible.

Interactions with Other Drugs

    A. Effect of Other Drugs on Activity of Capreomycin
        1. Antibiotics ↑
            (Kanamycin, Streptomycin, Viomycin)
        2. General anesthetics (apnea) ↑
        3. Anticholinesterases ↓
        4. Corticosteroids ↓

References

Blacow, N. W. (Ed.): Martindale: The Extra Pharmacopoeia. 26th Ed., London, Pharmaceutical Press, 1972, pp. 1326–1327.
Davidson, S. I.: Reports of ocular adverse reactions. Trans. Ophthalmol. Soc. U. K. *93*:495, 1973.
Physicians' Desk Reference. 28th Ed., Oradell, N. J., Medical Economics Co., 1974, p. 891.

* * * * * * * * * * * * *

Generic Name: Cycloserine

Proprietary Name: Closina (Austral.), Oxamycin, Seromycin

Primary Use: This isoxazolidone is effective against certain gram-negative and gram-positive bacteria and *M. tuberculosis.*

Ocular Side Effects

    A. Systemic Administration
        1. Decreased vision
        2. Eyelids or conjunctiva
            a. Allergic reactions
            b. Photosensitivity
        3. Visual hallucinations
        4. Flickering vision

5. Subconjunctival or retinal hemorrhages secondary to drug-induced anemia
6. Decreased accommodation (?)
7. Optic neuritis (?)
8. Optic atrophy (?)

Clinical Significance: Even though ocular complications due to cycloserine are quite rare, this drug is primarily used in combination with other drugs so that to pinpoint cause for ocular side effects is most difficult. Optic nerve damage has been reported, but the data are not conclusive.

References

AMA Drug Evaluations. 2nd Ed., Acton, Mass., Publishing Sciences Group, 1973, p. 584.
Goodman, L. S., and Gilman, A. (Eds.): The Pharmacological Basis of Therapeutics. 4th Ed., New York, Macmillan, 1970, pp. 1328–1329.
Grant, W. M.: Toxicology of the Eye. 2nd Ed., Springfield, Charles C Thomas, 1974, pp. 345–346.
Physicians' Desk Reference. 28th Ed., Oradell, N. J., Medical Economics Co., 1974, p. 931.
Walsh, F. B., and Hoyt, W. F.: Clinical Neuro-Ophthalmology. 3rd Ed. Baltimore, Williams & Wilkins, Vol. III, 1969, p. 2680.

* * * * * * * * * * * *

Generic Name: Ethambutol

Proprietary Name: Miambutol (Ital.), Myambutol

Primary Use: Ethambutol is a tuberculostatic agent which is effective against *M. tuberculosis.*

Ocular Side Effects

A. Systemic Administration
1. Decreased vision
2. Visual fields
    a. Scotomas — annular or central
    b. Constriction
    c. Hemianopsia
3. Optic neuritis
4. Photophobia
5. Problems with color vision
    a. Dyschromatopsia
    b. Achromatopsia, red-green or blue-yellow defect
6. Retinal hemorrhages — primarily peripapillary
7. Papilledema
8. Macular edema
9. Retinal vasodilatation
10. Paresis of extraocular muscles
11. Optic atrophy
12. Peripapillary atrophy (?)
13. Macular pigmentary changes (?)

Clinical Significance: Ethambutol in dosages of 15 mg/kg per day has caused few, if any, cases of ocular toxicity and relatively few adverse effects with 25 mg/kg per day for only a few months as initial therapy. Most of the ocular side effects are transitory and reversible when use of the drug is discontinued. Documentation of irreversible visual field changes, optic atrophy, and blindness due to ethambutol has only recently been reported.

Interactions with Other Drugs

A. Effect of Other Drugs on Activity of Ethambutol
  1. Corticosteroids ↓

References

Barron, G. J., Tepper, L., and Iovine, G.: Ocular toxicity from ethambutol, Am. J. Ophthalmol. 77:256, 1974.
Carr, R. E., and Henkind, P.: Ocular manifestations of ethambutol. Arch. Ophthalmol. 67:566, 1962.
Deodati, F., et al.: Optic neuritis due to ethambutol. Rev. Otoneuroophtalmol. 46:191, 1974.
Friedmann, A.: Investigation of drug toxicity. In Rose, F. (Ed.): Adverse Drug Reactions. London, Chapman and Hall. To be published.
Leibold, J. E.: The ocular toxicity of ethambutol and its relation to dose. Ann. N. Y. Acad. Sci. 135:904, 1966.
Roussos, T., and Tsolkas, A.: The toxicity of myambutol on the human eye. Ann. Ophthalmol. 2:578, 1970.
Yonekura, Y., Mori, T., and Kondo, N.: Optic nerve complications of ethambutol. Folia Ophthalmol. Jap. 20:545, 1969.

* * * * * * * * * * * *

Generic Name: Ethionamide

Proprietary Name: Trecator, Trescatyl (G.B.)

Primary Use: This isonicotinic acid derivative is effective against *M. tuberculosis* and *M. leprae.* It is indicated in the treatment of patients when resistance to primary tuberculostatic drugs has developed.

Ocular Side Effects

A. Systemic Administration
  1. Decreased vision
  2. Diplopia
  3. Eyelids or conjunctiva
     a. Allergic reactions
     b. Erythema
     c. Exfoliative dermatitis
  4. Photophobia
  5. Problems with color vision
     a. Dyschromatopsia
     b. Heightened color perception
  6. Optic neuritis
  7. Loss of eyelashes or eyebrows (?)

Clinical Significance: The incidence of adverse ocular effects due to ethionamide is quite small and seldom of clinical significance. While certain adverse
effects occur at low dosage levels, they usually do not continue even if the
dosage is increased.

Interactions with Other Drugs

A. Effect of Ethionamide on Activity of Other Drugs
    1. Alcohol ↑
B. Effect of Other Drugs on Activity of Ethionamide
    1. Corticosteroids ↓

References

Blacow, N. W. (Ed.): Martindale: The Extra Pharmacopoeia. 26th Ed., London, Pharma-
ceutical Press, 1972, pp. 1870–1872.
Fox, W., et al.: A study of acute intolerance to ethionamide, including a comparison with
prothionamide, and of the influence of a vitamin B-complex additive in prophylaxis.
Tubercule 50:125, 1969.
Goodman, L. S., and Gilman, A. (Eds.): The Pharmacological Basis of Therapeutics. 4th Ed.,
New York, Macmillan, 1970, pp. 1331–1332.
Meyler, L., and Herxheimer, A. (Eds.): Side Effects of Drugs. Amsterdam, Excerpta Medica,
Vol. VII, 1972, p. 426.

* * * * * * * * * * * * *

Generic Name: Isoniazid

Proprietary Name: Hyzyd, INH, Isobicina (Ital.), Isonico, Isotinyl (Austral.),
Isozid (Germ.), Neoteben (Germ.), Nicetal (G.B.), Niconyl, Nicozide, Nydra-
zid, Pycazide (G.B.), Raumanon (Swed.), Rimifon, Triniad, Tyvid, Uniad

Primary Use: This hydrazide of isonicotinic acid is effective against *M. tuberculosis.*

Ocular Side Effects

A. Systemic Administration
    1. Decreased vision
    2. Optic neuritis
    3. Optic atrophy
    4. Visual fields
        a. Scotomas
        b. Constriction
        c. Hemianopsia
    5. Papilledema
    6. Problems with color vision
        a. Dyschromatopsia
        b. Achromatopsia, red-green defect
    7. Eyelids or conjunctiva
        a. Allergic reactions
        b. Angioneurotic edema

      c. Lupoid syndrome
      d. Exfoliative dermatitis
  8. Pupils
      a. Mydriasis
      b. Absence of reaction to light
  9. Paralysis of accommodation
10. Diplopia
11. Paresis of extraocular muscles
12. Keratitis
13. Nystagmus
14. Subconjunctival or retinal hemorrhages secondary to drug-induced anemia
15. Blindness
16. Visual hallucinations (?)

Clinical Significance: The true incidence or significance of isoniazid-induced ocular side effects is difficult to evaluate since they are seen most commonly in malnourished, chronic alcoholics and in individuals who are characteristically on multiple drugs. Many, if not almost all, of the neurologic side effects can be prevented by the daily administration of pyridoxine. Signs and symptoms other than the neuro-ophthalmic complications are usually insignificant and reversible.

Interactions with Other Drugs

  A. Effect of Isoniazid on Activity of Other Drugs
    1. Analgesics ↑
    2. Anticholinergics ↑
    3. Barbiturates ↑
    4. General anesthetics ↑
    5. Sedatives and hypnotics ↑
    6. Sympathomimetics ↑
    7. Tricyclic antidepressants ↑
  B. Effect of Other Drugs on Activity of Isoniazid
    1. Salicylates ↑
    2. Alcohol ↓
    3. Corticosteroids ↓
    4. Pyridoxine ↓
  C. Synergistic Activity
    1. Streptomycin

References

Dixon, G. J., Roberts, G. B. S., and Tyrrell, W. F.: The relationship of neuropathy to the treatment of tuberculosis with isoniazid. Scot. Med. J. 1:350, 1956.

Kalinowski, S. Z., Lloyd, T. W., and Moyes, E. N.: Complications in the chemotherapy of tuberculosis. A review with analysis of the experience of 3,148 patients. Am. Rev. Respir. Dis. 83:359, 1961.

Kass, I., et al.: Isoniazid as a cause of optic neuritis and atrophy. JAMA 164:1740, 1957.

Keeping, J. A., and Searle, C. W. A.: Optic neuritis following isoniazid therapy. Lancet 2:278, 1955.

Money, G. L.: Isoniazid neuropathies in malnourished tuberculosis patients. J. Trop. Med. Hyg. 62:198, 1959.
Sutton, P. H., and Beattie, P. H.: Optic atrophy after administration of isoniazid with P.A.S. Lancet 1:650, 1955.

* * * * * * * * * * * *

Generic Name: Streptomycin. See under *Class: Antibiotics.*

* * * * * * * * * * * *

II. Agents Affecting the Central Nervous System

Class: Analeptics

Generic Name: Pentylenetetrazol (Pentetrazol)

Proprietary Name: Cardiazol, Leptazol (G.B.), Metrazol

Primary Use: This CNS stimulant is used to enhance the mental and physical activity of elderly patients.

Ocular Side Effects

A. Systemic Administration
   1. Pupils
      a. Mydriasis
      b. Absence of reaction to light
      c. Hippus
   2. Problems with color vision
      a. Dyschromatopsia
      b. Objects have yellow tinge
   3. Blepharospasm
   4. Visual hallucinations
   5. Scintillating scotomas
   6. Extraocular muscles
      a. Abnormal conjugate deviations
      b. Strabismus

Clinical Significance: Ocular side effects due to pentylenetetrazol are rare when the drug is administered orally; however, they are not uncommon if the drug is given intravenously. Ocular side effects are transient, most are reversible, and recovery is rapid after use of the drug is discontinued.

References

AMA Drug Evaluations. 2nd Ed., Acton, Mass., Publishing Sciences Group, 1973, p. 379.
Grant, W. M.: Toxicology of the Eye. 2nd Ed., Springfield, Charles C Thomas, 1974, p. 797.
Lubeck, M. J.: Effects of drugs on ocular muscles. Int. Ophthalmol. Clin. *11*(2):35, 1971.
Reese, H. H., Vander Veer, A., and Wedge, A. H.: Effect on induced Metrazol convulsions on schizophrenic patients. J. Nerv. Ment. Dis. *87*:570, 1938.
Walsh, F. B., and Hoyt, W. F.: Clinical Neuro-Ophthalmology. 3rd Ed., Baltimore, Williams & Wilkins, Vol. III, 1969, pp. 2626–2627.

* * * * * * * * * * * *

Class: Anorexiants

Generic Name: 1. Amphetamine; 2. Dextroamphetamine (Dexamphetamine); 3. Methamphetamine; 4. Phenmetrazine

Proprietary Name: 1. Badrin (Austral.), Benzedrine; 2. Bontid (G.B.), Dexamed (G.B.), Dexamine (Austral.), Dexamphate (Austral.), Dexedrine, Obotan, Phetadex (Austral.); 3. Desoxyn, Efroxine, Emphet (Austral.), Fetamin, Isophen (Germ.), Madrine (Austral.), Methamine (Austral.), Methamphet (Austral.), Methedrine, Methylamphetamine (G.B.), Norodin, Pervitin (Germ.), Syndrox; 4. Anazine (Austral.), Anorex (Austral.), Apedine (Austral.), Marsin (Isr.), Neo-Zine (Canad.), Preludin, Redulan (Austral.)

Primary Use: These sympathomimetic amines are used in the management of exogenous obesity. Amphetamine, dextroamphetamine, and methamphetamine are also effective in narcolepsy and in the management of minimal brain dysfunction in children.

Ocular Side Effects

A. Systemic Administration
1. Decreased vision
2. Pupils
   a. Mydriasis — may precipitate narrow-angle glaucoma
   b. Decreased reaction to light
3. Widening of palpebral fissure
4. Decreased accommodation
5. Decreased convergence
6. Visual hallucinations
7. Problems with color vision — objects have blue tinge (amphetamine)
8. Posterior subcapsular cataracts (phenmetrazine)
9. Blepharospasm (?)
10. Retinal venous thrombosis (?)

Clinical Significance: Ocular side effects due to these sympathomimetic amines are seldom of consequence and are mainly seen in overdose situations. Blepharospasm and retinal venous thrombosis have only been reported at massive dosages in one instance. Probable posterior subcapsular cataracts were seen in two young females on a massive weight reduction program and were extensive enough to require cataract extraction.

Interactions with Other Drugs

A. Effect of Sympathomimetics on Activity of Other Drugs
1. Analgesics ↑
2. Local anesthetics ↑
3. Adrenergic blockers ↓

B. Effect of Other Drugs on Activity of Sympathomimetics
    1. Antacids ↑
    2. Carbonic anhydrase inhibitors ↑
    3. Diuretics ↑
    4. Local anesthetics ↑
    5. Monoamine oxidase inhibitors ↑
    6. Tricyclic antidepressants ↑
    7. Ascorbic acid ↓
    8. Phenothiazines ↓

References

Bartholomew, A. A., and Marley, E.: Toxic response to 2-phenyl-3-methyl-tetrahydro-1, 4-oxazine hydrochloride "Preludin" in humans. Psychopharmacologia 1:124, 1959.
LeGrand, J., and Chevannes, H.: Les opacifications du cristallin dans les traitements contre l' obesité. Bull. Soc. Ophtalmol. Fr. 65:943, 1965.
McCormick, T. C., Jr.: Toxic reactions to amphetamines. Dis. Nerv. Syst. 23:219, 1962.
Walsh, F. B., and Hoyt, W. F.: Clinical Neuro-Ophthalmology. 3rd Ed., Baltimore, Williams & Wilkins, Vol. III, 1969, pp. 2618, 2660–2661.
Waud, S. P.: The effects of toxic doses of benzyl methyl carbinamine (Benzedrine) in man. JAMA 110:206, 1938.

* * * * * * * * * * * *

Generic Name: 1. Benzphetamine; 2. Chlorphentermine; 3. Diethylpropion; 4. Phendimetrazine; 5. Phentermine

Proprietary Name: 1. Didrex; 2. Lucofen (G.B.), Pre-Sate; 3. Dobesin (Swed.), Frekentine (Neth.), Tenuate, Tepanil; 4. Bacarate, Bontril PDM, Dietrol (Canad.), Melfiat, Plegine, Statobex, Tanorex; 5. Duromine (G.B.), Fastin, Ionamin, Linyl (Fr.), Wilpo

Primary Use: These sympathomimetic amines are used in the treatment of exogenous obesity.

Ocular Side Effects

A. Systemic Administration
    1. Decreased vision
    2. Mydriasis — may precipitate narrow-angle glaucoma
    3. Decreased accommodation
    4. Eyelids or conjunctiva
        a. Erythema
        b. Urticaria
    5. Retinal venous thrombosis (?)
    6. Loss of eyelashes or eyebrows (?)

Clinical Significance: Ocular side effects due to these sympathomimetic amines are rare and seldom of clinical significance.

Interactions with Other Drugs
- A. Effect of Sympathomimetics on Activity of Other Drugs
     1. Adrenergic blockers ↓
- B. Effect of Other Drugs on Activity of Sympathomimetics
     1. Monoamine oxidase inhibitors ↑
     2. Phenothiazines ↓

References

Council on Drugs: Evaluation of an anorexiant drug chlorphentermine hydrochloride (Pre-Sate). JAMA *196*:165, 1966.
Grant, W. M.: Toxicology of the Eye. 2nd Ed., Springfield, Charles C Thomas, 1974, pp. 281, 384, 814.
Physicians' Desk Reference. 28th Ed., Oradell, N. J., Medical Economics Co., 1974, pp. 605, 1193, 1466, 1495, 1541.
Rubin, R. T.: Acute psychotic reaction following ingestion of phentermine. Am. J. Psychiatry *120*:1124, 1964.

* * * * * * * * * * * *

Class: Antianxiety Agents

Generic Name: 1. Carisoprodol; 2. Meprobamate

Proprietary Name: 1. Carisoma (G.B.), Flexartal (Fr.), Rela, Soma, Sanoma (Germ.); 2. Equanil, Kesso-Bamate, Mepavlon (G.B.), Meprate (G.B.), Mepromate (Austral.), Mepron (Austral.), Meprospan, Meprotabs, Miltown, Pimal (Austral.), SK-Bamate, Tranmep

Primary Use: These agents are used to treat skeletal muscle spasms. In addition, meprobamate is used as a psychotherapeutic sedative in the treatment of nervous tension, anxiety, and simple insomnia.

Ocular Side Effects
- A. Systemic Administration
     1. Decreased accommodation
     2. Decreased vision
     3. Diplopia
     4. Paralysis of extraocular muscles
     5. Decreased corneal reflex
     6. Constriction of visual fields
     7. Periorbital edema
     8. Eyelids or conjunctiva
        a. Allergic reactions

        b. Angioneurotic edema
        c. Stevens-Johnson syndrome
        d. Exfoliative dermatitis
    9. Pupils
        a. Mydriasis
        b. Miosis
        c. Decreased or absent reaction to light
    10. Subconjunctival or retinal hemorrhages secondary to drug-induced
         anemia
    11. Random ocular movements
    12. Blindness
    13. Decreased intraocular pressure (?)

Clinical Significance: Significant ocular side effects due to these drugs are
uncommon and transitory. At normal dosage levels decreased accommodation,
diplopia, and paralysis of extraocular muscles may be found. Pupillary
responses are variable even in drug-induced coma.

Interactions with Other Drugs

  A. Effect of Carisoprodol or Meprobamate on Activity of Other Drugs
      1. Alcohol ↑
      2. Barbiturates ↑
      3. Monoamine oxidase inhibitors ↑
      4. Sedatives and hypnotics ↑
      5. Tricyclic antidepressants ↑
  B. Effect of Other Drugs on Activity of Carisoprodol or Meprobamate
      1. Alcohol ↑
      2. Monoamine oxidase inhibitors ↑
      3. Phenothiazines ↑
      4. Tricyclic antidepressants ↑
      5. Barbiturates ↓
      6. Sedatives and hypnotics ↓

References

Charkes, N. D.: Meprobamate idiosyncrasy. Arch. Intern. Med. *102*:584, 1958.
Friedman, H. T., and Marmelzat, W. L.: Adverse reactions to meprobamate. JAMA
    162:628, 1956.
Hermans, G.: Les psychotropes. Bull. Soc. Belge Ophtalmol. *160*:15, 1972.
Physicians' Desk Reference. 28th Ed., Oradell, N. J., Medical Economics Co., 1974, pp. 954,
    1322, 1372, 1519, 1522, 1526, 1603.
Walsh, F. B., and Hoyt, W. F.: Clinical Neuro-Ophthalmology. 3rd Ed., Baltimore, Williams
    & Wilkins, Vol. III, 1969, pp. 2633–2634.

* * * * * * * * * * * *

Generic Name: 1. Chlordiazepoxide; 2. Diazepam; 3. Flurazepam

Proprietary Name: 1. Elenium (Pol.), Libritabs, Librium; 2. Relanium (Pol.), Valium; 3. Dalmane

Primary Use: These benzodiazepine derivatives are effective in the management of psychoneurotic states manifested by anxiety, tension, or agitation. They are also used as adjunctive therapy in the relief of skeletal muscle spasms and as preoperative medications.

Ocular Side Effects

A. Systemic Administration
  1. Decreased vision
  2. Decreased corneal reflex
  3. Extraocular muscles
     a. Oculogyric crises
     b. Decreased spontaneous movements
     c. Abnormal conjugate deviations
     d. Jerky pursuit movements
  4. Decreased accommodation
  5. Decreased depth perception
  6. Diplopia
  7. Nystagmus
  8. Decreased intraocular pressure
  9. Visual hallucinations
  10. Subconjunctival or retinal hemorrhages secondary to drug-induced anemia
  11. Photosensitivity
  12. Nonspecific ocular irritation (flurazepam)
  13. Mydriasis — may precipitate narrow-angle glaucoma (?) (diazepam)
  14. Brown lens deposits (?) (diazepam)
  15. Paralysis of extraocular muscles (?) (diazepam)
  16. Photophobia (?) (diazepam)

Clinical Significance: In general, significant ocular side effects due to these benzodiazepine derivatives are rare and reversible. At therapeutic dosage levels, these agents may cause decreased corneal reflex, decreased accommodation, decreased depth perception, and abnormal extraocular muscle movements. Nystagmus and diplopia are more frequently seen secondary to diazepam rather than with chlordiazepoxide or flurazepam. To what degree diazepam causes pupillary dilatation is uncertain; however, drug manufacturers advise against its use in patients predisposed to narrow-angle glaucoma. Flurazepam has only been reported to have caused decreased vision, decreased accommodation, and nonspecific ocular irritation.

Interactions with Other Drugs

A. Effect of Benzodiazepine Derivatives on Activity of Other Drugs
  1. Alcohol ↑
  2. Analgesics ↑
  3. Anticholinergics ↑

    4. Antihistamines ↑
    5. Barbiturates ↑
    6. Monoamine oxidase inhibitors ↑
    7. Phenothiazines ↑
    8. Sedatives and hypnotics ↑
    9. Tricyclic antidepressants ↑
   10. Succinylcholine ↓
  B. Effect of Other Drugs on Activity of Benzodiazepine Derivatives
    1. Alcohol ↑
    2. Analgesics ↑
    3. Barbiturates ↑
    4. Monoamine oxidase inhibitors ↑
    5. Phenothiazines ↑
    6. Sedatives and hypnotics ↑
    7. Tricyclic antidepressants ↑

References

Davidson, S. I.: Report of ocular adverse reactions. Trans. Ophthalmol. Soc. U. K. *93*:495, 1973.

Keats, S., Morgese, A., and Nordlund, T.: Symposium on diazepam. Western Med. (Suppl. 1) *4*:22, 1963.

Miller, J. G.: Objective measurements of the effects of drugs on driver behavior. JAMA *179*:940, 1962.

Murray, N.: Covert effects of chlordiazepoxide therapy. J. Neuropsychiatry *3*:168, 1962.

Orbell, G.: Headaches and migraine associated with eyestrain. Preliminary report of a trial of chlordiazepoxide. Br. J. Ophthalmol. *47*:246, 1963.

Roberts, W.: The use of psychotropic drugs in glaucoma. Dis. Nerv. Syst. (Suppl.) *29*:40, 1968.

Walsh, F. B., and Hoyt, W. F.: Clinical Neuro-Ophthalmology. 3rd Ed., Baltimore, Williams & Wilkins, Vol. III, 1969, pp. 2631–2632.

* * * * * * * * * * * * *

Generic Name: Doxepin. See under *Class: Antidepressants.*

* * * * * * * * * * * * *

Class: Anticonvulsants

Generic Name: Diphenylhydantoin (Phenytoin)

Proprietary Name: Dilantin, Ditoin (Austral.), Ekko, Epanutin (G.B.), Epiphen (G.B.), Kessodanten, Phentoin (Austral.), Toin

Primary Use: This hydantoin is effective in the prophylaxis and treatment of chronic epilepsy and Parkinson's disease.

Ocular Side Effects

A. Systemic Administration
1. Nystagmus
2. Diplopia
3. Decreased vision
4. Mydriasis — may precipitate narrow-angle glaucoma
5. Oscillopsia
6. Orbital or periorbital pain
7. Myasthenic neuromuscular blocking effect
   a. Paralysis of extraocular muscles
   b. Ptosis
8. Decreased accommodation
9. Decreased convergence
10. Visual hallucinations
11. Visual sensations
    a. Glare phenomenon — objects appear covered with white snow
    b. Flashing lights
12. Blindness
13. Problems with color vision
    a. Objects have white tinge
    b. Colors appear faded
14. Eyelids or conjunctiva
    a. Allergic reactions
    b. Ulceration
    c. Purpura
    d. Lupoid syndrome
    e. Erythema multiforme
    f. Stevens-Johnson syndrome
    g. Exfoliative dermatitis
    h. Lyell's syndrome
15. Subconjunctival or retinal hemorrhages secondary to drug-induced anemia
16. Esotropia
17. Decreased intraocular pressure (?)
18. Ocular teratogenic effects (?)

Clinical Significance: Nearly all ocular side effects due to diphenylhydantoin are reversible after discontinuation of use of the drug. The first sign of systemic diphenylhydantoin toxicity is nystagmus and is directly related to the blood levels of the drug. Instances of nystagmus persisting for 20 months or longer after discontinued use of the drug have been reported. Paralysis of extraocular muscles is uncommon, reversible, and only found in the most toxic states.

Interactions with Other Drugs

A. Effect of Diphenylhydantoin on Activity of Other Drugs
1. Analgesics ↑
2. Barbiturates ↑

      3. Corticosteroids ↓
      4. Vitamin D ↓
  B. Effect of Other Drugs on Activity of Diphenylhydantoin
      1. Analgesics ↑
      2. Chloramphenicol ↑
      3. Oxyphenbutazone ↑
      4. Phenothiazines ↑
      5. Phenylbutazone ↑
      6. Salicylates ↑
      7. Sulfonamides ↑
      8. Tricyclic antidepressants ↑↓
      9. Adrenergic blockers ↓
    10. Alcohol ↓
    11. Antihistamines ↓
    12. Barbiturates ↓
    13. Sedatives and hypnotics ↓
  C. Cross Sensitivity
      1. Barbiturates

References

Bender, M. B.: Oscillopsia. Arch. Neurol. *13*:204, 1965.
Kutt, H., et al.: Diphenylhydantoin metabolism, blood levels, and toxicity. Arch. Neurol. *11*:642, 1964.
Manlapaz, J. S.: Abducens nerve palsy in Dilantin intoxication. J. Pediatr. *55*:73, 1959.
Morris, J. V., Fischer, E., and Bergin, J. T.: Rare complications of phenytoin sodium treatment. Br. Med. J. *2*:1529, 1956.
Orth, D. N., et al.: Ophthalmoplegia resulting from diphenylhydantoin and primidone intoxication. JAMA *201*:485, 1967.
Van Huyssteen, M. P.: Conjunctival ulceration as a complication in the treatment of epilepsy. S. Afr. Med. J. *27*:626, 1953.

* * * * * * * * * * * * *

Generic Name: 1. Ethosuximide; 2. Methsuximide; 3. Phensuximide

Proprietary Name: 1. Capitus (G.B.), Emeside (G.B.), Zarontin; 2. Celontin; 3. Milontin

Primary Use: These succinimides are effective in the management of petit mal seizures.

Ocular Side Effects

  A. Systemic Administration
      1. Decreased vision
      2. Diplopia
      3. Photophobia
      4. Myopia
      5. Periorbital edema or hyperemia

6. Subconjunctival or retinal hemorrhages secondary to drug-induced anemia
7. Eyelids or conjunctiva
    a. Allergic reactions
    b. Angioneurotic edema
    c. Lupoid syndrome
    d. Erythema multiforme
    e. Stevens-Johnson syndrome
    f. Exfoliative dermatitis

Clinical Significance: Methsuximide induces ocular side effects more frequently than ethosuximide or phensuximide. All adverse ocular reactions other than those due to anemias or dermatologic conditions are reversible after discontinuation of the drug.

References

AMA Drug Evaluations. 2nd Ed., Acton, Mass., Publishing Sciences Group, 1973, p. 354.

Council on Drugs. New and nonofficial drugs: Methsuximide. JAMA 171:1506, 1959.

Millichap, J. G.: Anticonvulsant drugs. Clinical and electroencephalographic indications, efficacy and toxicity. Postgrad. Med. 37:22, 1965.

Physicians' Desk Reference. 28th Ed., Oradell, N. J., Medical Economics Co., 1974, pp. 1088, 1111, 1126.

Walsh, F. B., and Hoyt, W. F.: Clinical Neuro-Ophthalmology. 3rd Ed., Baltimore, Williams & Wilkins, Vol. III, 1969, p. 2645.

* * * * * * * * * * * *

Generic Name: 1. Ethotoin; 2. Mephenytoin

Proprietary Name: 1. Peganone; 2. Mesantoin, Mesontoin (G.B.), Methoin (G.B.)

Primary Use: These hydantoins are effective in the management of psychomotor and grand mal seizures.

Ocular Side Effects

A. Systemic Administration
    1. Nystagmus
    2. Diplopia
    3. Photophobia
    4. Eyelids or conjunctiva
        a. Allergic reactions
        b. Conjunctivitis — nonspecific
        c. Angioneurotic edema
        d. Erythema multiforme
        e. Stevens-Johnson syndrome
        f. Exfoliative dermatitis
    5. Subconjunctival or retinal hemorrhages secondary to drug-induced anemia

6. Corneal or lens opacities (?)
7. Myasthenic neuromuscular blocking effect (?)
   a. Paresis of extraocular muscles (?)
8. Loss of eyelashes or eyebrows (?)

Clinical Significance: These hydantoin agents have fewer adverse ocular reactions than diphenylhydantoin. Ocular side effects are seen more frequently with mephenytoin than with ethotoin and are reversible either by decreasing the dosage or discontinuing use of the drug. As with diphenylhydantoin, nystagmus may persist for some time after use of the drug is stopped. Corneal or lens opacities and myasthenic neuromuscular blocking effect have been reported in only one series.

Interactions with Other Drugs

A. Effect of Hydantoins on Activity of Other Drugs
   1. Analgesics ↑
   2. Barbiturates ↑
   3. Corticosteroids ↓
   4. Vitamin D ↓
B. Effect of Other Drugs on Activity of Hydantoins
   1. Analgesics ↑
   2. Chloramphenicol ↑
   3. Oxyphenbutazone ↑
   4. Phenothiazines ↑
   5. Phenylbutazone ↑
   6. Salicylates ↑
   7. Sulfonamides ↑
   8. Tricyclic antidepressants ↑↓
   9. Adrenergic blockers ↓
   10. Alcohol ↓
   11. Antihistamines ↓
   12. Barbiturates ↓
   13. Sedatives and hypnotics ↓
C. Cross Sensitivity
   1. Barbiturates

References

Goodman, L. S., and Gilman, A.: The Pharmacological Basis of Therapeutics. 4th Ed., New York, Macmillan, 1970, pp. 212–213.
Hermans, G.: Les anticonvulsivants. Bull. Soc. Belge Ophtalmol. *160*:89, 1972.
Livingston, S.: Drug Therapy for Epilepsy. Springfield, Charles C Thomas, 1966.
Physicians' Desk Reference. 28th Ed., Oradell, N. J., Medical Economics Co., 1974, pp. 533, 1275.
Walsh, F. B., and Hoyt, W. F.: Clinical Neuro-Ophthalmology. 3rd Ed., Baltimore, Williams & Wilkins, Vol. III, 1969, p. 2644.

* * * * * * * * * * * *

Generic Name: 1. Paramethadione; 2. Trimethadione

Proprietary Name: 1. Paradione; 2. Tridione, Troxidone (G.B.)

Primary Use: These oxazolidinediones are used primarily in the treatment of refractory petit mal seizures and myoclonic contractions.

Ocular Side Effects

A.   Systemic Administration
1.   Glare phenomenon — objects appear covered with white snow
2.   Photophobia
3.   Night blindness
4.   Diplopia
5.   Gaze evoked nystagmus
6.   Problems with color vision
   a.   Dyschromatopsia
   b.   Objects have dazzling white tinge
   c.   Achromatopsia, red-green or yellow-blue defect
   d.   Colored haloes around lights — mainly white
   e.   Colors appear faded
7.   Scotomas
8.   Eyelids or conjunctiva
   a.   Allergic reactions
   b.   Photosensitivity
   c.   Angioneurotic edema
   d.   Lupoid syndrome
   e.   Erythema multiforme
   f.   Stevens-Johnson syndrome
   g.   Exfoliative dermatitis
   h.   Lyell's syndrome
9.   Subconjunctival or retinal hemorrhages secondary to drug-induced anemia
10.   Loss of eyelashes or eyebrows (?)
11.   Myasthenic neuromuscular blocking effect (?)
   a.   Paralysis of extraocular muscles
   b.   Ptosis

Clinical Significance: The oxazolidinediones have the unusual side effect of causing a prolonged "dazzle" when the eyes are exposed to light. This includes decreased vision, momentary blindness, and loss of color perception. This toxic effect seems to be specific for retinal cones and in all but two instances has been reversible. Symptoms may even continue for a number of weeks after use of the drug is discontinued. Paramethadione has significantly fewer and less prolonged ocular side effects than trimethadione.

References

Dekking, H. M.: Visual disturbances due to Tridione. Acta Cong. Ophthalmol. *1*:465, 1950.
Goodman, L. S., and Gilman, A.: The Pharmacological Basis of Therapeutics. 4th Ed., New York, Macmillan, 1970, pp. 215–219.

Peterson, H. deC.: Association of trimethadione therapy and myasthenia gravis. N. Engl. J. Med. *274*:506, 1966.

Sloan, L. L., and Gilger, A. P.: Visual effects of Tridione. Am. J. Ophthalmol. *30*:1387, 1947.

Walsh, F. B., and Hoyt, W. F.: Clinical Neuro-Ophthalmology. 3rd Ed., Baltimore, Williams & Wilkins, Vol. III, 1969, pp. 2562, 2639, 2655–2656.

* * * * * * * * * * * *

Class: Antidepressants

Generic Name: 1. Amitriptyline; 2. Desipramine; 3. Imipramine; 4. Nortriptyline; 5. Protriptyline

Proprietary Name: 1. Elavil, Laroxyl (G.B.), Lentizol (G.B.), Saroten (G.B.), Tryptizol (G.B.); 2. Norpramin, Pertofran (G.B.), Pertofrane; 3. Anpramine (G.B.), Berkomine (G.B.), Censtim (Austral.), Co-Caps Imipramine (G.B.), Dimipressin (G.B.), Ia-pram (G.B.), Imiprin (Austral.), Impamin (G.B.), Iramil (Austral.), Melipramine (Austral.), Oppanyl (G.B.), Praminil (G.B.), Presamine, Tofranil; 4. Acetexa (Germ.), Allergron (G.B.), Altilev (G.B.), Aventyl, Nortrilen (Germ.), Sensaval (Swed.); 5. Concordin (G.B.), Triptil (Austral.), Vivactil

Primary Use: These tricyclic antidepressants are effective in the relief of symptoms of mental depression. Imipramine is also used in the management of enuresis.

Ocular Side Effects

A. Systemic Administration
1. Decreased vision
2. Paralysis of accommodation
3. Pupils
    a. Mydriasis — may precipitate narrow-angle glaucoma
    b. Absence of reaction to light
4. Diplopia
5. Photosensitivity
6. Visual hallucinations
7. Extraocular muscles
    a. Paresis or paralysis — primarily lateral rectus
    b. Oculogyric crises
    c. Decreased spontaneous movements
    d. Abnormal conjugate deviations
    e. Jerky pursuit movements
8. Decreased lacrimation
9. Decreased corneal reflex

     10. Retinal vasospasms
     11. Retrobulbar or optic neuritis
     12. Subconjunctival or retinal hemorrhages secondary to drug-induced anemia
     13. Loss of eyelashes or eyebrows (?)
     14. Blindness (?)
     15. Problems with color vision — dyschromatopsia (?)
  B. Local Ophthalmic Use or Exposure — protriptyline
     1. Decreased intraocular pressure — especially if in combination with sympathomimetics
     2. Mydriasis — may precipitate narrow-angle glaucoma
     3. Corneal opacities

Clinical Significance: All adverse ocular reactions due to these tricyclic antidepressants are reversible, transitory, and in most cases, of little clinical significance. The most common ocular side effects are mydriasis and cycloplegia. A number of cases of narrow-angle glaucoma precipitated by amitriptyline have been reported. Extrapyramidal symptoms are primarily seen with imipramine. Topical ocular protriptyline has been used as an antiglaucoma agent, but it has not been marketed since it can cause corneal opacities of unknown composition. These agents probably cause few ocular sicca problems in normal tear producers. However, in patients with an already compromised tear production, all of these drugs have the potential to aggravate latent or manifested keratitis sicca.

Interactions with Other Drugs

  A. Effect of Tricyclic Antidepressants on Activity of Other Drugs
     1. Alcohol ↑
     2. Analgesics ↑
     3. Anticholinergics ↑
     4. Barbiturates ↑
     5. Monoamine oxidase inhibitors ↑
     6. Phenothiazines ↑
     7. Sedatives and hypnotics ↑
     8. Sympathomimetics ↑
     9. Adrenergic blockers ↓
  B. Effect of Other Drugs on Activity of Tricyclic Antidepressants
     1. Adrenergic blockers ↑
     2. Analgesics ↑
     3. Monoamine oxidase inhibitors ↑
     4. Phenothiazines ↑
     5. Sedatives and hypnotics ↑

References

Azima, H., Silver, A., and Arthurs, D.: Effects of G33040 (Ensidon) and G35020 (Petrofrane) on depressive states. Can. Med. Assoc. J. *87*:1224, 1962.
Davidson, S. I.: Reports of ocular adverse reactions. Trans. Ophthalmol. Soc. U. K. *93*:495, 1973.

Kitazawa, Y., and Langham, M. E.: Influence of an adrenergic potentiator on the ocular
  response of catecholamines in primates and man. Nature 219:1376, 1968.
Physicians' Desk Reference. 28th Ed., Oradell, N. J., Medical Economics Co., 1974, pp. 783,
  823, 888, 1038, 1481.
Steel, C. M., O'Duffy, J., and Brown, S. S.: Clinical effects and treatment of imipramine and
  amitriptyline poisoning in children. Br. Med. J. 3:663, 1967.
Walsh, F. B., and Hoyt, W. F.: Clinical Neuro-Ophthalmology. 3rd Ed., Baltimore, Williams
  & Wilkins, Vol. III, 1969, pp. 2621–2622, 2632.

* * * * * * * * * * * * *

Generic Name: Carbamazepine

Proprietary Name: Tegretol

Primary Use: This iminostilbene derivative is used in the treatment of pain associated with trigeminal neuralgia.

Ocular Side Effects

  A. Systemic Administration
      1. Decreased vision
      2. Diplopia
      3. Nystagmus
      4. Decreased spontaneous eye movements
      5. Visual hallucinations
      6. Eyelids or conjunctiva
         a. Allergic reactions
         b. Conjunctivitis – nonspecific
         c. Photosensitivity
         d. Urticaria
         e. Lupoid syndrome
         f. Erythema multiforme
         g. Stevens-Johnson syndrome
         h. Exfoliative dermatitis
      7. Mydriasis – may precipitate narrow-angle glaucoma
      8. Decreased accommodation
      9. Subconjunctival or retinal hemorrhages secondary to drug-induced anemia
    10. Lens opacities (?)
    11. Loss of eyelashes or eyebrows (?)

Clinical Significance: Most ocular side effects due to carbamazepine are usually reversible and resolve spontaneously within a week on the usual or a reduced drug dosage. However, about 25 percent of patients receiving this drug develop neurologic or hematopoietic reactions, some of which are associated with eye abnormalities.

Interactions with Other Drugs

  A. Effect of Carbamazepine on Activity of Other Drugs

1. Alcohol ↑
2. Barbiturates ↑

References

AMA Drug Evaluations. 2nd Ed., Acton, Mass., Publishing Sciences Group, 1973, pp. 355, 900–902.
Hermans, G.: Les anticonvulsivants. Bull. Soc. Belge Ophtalmol. 160:89, 1972.
Livingston, S., et al.: Use of carbamazepine in epilepsy. JAMA 200:204, 1967.
Lubeck, M. J.: Effects of drugs on ocular muscles. Int. Ophthalmol. Clin. 11(2):35, 1971.
Physicians' Desk Reference. 28th Ed., Oradell, N. J., Medical Economics Co., 1974, p. 780.
Warot, P., et al.: Acute ataxia following massive ingestion of carbamazepine. Lille Med. 12:601, 1967.

* * * * * * * * * * * *

Generic Name: Doxepin

Proprietary Name: Adapin, Sinequan

Primary Use: This tricyclic antidepressant is used in the treatment of psychoneurotic anxiety or depressive reactions.

Ocular Side Effects

A. Systemic Administration
1. Decreased vision
2. Mydriasis — may precipitate narrow-angle glaucoma
3. Photophobia
4. Decreased accommodation
5. Photosensitivity

Clinical Significance: Adverse ocular reactions due to doxepin are seldom of major importance and often subside even if the medication is continued. Since this drug may be bound to ocular melanin, there is a potential for retinal damage; however, this side effect has not been reported.

Interactions with Other Drugs

A. Effect of Doxepin on Activity of Other Drugs
1. Alcohol ↑
2. Anticholinergics ↑
3. Barbiturates ↑
4. Sympathomimetics ↑
5. Adrenergic blockers ↓

References

AMA Drug Evaluations. 2nd Ed., Acton, Mass., Publishing Sciences Group, 1973, p. 363.
Grant, W. M.: Toxicology of the Eye. 2nd Ed., Springfield, Charles C Thomas, 1974, pp. 427–428.
Hermans, G.: Les psychotropes. Bull. Soc. Belge Ophtalmol. 160:15, 1972.
Hobbs, D. C.: Distribution and metabolism of doxepin. Biochem. Pharmacol. 18:1941, 1969.
Physicians' Desk Reference. 28th Ed., Oradell, N. J., Medical Economics Co., 1974, p. 1127.

* * * * * * * * * * * *

Generic Name: 1. Isocarboxazid; 2. Nialamide; 3. Phenelzine; 4. Tranylcypromine

Proprietary Name: 1. Marplan; 2. Niamid; 3. Nardelzine (Fr.), Nardil; 4. Parnate

Primary Use: These monoamine oxidase inhibitors are used in the symptomatic relief of reactive or endogenous depression.

Ocular Side Effects

A. Systemic Administration
   1. Decreased vision
   2. Pupils
      a. Mydriasis — may precipitate narrow-angle glaucoma
      b. Miosis
      c. Anisocoria
      d. Absence of reaction to light
   3. Ptosis
   4. Photophobia
   5. Problems with color vision
      a. Dyschromatopsia
      b. Achromatopsia, red-green defect
   6. Photosensitivity
   7. Nystagmus (phenelzine)
   8. Visual hallucinations (nialamide)
   9. Papilledema (?) (tranylcypromine)
   10. Optic neuritis (?) (nialamide)
   11. Blindness (?)

Clinical Significance: Most ocular side effects due to these monoamine oxidase inhibitors are reversible and insignificant. Pupillary reactions occur primarily in overdose situations. Nystagmus may be induced by phenelzine and visual hallucinations by nialamide therapy, but these symptoms have not been reported due to any other monoamine oxidase inhibitors. Blindness has always been reported to be associated with multiple medical problems, so there is a question of whether it is truly drug-induced.

Interactions with Other Drugs

A. Effect of Monoamine Oxidase Inhibitors on Activity of Other Drugs
   1. Analgesics ↑
   2. Anticholinergics ↑
   3. Antihistamines ↑
   4. Barbiturates ↑
   5. Diuretics ↑
   6. General anesthetics ↑
   7. Local anesthetics ↑
   8. Monoamine oxidase inhibitors ↑
   9. Phenothiazines ↑
   10. Sedatives and hypnotics ↑

11. Succinylcholine ↑
12. Sympathomimetics ↑
13. Tricyclic antidepressants ↑
B. Effect of Other Drugs on Activity of Monoamine Oxidase Inhibitors
1. Monoamine oxidase inhibitors ↑
2. Tricyclic antidepressants ↑
3. Analgesics ↑↓
4. Phenothiazines ↓

References

Grant, W. M.: Toxicology of the Eye. 2nd Ed., Springfield, Charles C Thomas, 1974, pp. 605, 718–719, 744–745, 805–806, 1029–1030.
Hermans, G.: Les psychotropes. Bull. Soc. Belge Ophtalmol. 160:15, 1972.
Leonard, J. W., Gifford, R. W., Jr., and Williams, G. H., Jr.: Tranylcypromine sulfate therapy. Occurrence of severe paroxysmal headache. JAMA 187:957, 1964.
Physicians' Desk Reference. 28th Ed., Oradell, N. J., Medical Economics Co., 1974, pp. 1368, 1538.
Solberg, C. O.: Phenelzine intoxication. JAMA 177:572, 1961.

* * * * * * * * * * * * *

Generic Name: Methylphenidate

Proprietary Name: Ritalin

Primary Use: This piperidine derivative is used in the treatment of mild depression and in the management of children with the hyperkinetic syndrome.

Ocular Side Effects

A. Systemic Administration
1. Eyelids or conjunctiva
    a. Urticaria
    b. Erythema multiforme
    c. Stevens-Johnson syndrome
    d. Exfoliative dermatitis
2. Mydriasis — may precipitate narrow-angle glaucoma
3. Subconjunctival or retinal hemorrhages secondary to drug-induced anemia
4. Increased intraocular pressure (?)

Clinical Significance: Ocular side effects due to methylphenidate are rare, reversible, and seldom clinically significant. Mydriasis rarely occurs except in overdose situations.

Interactions with Other Drugs

A. Effect of Methylphenidate on Activity of Other Drugs
1. Barbiturates ↑
2. Phenylbutazone ↑
3. Tricyclic antidepressants ↑
4. Adrenergic blockers ↓

B. Contraindications
   1. Monoamine oxidase inhibitors

References

American Hospital Formulary Service. Washington, D. C., American Society of Hospital Pharmacists, Vol. 1, 28:20, 1973.
Grant, W. M.: Toxicology of the Eye. 2nd Ed., Springfield, Charles C Thomas, 1974, p. 702.
Meyler, L., and Herxheimer, A.: Side Effects of Drugs. Amsterdam, Excerpta Medica, Vol. VII, 1972, p. 13.
Physicians' Desk Reference. 28th Ed., Oradell, N. J., Medical Economics Co., 1974, p. 693.

* * * * * * * * * * * *

Class: Antipsychotic Agents

Generic Name: 1. Acetophenazine; 2. Butaperazine; 3. Carphenazine; 4. Chlorpromazine; 5. Diethazine; 6. Ethopropazine (Profenamine); 7. Fluphenazine; 8. Mesoridazine; 9. Methdilazine; 10. Methotrimeprazine; 11. Perazine; 12. Pericyazine; 13. Perphenazine; 14. Piperacetazine; 15. Prochlorperazine; 16. Promazine; 17. Promethazine; 18. Propiomazine; 19. Thiethylperazine; 20. Thiopropazate; 21. Thioproperazine; 22. Thioridazine; 23. Trifluoperazine; 24. Triflupromazine; 25. Trimeprazine

Proprietary Name: 1. Tindal; 2. Randolectil (Austral., Germ.), Repoise; 3. Proketazine; 4. Aminazini (U.S.S.R.), Chlor-PZ, Largactil, Megaphen, Promacid (Austral.), Sonazine, Thorazine; 5. Diparcol (Fr.); 6. Lysivane (G.B.), Parsidol; 7. Anatensol (Austral.), Modecate (G.B.), Moditen (G.B.), Permitil, Prolixin; 8. Lidanil (Austral.), Serentil; 9. Dilosyn (G.B.), Tacaryl; 10. Levoprome, Nozinan (Fr.), Veractil (G.B.); 11. Taxilan (Germ.); 12. Neulactil (G.B.), Neuleptil (Fr.); 13. Fentazin (G.B.), Trilafon; 14. Quide; 15. Compazine, Stemetil (G.B.), Tementil (Fr.); 16. Sparine; 17. Avomine (G.B.), Fellowzine, Ganphen, Phenergan, Progan (Austral.), Prothazine (Austral.), Remsed, Zipan; 18. Largon, Propavan (Swed.); 19. Torecan; 20. Dartal, Dartalan (G.B.); 21. Majeptil (G.B.); 22. Mellaril, Sonapax (Pol.); 23. Stelazine, Terfluzine (Fr.); 24. Siquil (Austral.), Vesprin; 25. Panectyl (Canad.), Temaril, Theralene (Fr.), Vallergan (G.B.).

Primary Use: These phenothiazines are used in the treatment of depressive, involutional, senile, or organic psychoses and various forms of schizophrenia. Some of the phenothiazines are also used as adjuncts to anesthesia, antiemetics, and in the treatment of tetanus.

Ocular Side Effects

A. Systemic Administration
   Not all of the ocular side effects listed have been reported for each phenothiazine.

1. Decreased vision
2. Paralysis of accommodation
3. Night blindness
4. Problems with color vision
   a. Dyschromatopsia
   b. Objects have yellow or brown tinge
   c. Achromatopsia, red-green defect
   d. Colored haloes around lights
5. Punctate keratitis
6. Pupils
   a. Mydriasis — may precipitate narrow-angle glaucoma
   b. Miosis
7. Retinal pigmentary changes
8. Oculogyric crises
9. Visual fields
   a. Scotomas — annular, central, or paracentral
   b. Constriction
10. Pigmentary deposits
    a. Eyelids
    b. Conjunctiva
    c. Sclera
    d. Cornea
    e. Lens
    f. Retina
11. Stellate or polar lens changes
12. Retinal edema
13. Visual hallucinations
14. Lacrimation
    a. Increased
    b. Decreased — more common
15. Horner's syndrome
16. Diplopia
17. Corneal edema
18. Jerky pursuit movements
19. Photophobia
20. Optic atrophy
21. Papilledema
22. Myopia
23. Blindness
24. Eyelids or conjunctiva
    a. Allergic reactions
    b. Edema
    c. Angioneurotic edema
    d. Stevens-Johnson syndrome
    e. Exfoliative dermatitis
25. Subconjunctival or retinal hemorrhages secondary to drug-induced anemia
26. Ocular teratogenic effects (?)

Clinical Significance: The phenothiazines as a class are among the more widely used drugs in the practice of medicine today. The most commonly prescribed drug in this group is chlorpromazine, which has been so thoroughly investigated that over 10,000 publications alone deal with its actions. Even so, these drugs are remarkably safe compared to previously prescribed anti-psychotic agents. Their overall rate of all side effects is estimated at only 3 percent. However, if patients are on phenothiazine therapy for a number of years, a 30 percent rate of ocular side effects has been reported. If therapy continues over 10 years, the rate of ocular side effects increases to 100 percent. Side effects are dose- and drug-dependent, with the most significant side effects reported with chlorpromazine and thioridazine therapy, probably since they are the most often prescribed. Each phenothiazine has the potential to cause ocular side effects although it is unlikely to cause all of those mentioned. The basic problem is that pinpointing specific toxic effects to a specific phenothiazine is extremely difficult since most patients have been receiving more than one type. The most common adverse ocular effect with this group of drugs is decreased vision, probably due to anticholinergic inter-ference. Chlorpromazine, in chronic therapy, is the most common phenothia-zine to cause pigmentary deposits in or on the eye, with multiple reports claiming that other phenothiazines can cause this as well. These deposits are first seen on the lens surface in the pupillary aperture, later near Descemet's membrane, and only in extreme cases in the corneal epithelium. Retinopathy, optic nerve disease, and blindness are exceedingly rare at the recommended dosage levels and then they are only found in patients on chronic therapy. Retinal pigmentary changes are most frequently found with thioridazine. This reaction is dose-related and is seldom seen at recommended dosages. A phototoxic process has been postulated to be involved in both the increased ocular pigmentary deposits and the retinal degeneration. The phenothiazines combine with ocular and dermal pigment and are only slowly released. This slow release has in part been given as the reason why adverse ocular reactions may progress even after use of the drug is discontinued.

Interactions with Other Drugs

A. Effect of Phenothiazines on Activity of Other Drugs
1. Alcohol ↑
2. Analgesics ↑
3. Anticholinergics ↑
4. Antihistamines ↑
5. Barbiturates ↑
6. Diuretics ↑
7. General anesthetics ↑
8. Other phenothiazines ↑
9. Salicylates ↑
10. Sedatives and hypnotics ↑
11. Adrenergic blockers ↑↓
12. Sympathomimetics ↑↓
13. Monoamine oxidase inhibitors ↓
B. Effect of Other Drugs on Activity of Phenothiazines
1. Adrenergic blockers ↑

    2. Alcohol ↑
    3. Analgesics ↑
    4. Anticholinergics ↑
    5. Anticholinesterases ↑
    6. Diuretics ↑
    7. Sedatives and hypnotics ↑
    8. Tricyclic antidepressants ↑
    9. Antacids ↓
    10. Barbiturates ↓
    11. Monoamine oxidase inhibitors ↓
    12. Sympathomimetics ↓

References

AMA Drug Evaluations. 2nd Ed., Acton, Mass., Publishing Sciences Group, 1973, pp. 326–334.

Connell, M. M., Poley, B. J., and McFarlane, J. R.: Chorioretinopathy associated with thioridazine therapy. Arch. Ophthalmol. 71:816, 1964.

Delong, S. L., Poley, B. J., and McFarlane, J. R.: Ocular changes associated with long term chlorpromazine therapy. Arch. Ophthalmol. 73:611, 1965.

Grant, W. M.: Toxicology of the Eye. 2nd Ed., Springfield, Charles C Thomas, 1974, pp. 281–286, 1005–1010.

McClanahan, W. S., et al.: Ocular manifestations of chronic phenothiazine derivative administration. Arch. Ophthalmol. 75:319, 1966.

Potts, A. M.: Drug-induced macular disease. Trans. Am. Acad. Ophthalmol. Otolaryngol. 70:1054, 1966.

Satanove, A., and McIntosh, J. S.: Phototoxic reactions induced by high doses of chlorpromazine and thioridazine. JAMA 200:209, 1967.

Siddall, J. R.: Ocular complications related to phenothiazines. Dis. Nerv. Syst. (Suppl.) 29:10, 1968.

Walsh, F. B., and Hoyt, W. F.: Clinical Neuro-Ophthalmology. 3rd Ed., Baltimore, Williams & Wilkins, Vol. III, 1969, pp. 2634–2637.

Weekley, R. D., et al.: Pigmentary retinopathy in patients receiving high doses of a new phenothiazine. Arch. Ophthalmol. 64:65, 1960.

Wetterholm, D. H., Snow, H. L., and Winter, F. C.: A clinical study of pigmentary change in cornea and lens in chronic chlorpromazine therapy. Arch. Ophthalmol. 74:55, 1965.

* * * * * * * * * * * *

Generic Name: 1. Chlorprothixene; 2. Thiothixene

Proprietary Name: 1. Taractan, Tarasan (Canad.), Truxal (Denm.); 2. Navane, Orbinamon (Germ.)

Primary Use: These thioxanthene derivatives are used in the management of schizophrenia. Chlorprothixene is also used in agitation neuroses and as an antiemetic.

Ocular Side Effects

  A. Systemic Administration
    1. Decreased vision
    2. Decreased accommodation

   3. Oculogyric crisis
   4. Pupils
      a. Mydriasis — may precipitate narrow-angle glaucoma
      b. Miosis
   5. Diplopia
   6. Fine particulate matter or pigmentary deposits
      a. Cornea
      b. Lens
   7. Star-shaped lens opacities
   8. Keratitis
   9. Retinal pigmentary changes
 10. Eyelids or conjunctiva
      a. Allergic reactions
      b. Angioneurotic edema
      c. Exfoliative dermatitis
 11. Subconjunctival or retinal hemorrhages secondary to drug-induced anemia

Clinical Significance: In short-term therapy, ocular side effects due to these thioxanthene derivatives are reversible and usually insignificant. In long-term therapy, however, cases of corneal or lens deposits (chlorprothixene) or lens pigmentation (thiothixene) have been reported. Retinal pigmentary changes are exceedingly rare.

Interactions with Other Drugs

A. Effect of Thioxanthene Derivatives on Activity of Other Drugs
   1. Alcohol ↑
   2. Analgesics ↑
   3. Anticholinergics ↑
   4. Antihistamines ↑
   5. Barbiturates ↑
   6. Diuretics ↑
   7. General anesthetics ↑
   8. Phenothiazines ↑
   9. Salicylates ↑
 10. Sedatives and hypnotics ↑
 11. Adrenergic blockers ↑↓
 12. Sympathomimetics ↑↓
 13. Monoamine oxidase inhibitors ↓
B. Effect of Other Drugs on Activity of Thioxanthene Derivatives
   1. Adrenergic blockers ↑
   2. Alcohol ↑
   3. Analgesics ↑
   4. Anticholinergics ↑
   5. Anticholinesterases ↑
   6. Diuretics ↑
   7. Sedatives and hypnotics ↑
   8. Tricyclic antidepressants ↑

       9.   Antacids ↓
      10.   Barbiturates ↓
      11.   Monoamine oxidase inhibitors ↓
      12.   Sympathomimetics ↓
   C.   Cross Sensitivity
       1.   Phenothiazines

References

AMA Drug Evaluations. 2nd Ed., Acton, Mass., Publishing Sciences Group, 1973, pp. 334–335.
Council on Drugs: Evaluation of chlorprothixene (Taractan). JAMA 186:144, 1963.
Hermans, G.: Les psychotropes. Bull. Soc. Belge Ophtalmol. 160:15, 1972.
Physicians' Desk Reference. 28th Ed., Oradell, N. J., Medical Economics Co., 1974, pp. 1236, 1248.
Simpson, G. M.: Reactions following the intra-muscular administration of chlorprothixene. Am. J. Psychiatry 120:1021, 1964.

* * * * * * * * * * * *

Generic Name: 1. Droperidol; 2. Haloperidol; 3. Trifluperidol

Proprietary Name: 1. Droleptan (G.B.), Inapsine; 2. Haldol, Serenace (G.B.); 3. Triperidol (G.B.)

Primary Use: These butyrophenone derivatives are used in the management of acute and chronic schizophrenia, and manic depressive, involutional, senile, organic, and toxic psychoses. Droperidol is also used as an adjunct to anesthesia and as an antiemetic.

Ocular Side Effects

   A.   Systemic Administration
       1.   Decreased vision
       2.   Oculogyric crises
       3.   Decreased intraocular pressure
       4.   Pupils
            a.   Mydriasis — may precipitate narrow-angle glaucoma
            b.   Miosis
       5.   Decreased accommodation
       6.   Eyelids or conjunctiva
            a.   Allergic reactions
            b.   Photosensitivity
            c.   Angioneurotic edema
            d.   Exfoliative dermatitis
       7.   Visual hallucinations
       8.   Subconjunctival or retinal hemorrhages secondary to drug-induced anemia
       9.   Capsular cataracts (?)
      10.   Loss of eyelashes or eyebrows (?)

Clinical Significance: Ocular side effects due to these butyrophenone derivatives are often transient and reversible on withdrawal of the medication. The decreased intraocular pressure due to these drugs is not of a sufficient amount to be of clinical value.

Interactions with Other Drugs

A. Effect of Butyrophenones on Activity of Other Drugs
    1. Alcohol ↑
    2. Analgesics ↑
    3. Anticholinergics ↑
    4. Barbiturates ↑
    5. General anesthetics ↑
    6. Phenothiazines ↑
    7. Sedatives and hypnotics ↑
    8. Adrenergic blockers ↓
    9. Sympathomimetics ↓
B. Effect of Other Drugs on Activity of Butyrophenones
    1. Alcohol ↑
    2. Analgesics ↑
    3. Barbiturates ↑
    4. Monoamine oxidase inhibitors ↑
    5. Phenothiazines ↑
    6. Tricyclic antidepressants ↑
    7. Sympathomimetics ↓

References

AMA Drug Evaluations. 2nd Ed., Acton, Mass., Publishing Sciences Group, 1973, pp. 335–336.
Barton, D.: Side reactions of drugs in anesthesia. Int. Ophthalmol. Clin. 11(2):185, 1971.
Clark, M. M.: Droperidol in preoperative anxiety. Anaesthesia 24:36, 1969.
Ferrari, H. A., and Stephen, C. R.: Neuroleptanalgesia: Pharmacology and clinical experiences with droperidol and fentanyl. South. Med. J. 59:815, 1966.
Fink, M., et al.: Trifluperidol in the treatment of psychosis. J. New Drugs 6:174, 1966.
Freeman, J. E., Robertson, A. C., and Ngan, H.: Oculogyric crises due to phenothiazines. (Correspondence). Br. Med. J. 3:738, 1967.
Hermans, G.: Les psychotropes. Bull. Soc. Belge Ophtalmol. 160:15, 1972.
Honda, S.: Drug-induced cataract in mentally ill subjects. Rinsho Ganka 28:521, 1974.
LeVann, L. J.: Haloperidol in the treatment of behavioural disorders in children and adolescents. Can. Psychiatr. Assoc. J. 14:217, 1969.
Physicians' Desk Reference. 28th Ed., Oradell, N. J., Medical Economics Co., 1974, p. 969.
Pontinen, P. J., and Miettinen, P.: Neuroleptanalgesia in cataract surgery. Acta Ophthalmol. (Suppl.) 80:25, 1964.

* * * * * * * * * * * *

Generic Name: Lithium Carbonate

Proprietary Name: Camcolit (G.B.), Eskalith, Lithane, Lithonate, Lithotabs, Priadel (G.B.)

Primary Use: This lithium salt is used in the management of the manic phase of manic depressive psychosis.

Ocular Side Effects

A. Systemic Administration
 1. Decreased vision
 2. Nystagmus — horizontal or vertical
 3. Scotomas
 4. Extraocular muscles
  a. Oculogyric crises
  b. Decreased spontaneous movements
  c. Lateral conjugate deviations
  d. Jerky pursuit movements
 5. Eyelids or conjunctiva — edema
 6. Blindness

Clinical Significance: Ocular side effects due to lithium are reversible upon withdrawal of the drug. While blindness in toxic states has been reported, it is usually transitory and probably affects vision at the cortical level. Toxic drug responses are closely related to serum lithium blood levels.

Interactions with Other Drugs

A. Effect of Other Drugs on Activity of Lithium Carbonate
 1. Carbonic anhydrase inhibitors ↓
 2. Diuretics ↓
 3. Urea ↓

References

Baastrup, P. C., and Schou, M.: Lithium as a prophylactic agent. Arch. Gen. Psychiatry *16*:162, 1967.

Fann, W. E., Asher, H., and Luton, F. H.: Use of lithium in mania. Dis. Nerv. Syst. *30*:605, 1969.

Schlagenhauf, G., Tupin, J., and White, R. B.: Use of lithium carbonate in the treatment of manic psychoses. Am. J. Psychiatry *123*:201, 1966.

Schou, M., et al.: The treatment of manic psychoses by the administration of lithium salts. J. Neurol. Neurosurg. Psychiatry *17*:250, 1954.

Walsh, F. B., and Hoyt, W. F.: Clinical Neuro-Ophthalmology. 3rd Ed., Baltimore, Williams & Wilkins, Vol. III, 1969, pp. 2632–2633.

* * * * * * * * * * * *

Class: Psychedelic Agents

Proprietary Name: 1. Hashish; 2. Marihuana; 3. Tetrahydrocannabinol, THC

Street Name: 1. Bhang, Charas, Gram, Hash, Keif, Pot, Black Russian; 2. Ace, Acapulco gold, Baby, Belyando sprue, Bhang, Boo, Brown weed, Bush, Cannabis, Charas, Gage, Ganja, Gold, Grass, Gungeon, Hay, Hemp, Herb, Jay, Joint, Kick sticks, Lid, Locoweed, Mary Jane, Mexican green, MJ, Muggles, OJ (opium joint), Panama red, Pot, Rainy-day woman, Reefer, Roach, Rope, Stick, Tea, Twist, Weed, Wheat; 3. The one

Primary Use: These psychedelic agents are occasionally used as cerebral sedatives or narcotics commonly available on the illicit drug market.

Ocular Side Effects

A. Systemic Administration
  1. Visual hallucinations
  2. Problems with color vision
      a. Dyschromatopsia
      b. Objects have yellow or violet color
      c. Colored flashing lights
      d. Heightened color perception
  3. Nystagmus
  4. Nonspecific ocular irritation
      a. Hyperemia
      b. Photophobia
  5. Decreased accommodation
  6. Diplopia
  7. Decreased vision
  8. Blepharospasm
  9. Decreased intraocular pressure
  10. Abnormal conjugate deviations (?)
  11. Mydriasis (?)
  12. Ocular teratogenic effects (?)

Clinical Significance: Ocular side effects due to these drugs are transient and seldom of clinical importance. The mydriatic effect of marihuana is open to question and may in part be due to the multitude of preparations and the species of plants available. While these drugs are only occasionally used medically, they are in common social usage in many cultures.

References

Bromberg, W.: Marihuana intoxication; Clinical study of Cannabis sativa intoxication. Am. J. Psychiatry 91:303, 1934.
Cohen, S.: Psychotomimetic agents. Ann. Rev. Pharmacol. 7:301, 1967.
Duke-Elder, S.: Systems of Ophthalmology. St. Louis, C. V. Mosby, Vol. XIV, Part 2, 1972, pp. 1334–1335.
Goodman, L. S., and Gilman, A. (Eds.): The Pharamcological Basis of Therapeutics. 4th Ed., New York, Macmillan, 1970, pp. 298–300.
Grant, W. M.: Toxicology of the Eye. 2nd Ed., Springfield, Charles C Thomas, 1974, pp. 226–227.
Mohan, H., and Sood, G. C.: Conjugate deviation of the eyes after Cannabis indica intoxication. Br. J. Ophthalmol. 48:160, 1964.
Shapiro, D.: The ocular manifestations of the cannabinols. Ophthalmologica 168:366, 1974.
Stuart, K. L.: Ganja (Cannabis sativa L.). West Indian Med. J. 12:156, 1963.
Weil, A. T., Zinberg, N. E., and Nelsen, J. M.: Clinical and psychological effects of marihuana in man. Science 162:1234, 1968.

* * * * * * * * * * * *

Proprietary Name: 1. LSD, Lysergide; 2. Mescaline; 3. Psilocybin

Street Name: 1. Acid, Barrels, Big D, Blue acid, Brown dots, California sunshine, Crackers, Cubes, Cupcakes, Grape parfait, Green domes, Hawaiian sunshine, Lucy in the sky with diamonds, Micro dots, Purple barrels, Purple haze, Purple ozolone, Sunshine, The animal, The beast, The chief, The hawk, The ticket, Trips, Twenty-five, Yellow dimples; 2. Buttons, Cactus, Mesc, Peyote, The bad seed, Topi; 3. Magic mushroom

Primary Use: These experimental drugs are used in the treatment of chronic alcoholism, character neuroses, and sexual perversions.

Ocular Side Effects

A. Systemic Administration
  1. Pupils
     a. Mydriasis
     b. Anisocoria
     c. Decreased or absent reaction to light
  2. Visual hallucinations including micro- and macropsia
  3. Problems with color vision
     a. Dyschromatopsia
     b. Heightened color perception
  4. Prolongation of after image
  5. Decreased accommodation
  6. Decreased dark adaptation
  7. Ocular teratogenic effects (?)

Clinical Significance: Ocular side effects due to these drugs are common, but seldom of significant importance except when bizarre visual hallucinations aggravate an already disturbed sensorium. Some claim true visual hallucinations seldom occur with these drugs, but rather a complicated visual experience results from a perceptual disturbance. Lysergide is 100 times more potent than psilocybin, which in turn is 4000 times more potent than mescaline. While these drugs are only occasionally used medically, they are easily obtained through illicit channels.

References

Blacow, N. W. (Ed.): Martindale: The Extra Pharmacopoeia. 26th Ed., London, Pharmaceutical Press, 1972, pp. 1042–1047.

Carlson, V. R.: Individual pupillary reactions to certain centrally acting drugs in man. J. Pharmacol. Exp. Ther. 121:501, 1957.

Goodman, L. S., and Gilman, A. (Eds.): The Pharmacological Basis of Therapeutics. 4th Ed., New York, Macmillan, 1970, pp. 296–298.

Keeler, M. H.: The effects of psilocybin on a test of after-image perception. Psychopharmacologia 8:131, 1965.

Lyle, W. M.: Drugs and conditions which may affect color vision. Part 1. Drugs and chemicals. J. Am. Optometric Assoc. 45:47, 1974.

Payne, J. W.: LSD-25 and accommodative convergence ratios. Arch. Ophthalmol. 74:81, 1965.

* * * * * * * * * * * *

Class: Sedatives and Hypnotics

Generic Name: Alcohol (Ethanol)

Proprietary Name: Alcohol

Primary Use: This colorless liquid is used as a solvent, an antiseptic, a beverage, and as a nerve block in the management of certain types of intractable pain.

Ocular Side Effects

A. Systemic Administration — Acute Intoxication
   1. Diplopia
   2. Nystagmus
   3. Esophoria or exophoria
   4. Esotropia
   5. Decreased convergence
   6. Pupils
      a. Mydriasis
      b. Decreased or absent reaction to light
      c. Anisocoria
   7. Decreased vision
   8. Decreased accommodation
   9. Problems with color vision
      a. Dyschromatopsia
      b. Objects have blue tinge
   10. Decreased dark adaptation
   11. Decreased intraocular pressure
   12. Constriction of visual fields
   13. Decreased depth perception
   14. Decreased optokinetic nystagmus
   15. Visual hallucinations
   16. Blindness

B. Systemic Administration — Chronic Intoxication
   1. Paralysis of extraocular muscles
   2. Nystagmus
   3. Paralysis of accommodation
   4. Pupils
      a. Miosis
      b. Decreased or absent reaction to light
   5. Decreased vision
   6. Scotomas — central
   7. Problems with color vision
      a. Dyschromatopsia
      b. Achromatopsia, red-green defect
   8. Lacrimation
   9. Decreased intraocular pressure

      10. Visual hallucinations
      11. Blindness
C. Local Ophthalmic Use or Exposure — Retrobulbar Injection
      1. Irritation
         a. Hyperemia
         b. Ocular pain
         c. Edema
      2. Keratitis
      3. Paralysis of extraocular muscles
      4. Nystagmus
      5. Corneal ulceration
      6. Blindness
      7. Loss of eyelashes or eyebrows (?)
D. Inadvertent Ocular Exposure
      1. Irritation
         a. Lacrimation
         b. Hyperemia
         c. Ocular pain
         d. Edema
         e. Burning sensation
      2. Keratitis
      3. Corneal necrosis or opacities

Clinical Significance: The large number of adverse ocular effects reported due to ethyl alcohol is in part due to the fact that this agent is second only to water in the volume man consumes. Transient blindness lasting up to 5 days is well documented in both acute and chronic alcholism; however, permanent blindness directly caused by ethyl alcohol is debatable. So-called toxic alcohol amblyopia is probably secondary to a vitamin B deficiency, and if the alcoholic were taking vitamin supplements, it would probably not occur. Intraocular pressure may be significantly lowered in the glaucomatous patient after 40 to 60 ml. of ethyl alcohol; however, this effect lasts only for a few hours. Ethyl alcohol probably has little significant sensory effect on a person's ability to drive; however, nystagmus, diplopia, and incoordinated ocular movements may cause serious problems. The popularity of retrobulbar injections of alcohol is probably not as great today as it was in the past because of numerous untoward effects.

Interactions with Other Drugs

A. Effect of Alcohol on Activity of Other Drugs
      1. Anticholinesterases ↑
      2. Barbiturates ↑
      3. Adrenergic blockers ↑
      4. Phenothiazines ↑
B. Effect of Other Drugs on Activity of Alcohol
      1. Analgesics ↑
      2. Antihistamines ↑
      3. Barbiturates ↑
      4. Monoamine oxidase inhibitors ↑

5. Phenothiazines ↑
6. Tricylcic antidepressants ↑

References

Carney, M. W.: Alcoholic hallucinosis among servicemen in Cyprus. J. R. Army Med. Corps
   109:164, 1963.
Gramberg-Danielsen, B.: Ophthalmological findings after the use of alcohol. Zentralbl.
   Verkehrs-med. *11*:129, 1965.
Grant, W. M.: Toxicology of the Eye. 2nd Ed., Springfield, Charles C Thomas, 1974, pp.
   467–472.
Havener, W. H.: Ocular Pharmacology. 2nd Ed., St. Louis, C. V. Mosby, 1970, pp. 317–322.
Newman, H., and Fletcher, E.: Effects of alcohol on driving skill. JAMA *115*:1600, 1940.
Pergens, E.: Contribution a la connaissance de la cyanopsie. Ann. Oculist *120*:114, 1898.
Peters, H. B.: Changes in color fields occasioned by experimentally induced alcohol
   intoxication. J. Appl. Psychol. *26*:692, 1942.
Walsh, F. B., and Hoyt, W. F.: Clinical Neuro-Ophthalmology. 3rd Ed., Baltimore, Williams
   & Wilkins, Vol. III, 1969, pp. 2606–2610.

* * * * * * * * * * * *

Generic Name: 1. Allobarbital; 2. Amobarbital; 3. Aprobarbital; 4. Barbital;
5. Butabarbital; 6. Butalbital; 7. Butallylonal; 8. Butethal; 9. Cyclobarbital;
10. Cyclopentyl Allylbarbituric Acid; 11. Heptabarbital; 12. Hexethal;
13. Hexobarbital; 14. Mephobarbital; 15. Metharbital; 16. Methitural;
17. Methohexital; 18. Pentobarbital; 19. Phenobarbital; 20. Primidone;
21. Probarbital; 22. Secobarbital; 23. Talbutal; 24. Thiamylal; 25. Thiopental;
26. Vinbarbital

Proprietary Name: 1. Dial; 2. Amal (Austral.), Amsal (Austral.), Amylobarbi-
tone (G.B.), Amylosol (Austral.), Amytal, Mylosed (Austral.), Neur-Amyl
(Austral.), Pentymali (Scand.), Sedal (Austral.); 3. Alurate; 4. Barbitone
(G.B.), Hypnoral (Aust.), Neuronidia, Verodon (U.S.S.R.), Veronal; 5. Buta-
zem, Buticaps, Butisol; 6. Lotusate, Sandoptal; 7. Pernoston; 8. Bubal (Austral.), Butobarbitone (G.B.), Hyperbutal (Austral.), Neonal, Sonabarb
(Austral.), Soneryl (G.B.); 9. Amnosed (Austral.), Cybal (Austral.), Cyclobar-
bitone (G.B.), Fabadorm (Austral.), Phanodorm (G.B.), Phanodorn, Placyl
(Austral.), Rapidal (G.B.); 10. Cyclopal; 11. Medomin; 12. Ortal; 13. Evipal,
Hexobarbitone (G.B.), Noctivane (Fr.); 14. Mebaral, Menta-Bal, Methylpheno-
barbitone (G.B.), Prominal (G.B.), Promitone (Austral.); 15. Gemonil;
16. Neraval; 17. Brevital, Brietal (G.B.), Methohexitone (G.B.); 18. Aquabarb,
Barbopent (Austral.), Mebumali (Scand.), Nebralin, Nembutal, Penbarb
(Austral.), Penbon (Austral.), Pentobarbitone (G.B.), Pentone (Austral.), Petab
(Austral.), Sodepent (Austral.), Somnital (Austral.); 19. Barbita, Eskabarb,
Gardenal (G.B.), Luminal, Parabal (G.B.), Phenased (Austral.), Phenobarbitone
(G.B.), Somnolens (G.B.), Solfoton, Solu-Barb, Stental; 20. Elmidone (Aus-
tral.), Midone (Austral.), Mysoline; 21. Ipral; 22. Baqual (Austral.), Proquinal
(Austral.), QB (Austral.), Quinalbarbitone (G.B.), Quinaltone (Austral.),
Quinbar (Austral.), Seco-8, Seconal; 23. Lotusate; 24. Surital; 25. Intraval
(G.B.), Pentothal, Thiopentone (G.B.); 26. Delvinal, Diminal (Swed.)

Primary Use: These barbituric acid derivatives vary primarily in duration and intensity of action and are used as central nervous system depressants, hypnotics, sedatives, and anticonvulsants.

Ocular Side Effects

A. Systemic Administration
1. Eyelids
   a. Ptosis
   b. Blepharoclonus
   c. Symblepharon (?)
2. Pupils
   a. Mydriasis
   b. Miosis
   c. Decreased reaction to light
   d. Hippus
3. Extraocular muscles
   a. Jerky pursuit movements
   b. Random ocular movements
4. Diplopia
5. Decreased convergence
6. Paresis of extraocular muscles
7. Oscillopsia
8. Nystagmus
   a. Vertical
   b. Depressed or abolished optokinetic, latent, positional, voluntary, or congenital nystagmus
9. Decreased vision
10. Visual fields
    a. Scotomas
    b. Constriction
11. Problems with color vision
    a. Dyschromatopsia
    b. Objects have yellow or green tinge
12. Visual hallucinations
13. Eyelids or conjunctiva
    a. Allergic reactions
    b. Edema
    c. Photosensitivity
    d. Angioneurotic edema
    e. Stevens-Johnson syndrome
    f. Exfoliative dermatitis
    g. Lyell's syndrome
14. Decreased intraocular pressure
15. Blindness
16. Retinal vasoconstriction
17. Optic nerve disorders
    a. Retrobulbar or optic neuritis
    b. Papilledema
    c. Optic atrophy

18. Subconjunctival or retinal hemorrhages secondary to drug-induced anemia
19. Cortical blindness (?) (thiopental)
20. Ocular teratogenic effects (?) (primidone)

Clinical Significance: Numerous adverse ocular side effects have been attributed to barbiturate usage, yet nearly all significant ocular side effects are found in habitual users or in barbiturate poisoning. Few toxic ocular reactions are found due to barbiturate usage at therapeutic dosages or on short-term therapy. The most common ocular abnormalities are disturbances of ocular movement such as decreased convergence, paresis of extraocular muscles. or nystagmus. The pupillary response to barbiturate intake is quite variable, but usually miosis occurs except in the most toxic states when mydriasis is the most frequent side effect. Transient or permanent visual loss is primarily found in patients who are in barbiturate coma. Barbital and phenobarbital have the most frequently reported ocular side effects; however, all barbiturates may produce adverse ocular effects. Chronic barbiturate users have a "tattle tale" ptosis and blepharoclonus. Normally, a tap on the glabella area of the head produces a few eyelid blinks, but in the barbiturate addict the response will be a rapid fluttering of the eyelids.

Interactions with Other Drugs

A. Effect of Barbiturates on Activity of Other Drugs
   1. Alcohol ↑
   2. Antibiotics ↑
      (Kanamycin, Neomycin, Streptomycin)
   3. General anesthetics ↑
   4. Sedatives and hypnotics ↑↓
   5. Analgesics ↓
   6. Antihistamines ↓
   7. Chloramphenicol ↓
   8. Corticosteroids ↓
   9. Local anesthetics ↓
   10. Phenothiazines ↓
   11. Phenylbutazone ↓
   12. Salicylates ↓
   13. Sulfonamides ↓
   14. Tricyclic antidepressants ↓
B. Effect of Other Drugs on Activity of Barbiturates
   1. Alcohol ↑
   2. Analgesics ↑
   3. Anticholinesterases ↑
   4. Ascorbic acid ↑
   5. Chloramphenicol ↑
   6. Corticosteroids ↑
   7. Monoamine oxidase inhibitors ↑
   8. Phenothiazines ↑
   9. Sulfonamides ↑
   10. Tricyclic antidepressants ↑

11. Antihistamines ↑↓
12. Phenylbutazone ↓

References

Bender, M. B., and Brown, C. A.: The character of the nystagmus induced by Amytal in chronic alcoholics. Am. J. Ophthalmol. 31:825, 1948.

Bender, M. B., and Gorman, W. F.: Vertical nystagmus on direct forward gaze with vertical oscillopsia. Am. J. Ophthalmol. 32:967, 1949.

Carlson, V. R.: Individual pupillary reactions to certain centrally acting drugs in man. J. Pharmacol. Exp. Ther. 121:501, 1957.

Carrillo, R., Malbran, J., and Chichilnisky, S.: Neuritis retrobulbar barbiturica (Intoxication por Luminal). Arch. de Oftal. Buenos Aires 13:370, 1938.

Committee on Alcoholism and Addiction and Council on Mental Health: Dependence on barbiturates and other sedative drugs. JAMA 193:673, 1965.

Rashbass, C.: Barbiturate nystagmus and the mechanisms of visual fixation. Nature 183:897, 1959.

Roth, J. H.: Luminal poisoning with conjunctival residue. Am. J. Ophthalmol. 9:533, 1926.

Westheimer, G.: Amphetamine, barbiturates, and accommodation-convergence. Arch. Ophthalmol. 70:830, 1963.

* * * * * * * * * * * * *

Generic Name: Bromide

Proprietary Name: Bromide

Primary Use: This nonbarbiturate sedative-hypnotic is primarily effective as an anticonvulsant in recalcitrant epilepsy.

Ocular Side Effects

A. Systemic Administration
1. Decreased vision
2. Pupils
   a. Mydriasis
   b. Miosis
   c. Decreased or absent reaction to light
   d. Anisocoria
3. Problems with color vision — dyschromatopsia
4. Visual hallucinations — mainly Lilliputian
5. Eyelids or conjunctiva
   a. Allergic reactions
   b. Erythema
   c. Blepharoconjunctivitis
   d. Stevens-Johnson syndrome
6. Decreased accommodation
7. Decreased convergence
8. Diplopia
9. Nystagmus
10. Extraocular muscles
    a. Decreased spontaneous movements
    b. Jerky pursuit movements

11. Photophobia
12. Decreased corneal reflex
13. Apparent movement of stationary objects
14. Scotomas
15. Papilledema (?)
16. Optic atrophy (?)

Clinical Significance: The medical use of bromides has been drastically reduced by newer agents since the therapeutic blood level of bromide is so close to its toxic level. Nearly all ocular side effects are reversible after use of the drug is discontinued.

Interactions with Other Drugs

A. Effect of Bromide on Activity of Other Drugs
  1. Phenothiazines ↑
  2. Tricyclic antidepressants ↑
  3. Analgesics ↓
  4. Antihistamines ↓
  5. Corticosteroids ↓
B. Effect of Other Drugs on Activity of Bromide
  1. Antihistamines ↑
  2. Corticosteroids ↑
  3. Monoamine oxidase inhibitors ↑
  4. Tricyclic antidepressants ↑

References

Barbour, R. F., Pilkington, F., and Sargant, W.: Bromide intoxication. Br. Med. J. 2:957, 1936.
Bucy, P. C., Weaver, T. A., and Camp, E. H.: Bromide intoxication of unusual severity and chronicity resulting from self medication with bromoseltzer. JAMA 117:1256, 1941.
Levin, M.: Eye disturbances in bromide intoxication. Am. J. Ophthalmol. 50:478, 1960.
Perkins, H. A.: Bromide intoxication: Analysis of cases from a general hospital. Arch. Intern. Med. 85:783, 1950.
Walsh, F. B., and Hoyt, W. F.: Clinical Neuro-Ophthalmology. 3rd Ed., Baltimore, Williams & Wilkins, Vol. III, 1969, pp. 2541, 2618, 2641.

* * * * * * * * * * * *

Generic Name: 1. Bromisovalum; 2. Carbromal

Proprietary Name: 1. Bromural, Bromvaletone (G.B.); 2. Caral (Austral.)

Primary Use: These brominated monoureides are effective in the management of mild insomnia.

Ocular Side Effects

A. Systemic Administration
  1. Decreased vision
  2. Nystagmus – horizontal or vertical
  3. Pupils
      a. Mydriasis

      b. Miosis
      c. Decreased reaction to light
      d. Anisocoria
    4. Visual fields
      a. Scotomas — central
      b. Constriction
    5. Retrobulbar or optic neuritis
    6. Eyelids or conjunctiva — Stevens-Johnson syndrome
    7. Diplopia (bromisovalum)
    8. Decreased convergence (bromisovalum)
    9. Ptosis (carbromal)
   10. Cataracts (?) (carbromal)

Clinical Significance: Adverse ocular side effects due to these agents are rare except in overdose situations. Except for signs or symptoms related to optic nerve disease, the effects are reversible. Both drugs can elevate serum bromide levels, and this in part may account for some adverse ocular side effects. It is said that nystagmus and diplopia are seen more frequently with bromide poisoning than with these brominated monoureides. Only one case of acute reversible cataracts was reported.

Interactions with Other Drugs

A. Effect of Brominated Monoureides on Activity of Other Drugs
    1. Phenothiazines ↑
    2. Tricyclic antidepressants ↑
    3. Analgesics ↓
    4. Antihistamines ↓
    5. Corticosteroids ↓
B. Effect of Other Drugs on Activity of Brominated Monoureides
    1. Analgesics ↑
    2. Antihistamines ↑
    3. Corticosteroids ↑
    4. Monoamine oxidase inhibitors ↑
    5. Phenothiazines ↑
    6. Tricyclic antidepressants ↑

References

Blacow, N. W. (Ed.): Martindale: The Extra Pharmacopoeia. 26th Ed., London, Pharmaceutical Press, 1972, pp. 896–897.
Copas, D. E., Kay, W. W., and Longman, V. H.: Carbromal intoxication. Lancet 1:703, 1959.
Crawford, R.: Toxic cataract. Br. Med. J. 2:1231, 1959.
Harenko, A.: Irreversible cerebello-bulbar syndrome as the sequela of bromisovalum poisoning. Ann. Med. Interne. Fenn. 56:29, 1967.
Harenko, A.: Neurologic findings in chronic bromisovalum poisoning. Ann. Med. Interne Fenn. 56:181, 1967.
Sattler, C. H.: Bromural und Adalinvergiftung des Auges. Klin. Monatsbl. Augenheilkd. 70:149, 1923.
Stohr, G.: Adalin-Schadigungen. Arztl. Wchnschr. 6:1097, 1951.

* * * * * * * * * * * * *

Generic Name: Chloral Hydrate

Proprietary Name: Aquachoral, Chloradorm (Austral.), Chloralate (Austral.), Chlorhydrate Dormel (Austral.), Elix-Nocte (Austral.), Felsules, Kessodrate, Noctec, Rectules, Somnos

Primary Use: This nonbarbiturate sedative-hypnotic is effective in the treatment of insomnia.

Ocular Side Effects
A. Systemic Administration
1. Decreased vision
2. Pupils
a. Mydriasis
b. Miosis
3. Visual hallucinations – mainly Lilliputian
4. Ptosis
5. Decreased convergence
6. Eyelids or conjunctiva
a. Allergic reactions
b. Hyperemia
c. Edema
7. Lacrimation
8. Nonspecific ocular irritation
9. Nystagmus
10. Paralysis of extraocular muscles
11. Optic neuritis (?)
12. Blindness (?)

Clinical Significance: While the more serious ocular side effects due to chloral hydrate occur at excessive dosage levels, decreased convergence, miosis, and occasionally ptosis are seen even at recommended therapeutic dosages. Lilliputian hallucinations (in which objects appear smaller than their actual size) are said to be almost characteristic for chloral hydrate-induced delirium. Mydriasis only occurs in severely toxic states.

Interactions with Other Drugs
A. Effect of Chloral Hydrate on Activity of Other Drugs
1. Alcohol ↑
2. Phenothiazines ↑
3. Tricyclic antidepressants ↑
4. Analgesics ↓
5. Antihistamines ↓
6. Corticosteroids ↓
7. Phenylbutazone ↓
8. Sedatives and hypnotics ↓
B. Effect of Other Drugs on Activity of Chloral Hydrate
1. Alcohol ↑
2. Analgesics ↑

3.   Antihistamines ↑
4.   Corticosteroids ↑
5.   Monoamine oxidase inhibitors ↑
6.   Phenothiazines ↑
7.   Tricyclic antidepressants ↑

References

de Schweinitz, G. E.: Toxic Amblyopias. Philadelphia, Lea Brothers, 1896.
Goldstein, J. H.: Effects of drugs on cornea, conjunctiva, and lids. Int. Ophthalmol. Clin. *11*(2):13, 1971.
Hermans, G.: Les psychotropes. Bull. Soc. Belge Ophtalmol. *160*:15, 1972.
Lubeck, M. J.: Effects of drugs on ocular muscles. Int. Ophthalmol. Clin. *11*(2):35, 1971.
Margetts, E. L.: Chloral delirium. Psychiatr. Q. *24*:278, 1950.
Walsh, F. B., and Hoyt, W. F.: Clinical Neuro-Ophthalmology. 3rd Ed., Baltimore, Williams & Wilkins, Vol. III, 1969, p. 2619.

* * * * * * * * * * * *

Generic Name: Ethchlorvynol

Proprietary Name: Arvynol (G.B.), Placidyl, Serenesil (G.B.)

Primary Use: This nonbarbiturate sedative-hypnotic is effective in the treatment of simple insomnia. It is also used as a daytime sedative.

Ocular Side Effects

A.   Systemic Administration
1.   Decreased vision
2.   Diplopia
3.   Nystagmus
4.   Visual hallucinations
5.   Problems with color vision – dyschromatopsia
6.   Visual fields
a.   Scotomas – central or centrocecal
b.   Constriction
7.   Decreased accommodation
8.   Blindness
9.   Anisocoria
10.   Optic neuritis

Clinical Significance: Nearly all ocular side effects due to ethchlorvynol are reversible, after discontinuation of the drug. Upon withdrawal of the drug, visual hallucinations are common in patients who have been receiving high doses.

Interactions with Other Drugs

A.   Effect of Ethchlorvynol on Activity of Other Drugs
1.   Phenothiazines ↑
2.   Tricyclic antidepressants ↑
3.   Analgesics ↓

    4. Antihistamines ↓
    5. Corticosteroids ↓
  B. Effect of Other Drugs on Activity of Ethchlorvynol
    1. Alcohol ↑
    2. Analgesics ↑
    3. Antihistamines ↑
    4. Barbiturates ↑
    5. Corticosteroids ↑
    6. Monoamine oxidase inhibitors ↑
    7. Phenothiazines ↑
    8. Tricyclic antidepressants ↑

References

Brown, E., and Meyer, G. G.: Toxic amblyopia and peripheral neuropathy with ethchlorvynol abuse. Am. J. Psychiatry *126*:882, 1969.
Grant, W. M.: Toxicology of the Eye. 2nd Ed., Springfield, Charles C Thomas, 1974, pp. 463–464.
Haining, W. M., and Beveridge, G. W.: Toxic amblyopia in a patient receiving ethchlorvynol as a hypnotic. Br. J. Ophthalmol. *48*:598, 1964.
Hudson, H. S., and Walker, H. I.: Withdrawal symptoms following ethchlorvynol (Placidyl) dependence. Am. J. Psychiatry *118*:361, 1961.
Millhouse, J., Davies, D. M., and Wraith, S. R.: Chronic ethchlorvynol intoxication. Lancet *2*:1251, 1966.

* * * * * * * * * * * * *

Generic Name: 1. Glutethimide; 2. Methyprylon

Proprietary Name: 1. Doriden, Glimid (Pol.), Gludorm (Austral.); 2. Methyprylone (G.B.), Noludar

Primary Use: These piperidinedione derivatives are effective in the treatment of simple insomnia or as a mild daytime sedative.

Ocular Side Effects

  A. Systemic Administration
    1. Decreased vision
    2. Pupils
      a. Mydriasis
      b. Miosis (methyprylon)
      c. Decreased or absent reaction to light
    3. Nystagmus — horizontal or vertical
    4. Diplopia
    5. Decreased accommodation
    6. Visual hallucinations
    7. Eyelids or conjunctiva
      a. Allergic reactions
      b. Exfoliative dermatitis
    8. Subconjunctival or retinal hemorrhages secondary to drug-induced anemia
    9. Decreased corneal reflex
   10. Papilledema

Clinical Significance: At the recommended dosage, few ocular side effects due to these agents are seen; however, in overdose situations ocular side effects, especially with glutethimide, are common. Papilledema and dilated fixed pupils have only been found in near terminal patients.

Interactions with Other Drugs

A. Effect of Piperidinedione Derivatives on Activity of Other Drugs
   1. Phenothiazines ↑
   2. Tricyclic antidepressants ↑
   3. Analgesics ↓
   4. Antihistamines ↓
   5. Corticosteroids ↓
   6. Sedatives and hypnotics ↓
B. Effect of Other Drugs on Activity of Piperidinedione Derivatives
   1. Alcohol ↑
   2. Antihistamines ↑
   3. Barbiturates ↑
   4. Corticosteroids ↑
   5. Monoamine oxidase inhibitors ↑
   6. Tricyclic antidepressants ↑

References

DeMyttenaere, M., Schoenfeld, L., and Maher, J. F.: Treatment of glutethimide poisoning. JAMA 203:885, 1968.
Hermans, G.: Les psychotropes, Bull. Soc. Belge Ophtalmol. 160:15, 1972.
Maher, J. F., Schreiner, G. E., and Westervelt, F. B.: Acute glutethimide intoxication. Am. J. Med. 33:70, 1962.
Medgyaszay, A.: Impairment of adaptation in response to Noxyron. Szemeszet 100:228, 1963 (Am. J. Ophthalmol. 57:1073, 1964).
Walsh, F. B., and Hoyt, W. F.: Clinical Neuro-Ophthalmology. 3rd Ed., Baltimore, Williams & Wilkins, Vol. III, 1969, pp. 2647–2648.

* * * * * * * * * * * * *

Generic Name: Methaqualone

Proprietary Name: Barbitrax (Austral.), Dormir (Austral.), Melsed (G.B.), Melsedin (G.B.), Mequal (Austral.), Mequelon (Canad.), Methalone (Austral.), Methased (Austral.), Parest, Paxidorm (G.B.), Quaalude, Revonal (G.B.), Roulone (Austral.), Sedaquin (G.B.), Sleepinal (Austral.), Somnafac, Sopor, Thendorm (Austral.), Toraflon (Fr.)

Primary Use: This nonbarbiturate sedative-hypnotic is effective in the treatment of simple insomnia or as a daytime sedative.

Ocular Side Effects

A. Systemic Administration
   1. Nystagmus
   2. Lacrimation
   3. Pupils

    a. Mydriasis (?)
    b. Miosis (?)
    c. Decreased reaction to light
    d. Anisocoria (?)
4. Diplopia
5. Decreased vision
6. Problems with color vision — objects have yellow tinge
7. Subconjunctival or retinal hemorrhages secondary to drug-induced anemia
8. Decreased accommodation (?)

Clinical Significance: All ocular side effects due to methaqualone are transient and reversible. Unfortunately, a number of patients were also taking other drugs, such as meprobamate, when toxic ocular side effects occurred. However, the aforementioned ocular side effects have been reported as being due to this drug alone.

Interactions with Other Drugs

A. Effect of Methaqualone on Activity of Other Drugs
    1. Phenothiazines ↑
    2. Tricyclic antidepressants ↑
    3. Analgesics ↓
    4. Antihistamines ↓
    5. Corticosteroids ↓
B. Effect of Other Drugs on Activity of Methaqualone
    1. Alcohol ↑
    2. Analgesics ↑
    3. Antihistamines ↑
    4. Barbiturates ↑
    5. Corticosteroids ↑
    6. Monoamine oxidase inhibitors ↑
    7. Phenothiazines ↑
    8. Sedatives and hypnotics ↑
    9. Tricyclic antidepressants ↑

References

American Hospital Formulary Service. Washington, D. C., American Society of Hospital Pharmacists, Vol. 1, 28:24, 1970.

Davidson, S. I.: Reports of ocular adverse reactions. Trans. Ophthalmol. Soc. U. K. 93:495, 1973.

Gitelson, S.: Methaqualone-meprobamate poisoning. JAMA 201:977, 1967.

Grant, W. M.: Toxicology of the Eye. 2nd Ed., Springfield, Charles C Thomas, 1974, pp. 676–677.

MacDonald, H. R. F., and Lakshman, A. D.: Poisoning with Mandrax. Br. Med. J. 1:500, 1967.

Physicians' Desk Reference. 28th Ed., Oradell, N. J., Medical Economics Co., 1974, p. 562.

* * * * * * * * * * * * *

Generic Name: Methylpentynol

Proprietary Name: Insomnol (G.B.), Oblivon (G.B.), N-Oblivon (Fr.)

Primary Use: This nonbarbiturate sedative-hypnotic is effective in the treatment of insomnia and as a premedication for minor surgical procedures.

Ocular Side Effects

A. Systemic Administration
1. Nystagmus
2. Diplopia
3. Conjunctival edema
4. Mydriasis — may precipitate narrow-angle glaucoma
5. Visual hallucinations
6. Ptosis

Clinical Significance: Ocular side effects are commonly seen with methylpentynol, especially nystagmus. Seldom are adverse ocular symptoms of major clinical importance, since this drug is short-acting and is not used for prolonged periods.

Interactions with Other Drugs

A. Effect of Methylpentynol on Activity of Other Drugs
1. Phenothiazines ↑
2. Tricyclic antidepressants ↑
3. Analgesics ↓
4. Antihistamines ↓
5. Corticosteroids ↓
B. Effect of Other Drugs on Activity of Methylpentynol
1. Analgesics ↑
2. Antihistamines ↑
3. Corticosteroids ↑
4. Monoamine oxidase inhibitors ↑
5. Phenothiazines ↑
6. Tricyclic antidepressants ↑

References

Bartholomew, A. A., et al.: Methylpentynol carbamate and liver function. Lancet *1*:346, 1958.

Blacow, N. W. (Ed.): Martindale: The Extra Pharmacopoeia. 26th Ed., London, Pharmaceutical Press, 1972, pp. 910–911.

Hermans, G.: Les psychotropes. Bull. Soc. Belge Ophtalmol. *160*:15, 1972.

Hitzschke, B., and Herbst, A.: Beobachtungen bei Missbrauch von Methylpentinol. Psychiatr. Neurol. (Basel) *153*:308, 1967.

Meyler, L., and Herxheimer, A.: Side Effects of Drugs. Amsterdam, Excerpta Medica, Vol. VII, 1972, p. 57.

* * * * * * * * * * * *

Generic Name: Paraldehyde

Proprietary Name: Paral

Primary Use: This nonbarbiturate sedative-hypnotic is also effective as an anticonvulsant in epilepsy and in alcohol withdrawal.

Ocular Side Effects

A. Systemic Administration
1. Pupils
   a. Mydriasis
   b. Miosis
2. Decreased vision
3. Visual hallucinations
4. Decreased corneal reflex
5. Hemianopsia (?)

Clinical Significance: Ocular side effects due to paraldehyde are common but seldom significant. At therapeutic dosage levels paraldehyde causes miosis; however, at toxic blood levels mydriasis may occur. Visual hallucinations occur primarily during withdrawal of the drug. In one instance of drug withdrawal, a homonymous hemianopsia with loss of corneal reflex occurred.

Interactions with Other Drugs

A. Effect of Paraldehyde on Activity of Other Drugs
1. Phenothiazines ↑
2. Tricyclic antidepressants ↑
3. Analgesics ↓
4. Antihistamines ↓
5. Corticosteroids ↓
6. Sulfonamides ↓
B. Effect of Other Drugs on Activity of Paraldehyde
1. Alcohol ↑
2. Analgesics ↑
3. Antihistamines ↑
4. Corticosteroids ↑
5. Monoamine oxidase inhibitors ↑
6. Phenothiazines ↑
7. Tricyclic antidepressants ↑

References

Grant, W. M.: Toxicology of the Eye. 2nd Ed., Springfield, Charles C Thomas, 1974, p. 786.
Heiman, M.: Visual hallucination during paraldehyde addiction. J. Nerv. Ment. Dis. 96:251, 1942.
Hermans, G.: Les psychotropes. Bull. Soc. Belge Ophtalmol. 160:15, 1972.
Lubeck, M. J.: Effects of drugs on ocular muscles. Int. Ophthalmol. Clin. 11(2):35, 1971.
Walsh, F. B., and Hoyt, W. F.: Clinical Neuro-Ophthalmology. 3rd Ed., Baltimore, Williams & Wilkins, Vol. III, 1969, pp. 2627–2628.

* * * * * * * * * * * * *

III. Analgesics, Narcotic Antagonists, and Agents Used to Treat Arthritis

Class: Agents Used to Treat Gout

Generic Name: Allopurinol

Proprietary Name: Zyloprim, Zyloric (G.B.)

Primary Use: This potent xanthine oxidase inhibitor is primarily used in the treatment of chronic hyperuricemia.

Ocular Side Effects

A. Systemic Administration
1. Decreased vision
2. Eyelids or conjunctiva
   a. Allergic reactions
   b. Stevens-Johnson syndrome
   c. Exfoliative dermatitis
3. Subconjunctival or retinal hemorrhages secondary to drug-induced anemia
4. Cataracts
5. Macular exudates (?)
6. Macular hemorrhages (?)
7. Macular degeneration (?)
8. Loss of eyelashes or eyebrows (?)

Clinical Significance: This potent drug has few reported ocular side effects; however, since it is still relatively new, additional adverse drug reactions are probably still to be discovered. Ocular side effects are usually not significant and are reversible with early discontinuation of the drug. Cataracts are probably caused by this drug, especially if they are associated with a severe drug-induced dermatitis. Macular changes due to allopurinol have been reported; however, they may have been coincidental.

Interactions with Other Drugs

A. Effect of Other Drugs on Activity of Allopurinol
1. Diuretics ↓

References

Davidson, S. I.: Reports of ocular adverse reactions. Trans. Ophthalmol. Soc. U. K. *93*:495, 1973.

Duke-Elder, S.: Systems of Ophthalmology. St. Louis, C. V. Mosby, Vol. XIV, Part 2, 1972, p. 1287.

Goodman, L. S., and Gilman, A. (Eds.): The Pharmacological Basis of Therapeutics. 4th Ed., New York, Macmillan, 1970, pp. 341–344.

Grant, W. M.: Toxicology of the Eye. 2nd Ed., Springfield, Charles C Thomas, 1974, pp. 101–102.

Laval, J.: Allopurinol and macular lesions. Arch. Ophthalmol. *80*:415, 1968.

March, W. F., Goren, S., and Shoch, D.: Action of allopurinol on the lens. In Leopold, I. H. (Ed.): Symposium on Ocular Therapy. St. Louis, C. V. Mosby, Vol. VII, 1974, pp. 83–95.

Physicians' Desk Reference. 28th Ed., Oradell, N. J., Medical Economics Co., 1974, p. 661.

Pinnas, G.: Possible association between macular lesions and allopurinol. Arch. Ophthalmol. *79*:786, 1968.

* * * * * * * * * * * *

Generic Name: Colchicine

Proprietary Name: Aqua-Colchin (Austral.), Colcin (Austral.), Colgout (Austral.), Coluric (Austral.)

Primary Use: This alkaloid is used in the prophylaxis and treatment of acute gout.

Ocular Side Effects

A. Systemic Administration
1. Paresis or paralysis of extraocular muscles
2. Diplopia
3. Subconjunctival or retinal hemorrhages secondary to drug-induced anemia
4. Keratitis (?)
5. Hypopyon (?)
6. Cataracts (?)
7. Loss of eyelashes or eyebrows (?)
B. Inadvertent Ocular Exposure
1. Decreased vision
2. Conjunctival hyperemia
3. Corneal clouding

Clinical Significance: Colchicine rarely causes adverse ocular side effects; however, when they do occur, they are usually insignificant and transitory. Major ocular side effects have occurred after a fatal overdose in one patient who developed paresis of extraocular muscles, keratitis, hypopyon, and cataracts. The lens changes may have been due to severe dehydration.

Interactions with Other Drugs

A. Effect of Colchicine on Activity of Other Drugs
1. Sympathomimetics ↑

References

American Hospital Formulary Service. Washington, D.C., American Society of Hospital Pharmacists, Vol. II, 92:00, 1973.

Estable, J. J.: The ocular effect of several irritant drugs applied directly to the conjunctiva. Am. J. Ophthalmol. 31:837, 1948.

Goodman, L. S., and Gilman, A. (Eds.): The Pharmacological Basis of Therapeutics. 4th Ed., New York, Macmillan, 1970, pp. 339–341.

Grant, W. M.: Toxicology of the Eye. 2nd Ed., Springfield, Charles C Thomas, 1974, pp. 304–305.

Walsh, F. B., and Hoyt, W. F.: Clinical Neuro-Ophthalmology. 3rd Ed., Baltimore, Williams & Wilkins, Vol. III, 1969, p. 2659.

* * * * * * * * * * * *

Class: Antirheumatic Agents

Generic Name: 1. Aurothioglucose; 2. Aurothioglycanide; 3. Gold Au^{198}; 4. Gold Sodium Thiomalate

Proprietary Name: 1. Solganal; 2. Lauron; 3. Aureotope, Aurocoloid-198; 4. Myochrysine, Myocrisin (G.B.)

Primary Use: These heavy metals are used in the treatment of active rheumatoid arthritis and nondisseminated lupus erythematosus. Radioactive gold (Au^{198}) is also employed for its radiation effects in treating neoplastic growths.

Ocular Side Effects

A. Systemic Administration
    1. Red, violet, purple, or brown gold deposits
        a. Eyelids
        b. Conjunctiva
        c. Cornea
        d. Surface of lens
    2. Eyelids or conjunctiva
        a. Allergic reactions
        b. Hyperemia — including ciliary body
        c. Erythema
        d. Blepharoconjunctivitis
        e. Edema
        f. Photosensitivity
        g. Symblepharon

        h. Stevens-Johnson syndrome
        i. Exfoliative dermatitis
        j. Lyell's syndrome
    3. Photophobia
    4. Keratitis — with or without ulceration
    5. Iritis
    6. Paralysis of extraocular muscles
    7. Ptosis
    8. Diplopia
    9. Nystagmus
   10. Blindness
   11. Cataracts
   12. Subconjunctival or retinal hemorrhages secondary to drug-induced anemia
   13. Papilledema (?)
   14. Phlyctenular keratoconjunctivitis (?)
B. Inadvertent Ocular Exposure
    1. Irritation
    2. Corneal clouding
    3. Iritis

Clinical Significance: The incidence of systemic adverse reactions associated with gold therapy ranges from 10 to 60 percent, depending on the series. Ocular side effects are common during long-term therapy, but they are seldom of major clinical significance. The highest incidence of systemic or ocular side effects occurs on the skin or mucous membranes. Deposits of gold in the cornea rarely cause visual complaints, since the particulate size is small and deposits are fewest in the visual axis. Significant corneal abnormalities are seldom present without a pathologic condition of the eyelid or conjunctiva. Ptosis, diplopia, and nystagmus due to gold therapy are extremely rare.

Interactions with Other Drugs

A. Contraindications
    1. Oxyphenbutazone
    2. Phenylbutazone

References

AMA Drug Evaluations. 2nd Ed., Acton, Mass., Publishing Sciences Group, 1973, pp. 300–301.

Goodman, L. S., and Gilman, A. (Eds.): The Pharmacological Basis of Therapeutics. 4th Ed., New York, Macmillan, 1970, pp. 969–974.

Grant, W. M.: Toxicology of the Eye. 2nd Ed., Springfield, Charles C Thomas, 1974, pp. 530–533.

Roberts, W. H., and Wolter, J. R.: Ocular chrysiasis. Arch. Ophthalmol. 56:48, 1956.

Sundelin, F.: Die Goldbehandlung der chronischen Arthritis unter besonderer Berucksichtigung der Komplikationen. Acta Med. Scand. (Suppl.) 117:1, 1941.

Walsh, F. B., and Hoyt, W. F.: Clinical Neuro-Ophthalmology. 3rd Ed., Baltimore, Williams & Wilkins, Vol. III, 1969, pp. 2651–2652, 2686–2687.

* * * * * * * * * * * *

Generic Name: Ibuprofen

Proprietary Name: Brufen (G.B.), Motrin

Primary Use: This antipyretic analgesic is used in the treatment of rheumatoid arthritis and osteoarthritis.

Ocular Side Effects

A. Systemic Administration
1. Decreased vision
2. Eyelids or conjunctiva
   a. Erythema
   b. Urticaria
   c. Purpura
   d. Edema
3. Visual fields
   a. Scotomas — centrocecal
   b. Hemianopsia (?)
4. Optic neuritis (?)
5. Blindness (?)
6. Papilledema (?)
7. Cataracts (?)
8. Paralysis of extraocular muscles (?)

Clinical Significance: While significant ocular side effects associated with ibuprofen have been seen, most have been in retrospective reports and are not proven. To date, nearly all ocular side effects due to ibuprofen have been reversible, including amblyopia. A prospective study did not show eye toxicity during a 24-week treatment period.

References

Blacow, N. W. (Ed.): Martindale: The Extra Pharmacopoeia. 26th Ed., London, Pharmaceutical Press, 1972, pp. 236–237.
Davidson, S. I.: Report of ocular adverse reactions. Trans. Ophthalmol. Soc. U. K. 93:495, 1973.
Melluish, J. W., et al.: Ibuprofen and visual function. Arch. Ophthalmol. 93:781, 1975.
Meyler, L., and Herxheimer, A. (Eds.): Side Effects of Drugs. Amsterdam, Excerpta Medica, Vol. VII, 1972, p. 173.

* * * * * * * * * * * *

Generic Name: Indomethacin

Proprietary Name: Amuno (Germ.), Inacid (Span.), Indacin (Jap.), Indocid (G.B.), Indocin, Indomee (Swed.), Metindol (Pol.), Mezolin (Jap.)

Primary Use: This indole compound is effective as an antipyretic, analgesic, and anti-inflammatory agent in the treatment of rheumatoid arthritis, rheumatoid spondylitis, and degenerative joint disease.

Ocular Side Effects

A. Systemic Administration
1. Decreased vision
2. Diplopia
3. Problems with color vision — dyschromatopsia
4. Visual hallucinations
5. Eyelids or conjunctiva — angioneurotic edema
6. Subconjunctival or retinal hemorrhages secondary to drug-induced anemia
7. Corneal deposits (?)
    a. Subepithelial whorl pattern
    b. Superficial
    c. Deep stromal
8. Retina (?)
    a. Pigmentary changes
    b. Cystoid degeneration
9. Macula (?)
    a. Edema
    b. Degeneration
    c. Central serous retinopathy
    d. Degeneration — paramacular
10. Night blindness (?)
11. Visual fields (?)
    a. Scotomas
    b. Constriction
    c. Enlarged blind spot
12. Orbital or periorbital pain (?)
13. Lacrimation (?)
14. Mydriasis (?)
15. Retinal hemorrhages (?)
16. Blindness (?)
17. Loss of eyelashes or eyebrows (?)

Clinical Significance: Systemic complications from indomethacin have been reported to occur in 35 to 50 percent of patients taking accepted therapeutic doses. The true role of indomethacin-induced ocular adverse effects is clouded by an almost equal number of contradictory reports. Unfortunately, much of the data implicating indomethacin is in retrospective studies. The clinician confronted with a possible adverse ocular effect must judge each case individually, fully aware that the possibility of drug-induced ocular toxic effects may exist. At our current stage of knowledge, however, many investigators feel that indomethacin causes a number of ocular side effects.

Interactions with Other Drugs

A. Effect of Indomethacin on Activity of Other Drugs
1. Corticosteroids ↑
2. Sulfonamides ↑
B. Effect of Other Drugs on Activity of Indomethacin
1. Salicylates ↓

References

Burns, C. A.: Indomethacin, reduced retinal sensitivity, and corneal deposits. Am. J. Ophthalmol. 66:825, 1968.

Carr, R. E., and Siegel, I. M.: Retinal function in patients treated with indomethacin. Am. J. Ophthalmol. 75:302, 1973.

Davidson, S. I.: Report of ocular adverse reactions. Trans. Ophthalmol. Soc. U. K. 93:495, 1973.

Henkes, H. E., van Lith, G. H. M., and Canta, L. R.: Indomethacin retinopathy. Am. J. Ophthalmol. 73:846, 1972.

Kelly, M.: Treatment of 193 rheumatic patients with indomethacin: A new antirheumatic drug. J. Am. Geriat. Soc. 14:48, 1966.

Palimeris, G., Koliopoulos, J., and Velissaropoulos, P.: Ocular side effects of indomethacin. Ophthalmologica 164:339, 1972.

Physicians' Desk Reference. 28th Ed., Oradell, N. J., Medical Economics Co., 1974, p. 1029.

* * * * * * * * * * * *

Generic Name: 1. Oxyphenbutazone; 2. Phenylbutazone

Proprietary Name: 1. Butapirone (Ital.), Floghene (Ital.), Idrobutazina (Austral.), Iridil (Ital.), Oxalid, Tandearil, Tanderil (G.B.), Visubutina (Ital.); 2. Anpuzone (G.B.), Artizin (Denm.), Artropan (Ital.), Azolid, Benzone (G.B.), Butacal (Austral.), Butalgin (Austral.), Butaphen (Austral., G.B.), Butapirazol (Pol.), Butarex (Austral.), Butazolidin, Butazone (G.B.), Butoroid (Austral.), Buzon (Austral.), Diossidone (Ital.), Ethibute (G.B.), Flexazone (G.B.), Ia-but (G.B.), Kadol (Ital.), Oppazone (G.B.), Phenybute (Austral.), Tetnor (G.B.), Ticinil (Ital.)

Primary Use: These pyrazolon derivatives are effective in the management of acute gout, ankylosing spondylitis, osteoarthritis, and musculoskeletal disorders.

Ocular Side Effects

A. Systemic Administration
1. Decreased vision
2. Eyelids or conjunctiva
    a. Allergic reactions
    b. Hyperemia
    c. Edema
    d. Urticaria
    e. Symblepharon
    f. Stevens-Johnson syndrome
    g. Exfoliative dermatitis
    h. Lyell's syndrome
3. Retinal hemorrhages
4. Paralysis of extraocular muscles
5. Diplopia
6. Problems with color vision — dyschromatopsia
7. Corneal vascularization — peripheral stroma
8. Corneal opacities
9. Keratitis

10. Blindness
11. Optic neuritis
12. Optic atrophy
13. Retinal detachment
14. Visual hallucinations
15. Subconjunctival or retinal hemorrhages secondary to drug-induced anemia

Clinical Significance: Ocular side effects due to these drugs are not uncommon and can be severe. At least 10 to 15 percent of patients taking these agents must discontinue their use due to toxic reactions. This is due in part to the high dosages necessary in some patients to control their disease. Unlike most drugs, these act so that the older the patient the more likely an untoward side effect. Side effects are so common in patients above the age of 60 that the manufacturers recommend treatment only at weekly intervals. The most common ocular side effect is decreased vision. It has been suggested that this is due to increased lens hydration. Eyelid or conjunctival change followed by retinal hemorrhages are the next most frequent adverse ocular reactions.

Interactions with Other Drugs

A. Effect of Pyrazolon Derivatives on Activity of Other Drugs
  1. Penicillins ↑
  2. Sulfonamides ↑
  3. Barbiturates ↓
  4. Corticosteroids ↓
B. Effect of Other Drugs on Activity of Pyrazolon Derivatives
  1. Antacids ↓
  2. Barbiturates ↓
  3. Salicylates ↓
  4. Tricyclic antidepressants ↓

References

Goodman, L. S., and Gilman, A. (Eds.): The Pharmacological Basis of Therapeutics. 4th Ed., New York, Macmillan, 1970, pp. 334–337.

Meyler, L., and Herxheimer, A. (Eds.): Side Effects of Drugs. Amsterdam, Excerpta Medica, Vol. VII, 1972, pp. 165–170.

Physicians' Desk Reference. 28th Ed., Oradell, N. J., Medical Economics Co., 1974, pp. 772, 1469, 1477.

Raymond, L. F.: Neovascularization of the cornea due to Butazolidin toxicity. Am. J. Ophthalmol. 43:287, 1957.

Tostevin, A. L.: Retinal haemorrhages associated with the administration of Butazolidin. Med. J. Aust. 1:69, 1961.

Walsh, F. B., and Hoyt, W. F.: Clinical Neuro-Ophthalmology. 3rd Ed., Baltimore, Williams & Wilkins, Vol. III, 1969, p. 2591.

* * * * * * * * * * * *

Class: Mild Analgesics

Generic Name: 1. Acetaminophen; 2. Acetanilid; 3. Phenacetin

Proprietary Name: 1. Anpamol (G.B.), Apamide, Calpol (G.B.), Capital, Ceetamol (Austral.), Cetadol (G.B.), Cetal (G.B.), Febrilix (G.B.), Febrolin, Nebs, Neopap, Nevrol (Austral.), Pamol (G.B.), Panacete (Austral.), Panadol (G.B.), Panok (G.B.), Paracetamol (G.B.), Parasin (Austral.), Parmol (Austral.), PCM (G.B.), Salzone (G.B.), SK-APAP, Tabalgin (G.B.), Temlo, Tempra, Tetmal (G.B.), Tylenol, Valadol; 2. Acetanilide (G.B.); 3. Phenacetin

Primary Use: These para-aminophenol derivatives are used in the control of fever and mild pain.

Ocular Side Effects

A. Systemic Administration
  1. Decreased vision
  2. Eyelids or conjunctiva
      a. Allergic reactions
      b. Conjunctivitis – nonspecific
      c. Angioneurotic edema
      d. Urticaria
      e. Erythema multiforme
      f. Stevens-Johnson syndrome
  3. Problems with color vision
      a. Dyschromatopsia
      b. Objects have yellow tinge
  4. Green discoloration of subconjunctival or retinal blood vessels
  5. Pupils
      a. Mydriasis
      b. Decreased reaction to light
  6. Subconjunctival or retinal hemorrhages secondary to drug-induced anemia
  7. Blindness

Clinical Significance: Ocular side effects due to these analgesics are quite rare; however, some adverse ocular reactions have occurred at quite low doses, implying a drug idiosyncrasy or a peculiar sensitivity. The most frequent toxic responses have been reported due to acetanilid, followed by phenacetin, and the fewest are due to acetaminophen. In chronic therapy, all of these drugs can produce sulfhemoglobinemia, which accounts for the greenish color change in the subconjunctival or retinal blood vessels.

Interactions with Other Drugs

A. Effect of Para-Aminophenol Derivatives on Activity of Other Drugs
    1. Penicillins ↑ (acetaminophen)
    2. Salicylates ↑ (acetaminophen)
    3. Sulfonamides ↑ (acetaminophen)
    4. Sympathomimetics ↑ (acetaminophen)
    5. Barbiturates ↓ (acetaminophen)
B. Effect of Other Drugs on Activity of Para-Aminophenol Derivatives
    1. Alcohol ↑ (acetaminophen)
    2. Chloramphenicol ↑ (acetanilid)
    3. Phenothiazines ↑ (acetaminophen)
    4. Barbiturates ↓ (acetaminophen, phenacetin)

References

AMA Drug Evaluations. 2nd Ed., Acton, Mass., Publishing Sciences Group, 1973, pp. 266–267.

American Hospital Formulary Service. Washington, D. C., American Society of Hospital Pharmacists, Vol. 1, 28:08, 1973.

Grant, W. M.: Toxicology of the Eye. 2nd Ed., Springfield, Charles C Thomas, 1974, pp. 76–77, 804.

Physicians' Desk Reference. 28th Ed., Oradell, N. J., Medical Economics Co., 1974, p. 1555.

Walsh, F. B., and Hoyt, W. F.: Clinical Neuro-Ophthalmology. 3rd Ed., Baltimore, Williams & Wilkins, Vol. III, 1969, pp. 2540–2541.

* * * * * * * * * * * * *

Generic Name: Antipyrine (Phenazone)

Proprietary Name: Phenazone (G.B.)

Primary Use: This pyrazolone derivative is used as a mild analgesic and antipyretic.

Ocular Side Effects

A. Systemic Administration
    1. Eyelids or conjunctiva
        a. Allergic reactions
        b. Conjunctivitis – nonspecific
        c. Edema
        d. Discoloration
        e. Urticaria
        f. Lyell's syndrome
    2. Decreased vision
    3. Keratitis
    4. Blindness
    5. Optic atrophy
    6. Subconjunctival or retinal hemorrhages secondary to drug-induced anemia

Clinical Significance: Adverse ocular reactions due to antipyrine are not uncommon, with allergic reactions being the most frequent. Fixed eruptions (those occurring at the same site on re-exposure) have also been reported. A transitory decrease in vision or even blindness may occur and last for a few minutes or a few days. Optic atrophy has been reported in two instances.

Interactions with Other Drugs

A. Effect of Antipyrine on Activity of Other Drugs
1. General anesthetics ↑
2. Penicillins ↑
3. Sulfonamides ↑
B. Effect of Other Drugs on Activity of Antipyrine
1. Alcohol ↑
2. General anesthetics ↑
3. Phenothiazines ↑
4. Barbiturates ↓
5. Sedatives and hypnotics ↓

References

Blacow, N. W. (Ed.): Martindale: The Extra Pharmacopoeia. 26th Ed., London, Pharmaceutical Press, 1972, pp. 249–250.

Goldstein, J. H.: Effects of drugs on cornea, conjunctiva, and lids. Int. Ophthalmol. Clin. *11*(2):13, 1971.

Hotz, F. C.: A case of antipyrin amaurosis induced by 130 grains taken in 48 hours. Arch. Ophthalmol. *35*:160, 1906.

Lucas, D. R., and Newhouse, J. P.: Action of metabolic poisons on the isolated retina. Br. J. Ophthalmol. *43*:147, 1959.

Walsh, F. B., and Hoyt, W. F.: Clinical Neuro-Ophthalmology. 3rd Ed., Baltimore, Williams & Wilkins, Vol. III, 1969, p. 2593.

* * * * * * * * * * * * *

Generic Name: 1. Aspirin (Acetylsalicylic Acid); 2. Sodium Salicylate

Proprietary Name: 1. A.S.A., Asagran (G.B.), Bayer Aspirin, Bi-prin (Austral.), Caprin (G.B.), Ecotrin, Measurin, Nu-seals Aspirin (G.B.); 2. Ancosal (Austral.), Ensalate (Austral.), Enterosalyl (Standard) (G.B.), Nu-seals Sodium Salicylate (G.B.), Rhumax (Austral.)

Primary Use: These salicylates are used as antipyretics, analgesics, and in the management of gout, acute rheumatic fever, rheumatoid arthritis, subacute thyroiditis, and renal calculi.

Ocular Side Effects

A. Systemic Administration
1. Eyelids or conjunctiva
a. Allergic reactions
b. Conjunctivitis — nonspecific

   c. Edema
   d. Angioneurotic edema
   e. Urticaria
  2. Decreased vision
  3. Problems with color vision
   a. Dyschromatopsia
   b. Objects have yellow tinge
   c. Achromatopsia, red-green defect
  4. Paralysis of extraocular muscles
  5. Diplopia
  6. Visual hallucinations
  7. Myopia
  8. Decreased intraocular pressure
  9. Nystagmus
 10. Pupils
   a. Mydriasis
   b. Decreased or absent reaction to light
 11. Visual fields
   a. Scotomas
   b. Constriction
   c. Hemianopsia
 12. Scintillating scotomas
 13. Papilledema
 14. Retinal edema
 15. Subconjunctival or retinal hemorrhages
 16. Blindness
 17. Keratoconjunctivitis
 18. Ocular teratogenic effects
   a. Anophthalmos
   b. Micro-ophthalmos
   c. Exophthalmos
 19. Optic atrophy
 20. Hyphema (traumatic) — increased rebleeds
 B. Inadvertent Ocular Exposure
  1. Conjunctival edema or scarring
  2. Keratitis with or without ulceration

Clinical Significance: While ocular side effects due to salicylates are quite rare, significant adverse effects may occur at therapeutic dosage levels. This is probably due to a drug idiosyncrasy or hypersensitivity. Adverse drug-induced ocular reactions are primarily due to acid-base imbalances, metabolic disturbances, toxic encephalopathy, hemorrhagic phenomena, or hypersensitivity reactions. Sodium salicylate appears to have more toxic ocular reactions than aspirin; however, aspirin has a much higher percentage of hypersensitivity reactions. Toxic responses are more frequent and more severe in infants and children. Neuro-ophthalmologic defects have been primarily seen with sodium salicylate and are much less frequent with aspirin. A transitory blindness which lasts hours, days, or even weeks may occur. Optic atrophy with permanent blindness has, however, also been reported. In a retrospective study of traumatic hyphemas, the incidence of rebleeding was significantly increased with aspirin administration. Topical ocular aspirin powder has been used for self-mutilation and has caused various degrees of conjunctival and corneal damage.

Interactions with Other Drugs

A. Effect of Salicylates on Activity of Other Drugs
1. Analgesics ↑
2. Penicillins ↑
3. Phenothiazines ↑
4. Phenylbutazone ↓
B. Effect of Other Drugs on Activity of Salicylates
1. Analgesics ↑
2. Pencillins ↑
3. Barbiturates ↓

References

Copenhaver, R. M.: A report of an unusual self-inflicted eye injury. Arch. Ophthalmol. 63:266, 1960.
Crawford, J. S., Lewandowski, R. L., and Chan, W.: The effect of aspirin on rebleeding in traumatic hyphema. Am. J. Ophthalmol. 80:543, 1975
Duke-Elder, S.: Systems of Ophthalmology. St. Louis, C. V. Mosby, Vol. XIV, Part 2, 1972, p. 1327.
Goldstein, J. H.: Effects of drugs on cornea, conjunctiva, and lids. Int. Ophthalmol. Clin. 11(2):13, 1971.
Goodman, L. S., and Gilman, A. (Eds.): The Pharmacological Basis of Therapeutics. 4th Ed., New York, Macmillan, 1970, pp. 314–329.
Grant, W. M.: Toxicology of the Eye. 2nd Ed., Springfield, Charles C Thomas, 1974, pp. 87, 890–892.
Meyler, L., and Herxheimer, A. (Eds.): Side Effects of Drugs. Amsterdam, Excerpta Medica, Vol. VII, 1972, pp. 140–152.

* * * * * * * * * * * * *

Generic Name: 1. Codeine; 2. Propoxyphene

Proprietary Name: 1. Codlin (Austral.); 2. Antalvic (Fr.), Darvon, Depromic (Germ.), Depronal SA (G.B.), Develin (Germ.), Dextropropoxyphene (G.B.), Dolene, Doloxene (G.B.), Erantin (Germ.), SK-65

Primary Use: These mild analgesics are used for the relief of mild to moderate pain. Codeine is also used as an antitussive agent.

Ocular Side Effects

A. Systemic Administration
1. Miosis
2. Decreased vision
3. Myopia (codeine)
4. Eyelids — exfoliative dermatitis

Clinical Significance: Neither codeine nor propoxyphene causes significant ocular side effects. While codeine frequently may produce miosis, propoxyphene does so only in overdose situations. Visual disturbances are usually insignificant. Codeine has been reported to cause transient myopia.

Interactions with Other Drugs

A. Effect of Codeine or Propoxyphene on Activity of Other Drugs
 1. Alcohol ↑
 2. Barbiturates ↑
 3. Monoamine oxidase inhibitors ↑
 4. Phenothiazines ↑
 5. Sedatives and hypnotics ↑
 6. Tricyclic antidepressants ↑
B. Effect of Other Drugs on Activity of Codeine or Propoxyphene
 1. Alcohol ↑
 2. Anticholinesterases ↑
 3. Chloramphenicol ↑ (codeine)
 4. Monoamine oxidase inhibitors ↑
 5. Phenothiazines ↑
 6. Tricyclic antidepressants ↑

References

AMA Drug Evaluations. 2nd Ed., Acton, Mass., Publishing Sciences Group, 1973, pp. 262–264.
Baron, A., et al.: Myopie spasmodique. Bull. Soc. Ophtalmol. Fr. 67:716, 1967.
Grant, W. M.: Toxicology of the Eye. 2nd Ed., Springfield, Charles C Thomas, 1974, p. 304.
Hermans, G.: Analgesiques majeurs. Bull. Soc. Belge Ophtalmol. 160:116, 1972.
Physicians' Desk Reference. 28th Ed., Oradell, N. J., Medical Economics Co., 1974, pp. 849, 897, 1376.

* * * * * * * * * * * * *

Generic Name: Mefenamic Acid

Proprietary Name: Coslan (Span.), Parkemed (Germ.), Ponstan (G.B.), Ponstel

Primary Use: This anthranilic acid derivative is used for the relief of mild to moderate pain.

Ocular Side Effects

A. Systemic Administration
 1. Decreased vision
 2. Problems with color vision — dyschromatopsia
 3. Nonspecific ocular irritation
 4. Subconjunctival or retinal hemorrhages secondary to drug-induced anemia

Clinical Significance: Ocular side effects due to mefenamic acid are rare, transitory, and seldom require discontinuation of the use of the drug.

Interactions with Other Drugs

A. Effect of Mefenamic Acid on Activity of Other Drugs
1. Corticosteroids ↑
2. Phenylbutazone ↑
3. Salicylates ↑

References

AMA Drug Evaluations. 2nd Ed., Acton, Mass., Publishing Sciences Group, 1973, pp. 267–268.
American Hospital Formulary Service. Washington, D. C., American Society of Hospital Pharmacists, Vol. 1, 28:08, 1967.
Physicians' Desk Reference. 28th Ed., Oradell, N. J., Medical Economics Co., 1974, p. 1120.

* * * * * * * * * * * * *

Class: Narcotic Antagonists

Generic Name: 1. Levallorphan; 2. Nalorphine; 3. Naloxone

Proprietary Name: 1. Lorfan; 2. Lethidrone (G.B.), Nalline; 3. Narcan

Primary Use: These narcotic antagonists are used primarily in the management of narcotic-induced respiratory depression.

Ocular Side Effects

A. Systemic Administration
1. Pupils
a. Mydriasis — if a prior narcotic has been given
b. Miosis
2. Decreased vision
3. Visual hallucinations
4. Pseudoptosis
5. Lacrimation — withdrawal states
B. Local Ophthalmic Use or Exposure — nalorphine
1. Miosis

Clinical Significance: Although ocular side effects due to these narcotic antagonists are common, they have little clinical significance other than as a screening test to discover narcotic users. These narcotic antagonists produce either a miosis or no effect on the pupils when administered to nonaddicts; however, in addicts, they cause mydriasis. Vivid visual hallucinations are seen both as an adverse ocular reaction and as a withdrawal symptom. Naloxone has only been reported to cause pupillary changes.

Interactions with Other Drugs

    A. Effect of Narcotic Antagonists on Activity of Other Drugs
        1. Alcohol ↑
        2. Barbiturates ↑
        3. Sedatives and hypnotics ↑
        4. Analgesics ↓

References

AMA Drug Evaluations. 2nd Ed., Acton, Mass., Publishing Sciences Group, 1973, pp. 278–279.

Goodman, L. S., and Gilman, A. (Eds.): The Pharmacological Basis of Therapeutics. 4th Ed., New York, Macmillan, 1970, pp. 264–269.

Grant, W. M.: Toxicology of the Eye. 2nd Ed., Springfield, Charles C Thomas, 1974, pp. 629, 732–733.

Jasinski, D. R., Martin, W. R., and Haertzen, C.: The human pharmacology and abuse potential of N-Allylnoroxymorphone. (Naloxone). J. Pharmacol. Exp. Ther. *157*:420, 1967.

Martin, W. R.: Opioid antagonists. Pharmacol. Rev. *19*:463, 1967.

* * * * * * * * * * * *

Class: Strong Analgesics

Generic Name: 1. Hydromorphone; 2. Oxymorphone

Proprietary Name: 1. Dilaudid; 2. Numorphan

Primary Use: These hydrogenated ketones of morphine are used for the relief of moderate to severe pain.

Ocular Side Effects

    A. Systemic Administration
        1. Decreased vision
        2. Decreased accommodation
        3. Pupils
            a. Miosis
            b. Pinpoint pupils — toxic states
            c. Mydriasis — hypoxic states
        4. Eyelids or conjunctiva
            a. Allergic reactions
            b. Urticaria

Clinical Significance: Adverse ocular effects due to these drugs, although not uncommon, are rarely significant. All ocular side effects are reversible and transitory. Difficulty in focusing is probably the most frequent complaint.

Interactions with Other Drugs

A. Effect of Morphine Derivatives on Activity of Other Drugs
   1. Alcohol ↑
   2. Monoamine oxidase inhibitors ↑
   3. Phenothiazines ↑
   4. Sedatives and hypnotics ↑
   5. Tricyclic antidepressants ↑
B. Effect of Other Drugs on Activity of Morphine Derivatives
   1. Monoamine oxidase inhibitors ↑
   2. Phenothiazines ↑
   3. Tricyclic antidepressants ↑

References

AMA Drug Evaluations. 2nd Ed., Acton, Mass., Publishing Sciences Group, 1973, p. 253.
Blacow, N. W. (Ed.): Martindale: The Extra Pharmacopoeia. 26th Ed., London, Pharmaceutical Press, 1972, pp. 1122–1123, 1129.
Goodman, L. S., and Gilman, A. (Eds.): The Pharmacological Basis of Therapeutics. 4th Ed., New York, Macmillan, 1970, pp. 237–255.
Physicians' Desk Reference. 28th Ed., Oradell, N. J., Medical Economics Co., 1974, p. 812.

* * * * * * * * * * * *

Generic Name: Meperidine (Pethidine)

Proprietary Name: Demerol, Dolantin, Dolantol, Dolosal (Fr.), Eudolal, Pethoid (Austral.), Suppolosal (Fr.)

Primary Use: This phenylpiperidine narcotic analgesic is used for the relief of pain, as a preoperative medication, and to supplement surgical anesthesia.

Ocular Side Effects

A. Systemic Administration
   1. Pupils
      a. Mydriasis
      b. Miosis
      c. Decreased reaction to light
   2. Decreased intraocular pressure
   3. Decreased vision
   4. Corneal deposits (?)
B. Inadvertent Ocular Exposure
   1. Blepharitis
   2. Conjunctivitis — nonspecific

Clinical Significance: None of the ocular side effects due to meperidine are of major importance, and all are transitory. Miosis is uncommon at therapeutic dosages and seldom significant. Mydriasis and decreased pupillary light reflexes are only seen in acute toxicity or in long-term addicts. Ocular side effects such as blepharitis or conjunctivitis have been seen secondary to meperidine dust.

Interactions with Other Drugs

A. Effect of Meperidine on Activity of Other Drugs
  1. Anticholinergics ↑
  2. Anticholinesterases ↓
B. Effect of Other Drugs on Activity of Meperidine
  1. Alcohol ↑
  2. Analgesics ↑
  3. Antacids ↑
  4. Anticholinesterases ↑
  5. General anesthetics ↑
  6. Monoamine oxidase inhibitors ↑
  7. Phenothiazines ↑
  8. Sedatives and hypnotics ↑
  9. Tricyclic antidepressants ↑
  10. Barbiturates ↓

References

Bron, A. J.: Vortex patterns of the corneal epithelium. Trans. Ophthalmol. Soc. U. K. *93*:455, 1973.

Grant, W. M.: Toxicology of the Eye. 2nd Ed., Springfield, Charles C Thomas, 1974, pp. 800–801.

Hovland, K. R.: Effects of drugs on aqueous humor dynamics. Int. Ophthalmol. Clin. *11*(2):99, 1971.

Lubeck, M. J.: Effects of drugs on ocular muscles. Int. Ophthalmol. Clin. *11*(2):35, 1971.

Minton, J.: Occupational Eye Diseases and Injuries. New York, Grune, 1949.

Walsh, F. B., and Hoyt, W. F.: Clinical Neuro-Ophthalmology. 3rd Ed., Baltimore, Williams & Wilkins, Vol. III, 1969, pp. 2664–2665.

* * * * * * * * * * * * *

Generic Name: 1. Morphine; 2. Opium

Proprietary Name: 1. Duromorph (G. B.); 2. Pantopon

Primary Use: These opioids are used for the relief of severe pain. Morphine is the alkaloid that gives opium its analgesic action.

Ocular Side Effects

A. Systemic Administration
  1. Pupils
    a. Miosis
    b. Pinpoint pupils — toxic states
    c. Mydriasis — withdrawal or extreme toxic states
    d. Irregularity — withdrawal states
  2. Decreased vision
  3. Decreased accommodation
  4. Decreased convergence
  5. Decreased intraocular pressure
  6. Myopia

    7. Lacrimation
      a. Increased — withdrawal states
      b. Decreased
    8. Accommodative spasm
    9. Diplopia
   10. Eyelids or conjunctiva
      a. Allergic reactions
      b. Conjunctivitis — nonspecific
      c. Urticaria
   11. Ptosis (opium)
   12. Keratoconjunctivitis
   13. Problems with color vision (?)
      a. Dyschromatopsia
      b. Achromatopsia, red-green defect
   14. Visual fields (?)
      a. Scotomas
      b. Constriction
      c. Hemianopsia
   15. Blindness (?)
B. Local Ophthalmic Use or Exposure — Morphine
    1. Miosis
    2. Increased intraocular pressure (?)

Clinical Significance: These narcotics seldom cause significant ocular side effects, and all proven drug-induced toxic effects are transitory. Miosis is the most frequent ocular side effect and is seen routinely even at usual dosage levels. Ocular side effects reported in long-term addicts (#13–15 in the preceding list) are probably due to vitamin deficiency rather than to the drug itself. Withdrawal of morphine or opium in the addict may cause excessive tearing, irregular pupils, decreased accommodation, and diplopia.

Interactions with Other Drugs

A. Effect of Opioids on Activity of Other Drugs
    1. Alcohol ↑
    2. Analgesics ↑
    3. Antihistamines ↑
    4. Barbiturates ↑
    5. General anesthetics ↑
    6. Phenothiazines ↑
    7. Sedatives and hypnotics ↑
    8. Tricyclic antidepressants ↑
B. Effect of Other Drugs on Activity of Opioids
    1. Anticholinesterases ↑ (morphine)
    2. Monoamine oxidase inhibitors ↑
    3. Phenothiazines ↑ (morphine)
    4. Tricyclic antidepressants ↑ (opium)
    5. Anticholinergics ↓ (morphine)

C. Synergistic Activity
1. Adrenergic blockers
2. Alcohol
3. Anticholinergics

References

Duke-Elder, S.: Systems of Ophthalmology. St. Louis, C. V. Mosby, Vol. XIV, Part 2, 1972, pp. 1317, 1340–1341.
Goldstein, J. H.: Effects of drugs on cornea, conjunctiva, and lids. Int. Ophthalmol. Clin. *11*(2):13, 1971.
Grant, W. M.: Toxicology of the Eye. 2nd Ed., Springfield, Charles C Thomas, 1974, pp. 720–722, 767–768.
Hovland, K. R.: Effects of drugs on aqueous humor dynamics. Int. Ophthalmol. Clin. *11*(2):99, 1971.
von Oettingen, W. F.: Poisoning. A Guide to Clinical Diagnosis and Treatment. 2nd Ed., Philadelphia, W. B. Saunders, 1958.
Walsh, F. B., and Hoyt, W. F.: Clinical Neuro-Ophthalmology. 3rd Ed., Baltimore, Williams & Wilkins, Vol. III, 1969, pp. 2707–2709.

* * * * * * * * * * * *

Generic Name: Pentazocine

Proprietary Name: Fortal (Fr.), Fortalgesic (Swed., Switz.), Fortral (G.B.), Sosegon (Span.), Talwin, Win

Primary Use: This benzomorphan narcotic analgesic is used for the relief of pain, as a preoperative medication, and to supplement surgical anesthesia.

Ocular Side Effects

A. Systemic Administration
1. Miosis
2. Decreased vision
3. Visual hallucinations
4. Nystagmus
5. Diplopia
6. Lacrimation — abrupt withdrawal states
7. Decreased accommodation

Clinical Significance: Ocular side effects due to pentazocine are usually insignificant and reversible. Miosis is the most frequent one and is seen routinely even at usual dosage levels. All other ocular side effects are rare.

Interactions with Other Drugs

A. Effect of Pentazocine on Activity of Other Drugs
1. Analgesics ↓

References

AMA Drug Evaluations. 2nd Ed., Acton, Mass., Publishing Sciences Group, 1973, pp. 258–259.

American Hospital Formulary Service. Washington, D.C., American Society of Hospital Pharmacists, Vol. 1, 28:08, 1969.

Grant, W. M.: Toxicology of the Eye. 2nd Ed., Springfield, Charles C Thomas, 1974, p. 797.

Martin, W. R.: Opioid antagonists. Pharmacol. Rev. 19:463, 1967.

Physicians' Desk Reference. 28th Ed., Oradell, N. J., Medical Economics Co., 1974, p. 1596.

* * * * * * * * * * * * *

IV. Agents Used in Anesthesia

Class: Adjuncts to Anesthesia

Generic Name: 1. Dimethyl Tubocurarine Iodide; 2. Tubocurarine

Proprietary Name: 1. Metubine Iodide; 2. Tubarine

Primary Use: These neuromuscular blocking agents are used as adjuncts to anesthesia, primarily as skeletal muscle relaxants.

Ocular Side Effects

A. Systemic Administration
1. Decreased convergence
2. Diplopia
3. Nystagmus
4. Paresis or paralysis of extraocular muscles
5. Ptosis
6. Decreased intraocular pressure — minimal

Clinical Significance: The extraocular muscles, especially the abductors, are selectively affected as the first signs of toxicity due to these curare agents. These drugs, unlike succinylcholine, do not cause a transitory elevation of intraocular pressure, so they are safe to use if the globe is perforated.

Interactions with Other Drugs

A. Effect of Other Drugs on Activity of Neuromuscular Blocking Agents
1. Antibiotics (apnea) ↑
(Bacitracin, Colistin, Kanamycin, Neomycin, Polymyxin B, Streptomycin)
2. Diuretics ↑
3. Local anesthetics ↑
4. Monoamine oxidase inhibitors ↑
5. Anticholinesterases ↑↓
6. Adrenergic blockers ↓
7. Sympathomimetics ↓
B. Synergistic Activity
1. General anesthetics

References

Duke-Elder, S.: Systems of Ophthalmology. St. Louis, C. V. Mosby, Vol. XIV, Part 2, 1972, p. 1339.

Grant, W. M.: Toxicology of the Eye. 2nd Ed., Springfield, Charles C Thomas, 1974, p. 332.

Kornblueth, W., et al.: Influence of general anesthesia on intraocular pressure in man. Arch. Ophthalmol. 61:84, 1959.

Walsh, F. B., and Hoyt, W. F.: Clinical Neuro-Ophthalmology. 3rd Ed., Baltimore, Williams & Wilkins, Vol. III, 1969, pp. 2656–2657.

* * * * * * * * * * * *

Generic Name: Hyaluronidase

Proprietary Name: Alidase, Hyalase (G.B.), Hyason (Austral.), Hyazyme, Permease (Aust.), Wydase

Primary Use: This enzyme is added to local anesthetic solutions to enhance the effect of infiltrative anesthesia. It has also been used in paraphimosis, lepromatous nerve reactions, and in the management of carpal tunnel syndrome.

Ocular Side Effects

A. Local Ophthalmic Use or Exposure — Subconjunctival or Retrobulbar Injection
    1. Eyelids or conjunctiva
        a. Allergic reactions
        b. Conjunctivitis — follicular
    2. Irritation
    3. Myopia
    4. Astigmatism
    5. Decreases the duration of local anesthetic
    6. Increases the frequency of local anesthetic reactions

Clinical Significance: Adverse ocular reactions due to periocular injection of hyaluronidase are either quite rare or masked by the postoperative surgical reactions. Subconjunctival injection of this drug causes myopia and astigmatism secondary to changes in the corneal curvature. This is a transitory phenomenon with recovery occurring within a few weeks. Irritative or allergic reactions are often stated to be due to impurities in the preparation since pure hyaluronidase is felt to be nontoxic. Hyaluronidase decreases the duration of action of local anesthetic drugs by allowing them to diffuse out of the tissue more rapidly. Side effects of the local anesthetic are probably more frequent when it is used with hyaluronidase, since their absorption rate is increased.

114 IV. Agents Used in Anesthesia

Interactions with Other Drugs
  A. Effect of Hyaluronidase on Activity of Other Drugs
      1. Parenteral medications ↑
      2. Salicylates ↓

References

arton, D.: Side reactions to drugs in anesthesia. Int. Ophthalmol. Clin. *11*(2):185, 1971.
Blacow, N. W. (Ed.): Martindale: The Extra Pharmacopoeia. 26th Ed., London, Pharmaceutical Press, 1972, pp. 681–683.
Havener, W. H.: Ocular Pharmacology. 2nd Ed., St. Louis, C. V. Mosby, 1970, pp. 57–67.
Stanworth, A.: The ocular effects of local corticosteroids and hyaluronidase. In Paterson, G., Miller, S. J. H., and Paterson, G. D. (Eds.): Drug Mechanisms in Glaucoma. Boston, Little, Brown and Co., 1966, pp. 231–248.
Treister, G., Romano, A., and Stein, R.: The effect of subconjunctivally injected hyaluronidase on corneal refraction. Arch. Ophthalmol. *81*:645, 1969.

* * * * * * * * * * * *

Generic Name: Scopolamine (Hyoscine)

Proprietary Name: *Systemic:* Buscopan (G.B.), Genoscopolamine (Fr.), Methscopolamine, Methylscopolamine (Scand.), Neo-Avagal (Austral.), Pamine, Sereen (G.B.), SKopyl (G.B.). *Ophthalmic:* Hyoscine Hydrobromide Mimims (G.B.), Isopto Hyoscine, Scopolamine 0.2% S.O.P.

Primary Use: *Systemic:* This quaternary ammonium derivative is used as a preanesthetic medication to decrease bronchial secretions, as a sedative and an antispasmodic, and in the prophylaxis of motion sickness. *Ophthalmic:* This topical parasympatholytic mydriatic and cycloplegic agent is used in refractions, accommodative spasm, and in the management of uveitis.

Ocular Side Effects
  A. Systemic Administration
      1. Mydriasis — may precipitate narrow-angle glaucoma
      2. Decrease or paralysis of accommodation
      3. Decreased vision
      4. Decreased lacrimation
      5. Visual hallucinations
  B. Local Ophthalmic Use or Exposure
      1. Decreased vision
      2. Mydriasis — may precipitate narrow-angle glaucoma
      3. Decrease or paralysis of accommodation
      4. Eyelids or conjunctiva
          a. Allergic reactions
          b. Conjunctivitis — follicular
      5. Irritation
          a. Hyperemia
          b. Photophobia
          c. Edema

6. Increased intraocular pressure
7. Decreased lacrimation
8. Visual hallucinations

Clinical Significance: Ocular side effects from systemic scopolamine administration are common, seldom serious, and reversible. Mydriasis and paralysis of accommodation are intended ocular effects resulting from topical application of scopolamine. This drug may elevate the intraocular pressure in open-angle glaucoma and can precipitate narrow-angle glaucoma. Allergic reactions are not uncommon after topical ocular application.

Interactions with Other Drugs

A. Effect of Scopolamine on Activity of Other Drugs
   1. Phenothiazines ↑
B. Effect of Other Drugs on Activity of Scopolamine
   1. Antihistamines ↑
   2. Monoamine oxidase inhibitors ↑
   3. Phenothiazines ↑
   4. Tricyclic antidepressants ↑
   5. Adrenergic blockers ↓
C. Synergistic Activity
   1. Analgesics

References

Freund, M., and Merin, S.: Toxic effects of scopolamine eye drops. Am. J. Ophthalmol. 70:637, 1970.

Grant, W. M.: Toxicology of the Eye. 2nd Ed., Springfield, Charles C Thomas, 1974, pp. 899–902.

Harris, L. S.: Cycloplegic-induced intraocular pressure elevations. Arch. Ophthalmol. 79:242, 1968.

Leopold, I. H., and Comroe, J. H., Jr.: Effect of intramuscular administration of morphine, atropine, scopolamine and neostigmine on the human eye. Arch. Ophthalmol. 40:285, 1948.

Physicians' Desk Reference for Ophthalmology. 3rd Ed., Oradell, N. J., Medical Economics Co., 1974/75, pp. 204, 213.

* * * * * * * * * * * *

Generic Name: Succinylcholine (Suxamethonium)

Proprietary Name: Anectine, Brevidil E or M (G.B.), Celocurin-Klorid (Swed.), Lysthenon (Aust.), Midarine, Pantolax (Germ.), Quelicin, Scoline, Sucostrin

Primary Use: This neuromuscular blocking agent is used as an adjunct to general anesthesia to obtain relaxation of skeletal muscles.

Ocular Side Effects

A. Systemic Administration
    1. Extraocular muscles
        a. Eyelid retraction
        b. Enophthalmos
        c. Globe rotates inferiorly
    2. Intraocular pressure
        a. Increased — initial
        b. Decreased
    3. Paralysis of extraocular muscles
    4. Ptosis
    5. Eyelids or conjunctiva — allergic reactions

Clinical Significance: All ocular side effects due to succinylcholine are transitory; however, some have major clinical importance. A transient contraction of extraocular muscles may cause intraocular pressure elevations within one minute after succinylcholine is given from 5 to 15 mm Hg for as long as 1 to 4 minutes. While this short-term elevation of intraocular pressure has little or no effect in a glaucomatous eye, it has the potential to cause expulsion of the intraocular contents in a surgically opened or perforated globe. A slight decrease in intraocular pressure occurs in normal or glaucomatous eyes after this initial increase. Extraocular muscle contraction induced by succinylcholine may cause lid retraction or an enophthalmosis, which may cause the surgeon to misjudge the amount of resection needed in ptosis procedures. Eyelid retraction may be due to a direct action on Müller's muscle. Both eyelid retraction and enophthalmos seldom last for over 5 minutes after drug administration.

Interactions with Other Drugs

A. Effect of Other Drugs on Activity of Succinylcholine
    1. Antibiotics ↑
        (Bacitracin, Colistin, Kanamycin, Neomycin, Polymyxin B, Strepto-mycin)
    2. Anticholinesterases ↑
    3. EDTA ↑
    4. General anesthetics ↑
    5. Local anesthetics ↑
    6. Phenothiazines ↑

References

Bjork, A., Halldin, M., and Wahlin, A.: Enophthalmus elicited by succinylcholine. Acta Anaesthesiol. Scand. 1:41, 1957.
Hovland, K. R.: Effects of drugs on aqueous humor dynamics. Int. Ophthalmol. Clin. 11(2):99, 1971.
Katz, R. L., Eakins, K. E., and Lord, C. O.: The effects of hexafluorenium in preventing the increase in intraocular pressure produced by succinylcholine. Anesthesiology 29:70, 1968.
Lubeck, M. J.: Effects of drugs on ocular muscles. Int. Ophthalmol. Clin. 11(2):35, 1971.
Macri, F. J., and Grimes, P. A.: The effects of succinylcholine on the extraocular striate muscles and on the intraocular pressure. Am. J. Ophthalmol. 44:221, 1957.

Taylor, T. H., Mulcahy, M., and Nightingale, D. A.: Suxamethonium chloride in intraocular surgery. Br. J. Anaesthesiol. *40*:113, 1968.

* * * * * * * * * * * * *

Class: General Anesthetics

Generic Name: Chloroform (Anesthetic Chloroform)

Proprietary Name: Chloroform

Primary Use: This potent inhalation anesthetic, analgesic, and muscle relaxant is used in obstetrical anesthesia. It is also used as a solvent.

Ocular Side Effects

A. Systemic Administration
1. Pupils — dependent on plane of anesthesia
   a. Mydriasis — reactive to light (initial)
   b. Miosis — reactive to light (deep level of anesthesia)
   c. Mydriasis — nonreactive to light (coma)
2. Strabismus — convergent or divergent
3. Nystagmus
4. Decreased intraocular pressure
5. Decreased vision
6. Blindness
7. Cortical blindness (?)
B. Inadvertent Ocular Exposure
1. Irritation
   a. Hyperemia
   b. Ocular pain
   c. Edema
   d. Burning sensation
2. Keratitis
3. Corneal opacities
4. Corneal ulceration

Clinical Significance: Ocular side effects due to chloroform are common, transitory, and seldom of clinical significance other than as an aid in judging the level of anesthesia. During early levels of anesthesia induction, the eyes are convergent; however, with deeper levels they become divergent. Nystagmus most often occurs during the recovery phase of anesthesia. Blindness has been reported secondary to central anoxic episodes.

Interactions with Other Drugs

A. Effect of Chloroform on Activity of Other Drugs
    1. Adrenergic blockers ↑
    2. Analgesics ↑
    3. Antihistamines ↑
    4. Local anesthetics ↑
    5. Phenothiazines ↑
    6. Sympathomimetics ↑
B. Effect of Other Drugs on Activity of Chloroform
    1. Adrenergic blockers ↑
    2. Antihistamines ↑
    3. Monoamine oxidase inhibitors ↑
    4. Phenothiazines ↑

References

Duke-Elder, S.: Systems of Ophthalmology. St. Louis, C. V. Mosby, Vol. XIV, Part 2, 1972, pp. 1040, 1164, 1337, 1340.
Goodman, L. S., and Gilman, A. (Eds.): The Pharmacological Basis of Therapeutics. 4th Ed., New York, Macmillan, 1970, pp. 83–84.
Grant, W. M.: Toxicology of the Eye. 2nd Ed., Springfield, Charles C Thomas, 1974, pp. 135–136, 267–268.
Hovland, K. R.: Effects of drugs on aqueous humor dynamics. Int. Ophthalmol. Clin. *11*(2):99, 1971.
Howie, T. O.: Eye signs of anaesthesia. Br. Med. J. *1*:540, 1944.

* * * * * * * * * * * * *

Generic Name: Ether (Anesthetic Ether)

Proprietary Name: Ether

Primary Use: This potent inhalation anesthetic, analgesic, and muscle relaxant is used during induction of general anesthesia.

Ocular Side Effects

A. Systemic Administration
    1. Pupils — dependent on plane of anesthesia
        a. Mydriasis — reactive to light (initial)
        b. Miosis — reactive to light (deep level of anesthesia)
        c. Mydriasis — nonreactive to light (coma)
    2. Extraocular muscles — dependent on plane of anesthesia
        a. Slow oscillations (initial)
        b. Eccentric placement of globes (initial)
        c. Concentric placement of globes (coma)
    3. Nonspecific ocular irritation
    4. Conjunctival vasodilatation
    5. Lacrimal secretion — dependent on plane of anesthesia
        a. Increased (initial)
        b. Decreased (coma)
        c. Abolished (coma)

6. Decreased intraocular pressure
7. Decreased vision
8. Blindness
9. Cortical blindness (?)
B. Inadvertent Ocular Exposure
1. Irritation
2. Punctate keratitis
3. Corneal opacities

Clinical Significance: Adverse ocular reactions due to ether are common, reversible, and seldom of clinical importance other than in the determination of the plane of anesthesia. Ether vapor is an irritant to all mucous membranes, including the conjunctiva. Regardless of this irritant effect, ether vapor has, in addition, a vasodilator property. Permanent corneal opacities have been reported due to direct contact of liquid ether with the cornea. Blindness after induction of general anesthesia is probably due to asphyxic cerebral cortical damage.

Interactions with Other Drugs
A. Effect of Ether on Activity of Other Drugs
1. Adrenergic blockers ↑
2. Analgesics ↑
3. Local anesthetics ↑
4. Phenothiazines ↑
5. Sympathomimetics ↑
B. Effect of Other Drugs on Activity of Ether
1. Adrenergic blockers ↑
2. Antihistamines ↑
3. Monoamine oxidase inhibitors ↑
4. Phenothiazines ↑
5. Anticholinergics ↓

References
Blacow, N. W. (Ed.): Martindale: The Extra Pharmacopoeia. 26th Ed., London, Pharmaceutical Press, 1972, pp. 831–833.
Goodman, L. S., and Gilman, A. (Eds.): The Pharmacological Basis of Therapeutics. 4th Ed., New York, Macmillan, 1970, pp. 79–82.
Grant, W. M.: Toxicology of the Eye. 2nd Ed., Springfield, Charles C Thomas, 1974, pp. 135–136, 464–465.
Kornblueth, W., et al.: Influence of general anesthesia on intraocular pressure in man. Arch. Ophthalmol. 61:84, 1959.
Walsh, F. B., and Hoyt, W. F.: Clinical Neuro-Ophthalmology. 3rd Ed., Baltimore, Williams & Wilkins, Vol. III, 1969, pp. 2675–2676.

* * * * * * * * * * * *

Generic Name: Ketamine

Proprietary Name: Ketaject, Ketalar

Primary Use: This intravenous nonbarbiturate anesthetic is used for short-term diagnostic or surgical procedures. It may also be used as an adjunct to anesthesia.

Ocular Side Effects

A. Systemic Administration
1. Decreased vision
2. Diplopia
3. Horizontal nystagmus
4. Blindness
5. Increased intraocular pressure — minimal
6. Postsurgical visually induced "emergence reactions"
7. Extraocular muscles
   a. Abnormal conjugate deviations
   b. Random ocular movements
8. Lacrimation
9. Visual hallucinations

Clinical Significance: All ocular side effects due to ketamine are transient and reversible. "Emergence reactions" occur in 12 percent of patients and may consist of various psychological manifestations varying from pleasant dream-like states to irrational behavior. The incidence of these reactions is increased by visual stimulation as the effect of the drug is wearing off. Three cases of transient blindness following ketamine anesthesia have recently been reported. The blindness lasts about half an hour with complete restoration of sight and no apparent sequelae. This is thought to be a toxic cerebral-induced phenomenon. Ketamine is also being used by lay people for its psychedelic effect, and abusers may develop visual hallucinations, coarse horizontal nystagmus, abnormal conjugate eye deviations, and diplopia.

Interactions with Other Drugs

A. Effect of Ketamine on Activity of Other Drugs
1. Adrenergic blockers ↑
B. Effect of Other Drugs on Activity of Ketamine
1. Monoamine oxidase inhibitors ↑
2. Phenothiazines ↑

References

Barton, D.: Side reactions of drugs in anesthesia. Int. Ophthalmol. Clin. 11(2):185, 1971.
Corssen, G., and Hoy, J. E.: A new parenteral anesthetic. CI–581: Its effect on intraocular pressure. J. Pediatr. Ophthalmol. 4:20, 1967.
Fine, J., Weissman, J., and Finestone, S. C.: Side effects after ketamine anesthesia: Transient blindness. Anesth. Analg. 53:72, 1974.
Harris, J. E., Letson, R. D., and Buckley, J. J.: The use of CI–581. A new parenteral anesthetic in ophthalmic practice. Trans. Am. Ophthalmol. Soc. 66:206, 1968.
Hovland, K. R.: Effects of drugs on aqueous humor dynamics. Int. Ophthalmol. Clin. 11(2):99, 1971.
Shaffer, L. L.: Ketamine. JAMA 229:763, 1974.

* * * * * * * * * * * *

Generic Name: Methoxyflurane

Proprietary Name: Penthrane

Primary Use: This methyl ether is used as an inhalation anesthetic with good analgesic and muscle relaxant properties.

Ocular Side Effects

A. Systemic Administration
1. Decreased intraocular pressure
2. "Flecked retinal syndrome"

Clinical Significance: Ocular side effects due to methoxyflurane are rare, but recently a unique adverse ocular reaction has been reported. If this drug is used for an extended period of time, especially in a patient with renal insufficiency, irreversible renal failure may occur. Oxalosis occurs for unknown reasons, with calcium oxalate crystal deposits throughout the body including the retinal pigmentary epithelium. The deposition of these crystals in the retina gives the clinical picture of an apparent "flecked retinal syndrome."

Interactions with Other Drugs

A. Effect of Methoxyflurane on Activity of Other Drugs
1. Adrenergic blockers ↑
2. Analgesics ↑
3. Local anesthetics ↑
4. Phenothiazines ↑
5. Sympathomimetics ↑
B. Effect of Other Drugs on Activity of Methoxyflurane
1. Adrenergic blockers ↑
2. Antihistamines ↑
3. Barbiturates ↑
4. Monoamine oxidase inhibitors ↑
5. Phenothiazines ↑
6. Tetracyclines ↑
7. Anticholinergics ↓

References

Blacow, N. W. (Ed.): Martindale: The Extra Pharmacopoeia. 26th Ed., London, Pharmaceutical Press, 1972, pp. 840–842.

Bullock, J. D., and Albert, D. M.: Flecked retina. Arch. Ophthalmol. 93:26, 1975.

Goodman, L. S., and Gilman, A. (Eds.): The Pharmacological Basis of Therapeutics. 4th Ed., New York, Macmillan, 1970, pp. 87–88.

Grant, W. M.: Toxicology of the Eye. 2nd Ed., Springfield, Charles C Thomas, 1974, pp. 678–679.

Schettini, A., Owre, E. S., and Fink, A. I.: Effect of methoxyflurane anaesthesia on intraocular pressure. Can. Anaesth. Soc. J. 15:172, 1968.

* * * * * * * * * * * * *

Generic Name: Nitrous Oxide

Proprietary Name: Entonox (G.B.)

Primary Use: This inhalation anesthetic and analgesic is used in dentistry, in the second stage of labor in pregnancy, and during induction of general anesthesia.

Ocular Side Effects

A.   Systemic Administration
1.   Pupils — dependent on plane of anesthesia
     a.   Mydriasis — reactive to light (initial)
     b.   Miosis — reactive to light (deep level of anesthesia)
     c.   Mydriasis — nonreactive to light (coma)
2.   Intraocular pressure
     a.   Increased
     b.   Decreased
3.   Decreased vision
4.   Blindness
5.   Cortical blindness (?)

Clinical Significance: Pupillary changes due to nitrous oxide are common; however, other than aiding in determination of the anesthetic plane, they are seldom of importance. While decreased vision or blindness after induction of general anesthesia is quite rare, this phenomenon is more frequent with nitrous oxide than with most other general anesthetics. Visual loss is probably secondary to asphyxic cerebral cortical damage.

Interactions with Other Drugs

A.   Effect of Nitrous Oxide on Activity of Other Drugs
1.   Adrenergic blockers ↑
2.   Sympathomimetics ↑
B.   Effect of Other Drugs on Activity of Nitrous Oxide
1.   Monoamine oxidase inhibitors ↑
2.   Phenothiazines ↑

References

Grant, W. M.: Toxicology of the Eye. 2nd Ed., Springfield, Charles C Thomas, 1974, pp. 135–136, 759–760.
Hovland, K. R.: Effects of drugs on aqueous humor dynamics. Int. Ophthalmol. Clin. *11*(2):99, 1971.
Kornblueth, W., et al.: Influence of general anesthesia on intraocular pressure in man. Arch. Ophthalmol. *61*:84, 1959.
Walsh, F. B., and Hoyt, W. F.: Clinical Neuro-Ophthalmology. 3rd Ed., Baltimore, Williams & Wilkins, Vol. III, 1969, p. 2676.

* * * * * * * * * * * *

Generic Name: Trichloroethylene

Proprietary Name: Trethylene, Trilene

Primary Use: This potent inhalation anesthetic is used primarily for short-term diagnostic or surgical procedures and in obstetrics. It may also be used as an adjunct to anesthesia.

Ocular Side Effects

A. Systemic Administration
1. Paresis or paralysis of extraocular muscles
2. Diplopia
3. Ptosis
4. Decreased vision
5. Visual fields
    a. Scotomas — central or paracentral
    b. Constriction
    c. Enlarged blind spot
6. Photophobia
7. Extraocular muscles
    a. Pain on ocular movements
    b. Limitation of ocular movements
8. Paralysis of accommodation
9. Pupils
    a. Decrease or absence of reaction to light
    b. Anisocoria
10. Problems with color vision — dyschromatopsia
11. Horizontal nystagmus
12. Decreased lacrimation
13. Retrobulbar or optic neuritis
14. Optic atrophy
15. Blindness
16. Decreased intraocular pressure
17. Peripapillary hemorrhages
18. Decreased corneal reflex
19. Retinal edema
20. Retinal vasoconstriction
21. Visual hallucinations
22. Corneal anesthesia
23. Corneal ulceration

B. Inadvertent Ocular Exposure
1. Irritation
    a. Lacrimation
    b. Hyperemia
    c. Edema
    d. Burning sensation
2. Punctate keratitis
3. Corneal opacities

Clinical Significance: Ocular side effects due to trichloroethylene are uncommon since the discovery that most of the adverse reactions were due to toxic decomposition products of the drug. With adjustments in anesthetic equipment and technique such as using this drug for only short procedures, adverse ocular reactions are seldom seen. The most severe toxic response occurs in the central nervous system, and the cranial nerves are the most susceptible. Trichloroethylene may cause toxic ocular side effects from industrial exposure.

Interactions with Other Drugs

A. Effect of Trichloroethylene on Activity of Other Drugs
   1. Adrenergic blockers ↑
B. Effect of Other Drugs on Activity of Trichloroethylene
   1. Monoamine oxidase inhibitors ↑
   2. Phenothiazines ↑

References

Duke-Elder, S.: Systems of Ophthalmology. St. Louis, C. V. Mosby, Vol. XIV, Part 2, 1972, pp. 1165, 1315, 1337, 1344.

Hovland, K. R.: Effects of drugs on aqueous humor dynamics. Int. Ophthalmol. Clin. 11(2):99, 1971.

Humphrey, J. H., and McClelland, M.: Cranial nerve palsies with herpes following general anesthesia. Br. Med. J. 1:315, 1944.

Maloof, C. C.: Burns of the skin produced by trichloroethylene vapors at room temperature. J. Ind. Hyg. 31:295, 1949.

Smith, G. F.: Trichloroethylene: A review. Br. J. Ind. Med. 23:249, 1966.

Vernon, R. J., and Ferguson, R. K.: Effects of trichloroethylene on visual motor performance. Arch. Environ. Health 18:894, 1969.

* * * * * * * * * * * *

Class: Local Anesthetics

Generic Name: 1. Bupivacaine; 2. Chloroprocaine; 3. Lidocaine; 4. Mepivacaine; 5. Prilocaine; 6. Procaine; 7. Propoxycaine

Proprietary Name: 1. Carbostesin (Germ.), Marcain (G.B.), Marcaine; 2. Nesacaine; 3. Anestacon, Broncaine (G.B.), Evlocaine (Austral.), Lidothesin (G.B.), Lignocaine (G.B.), Lignostab (G.B.), Ultracaine, Xylocaine, Xylocard (G.B.), Xylotox (G.B.); 4. Carbocaine; 5. Citanest, Xylonest (Germ.); 6. Adrocaine (Austral.), Novocain, Novutox (G.B.), P45 (Austral.); 7. Blockaine

Primary Use: These amides or esters of para-aminobenzoic acid are used in infiltrative, epidural block, and peripheral or sympathetic nerve block anesthesia or analgesia.

Ocular Side Effects

A. Systemic Administration
1. Decreased vision
2. Miosis
3. Paresis or paralysis of extraocular muscles
4. Diplopia
5. Blepharoclonus
6. Retrobulbar neuritis (?)
7. Papilledema (?)
8. Optic atrophy (?)
9. Blindness (?)
B. Local Ophthalmic Use or Exposure — Retrobulbar Injection (Lidocaine, Procaine)
1. Blindness
2. Paresis or paralysis of extraocular muscles
3. Optic atrophy (?)
4. Retinal vasoconstriction (?)

Clinical Significance: Ocular side effects due to these drugs are directly dependent on their method of administration. Significant ocular side effects due to intravenous or spinal injections have been reported; however, nearly all are transitory. Cranial nerve paralyses of various kinds including extraocular muscle paralysis have been reported. The sixth cranial nerve has been the one most frequently affected, although the third and fourth nerves have occasionally also been involved. The paralysis may develop almost immediately, although it usually occurs a number of days later. Recovery usually occurs within a few days; however, in some instances it may take from 1 to 2 years. Exceptional cases of permanent optic nerve damage have also been seen and are probably due to impurities or other chemicals inadvertently administered. Transient loss of vision is practically routine from retrobulbar injections of lidocaine or procaine. Adverse ocular reactions from retrobulbar injections of local anesthetics have been difficult to prove since direct trauma from the needle pressure from a subdural injection on the optic nerve or from pressure from a traumatic hematoma may cause optic nerve damage mimicking a drug-induced toxicity.

Interactions with Other Drugs

A. Effect of Local Anesthetics on Activity of Other Drugs
1. Sulfonamides ↓
B. Effect of Other Drugs on Activity of Local Anesthetics
1. Anticholinesterases ↑

References

American Hospital Formulary Service. Washington, D. C., American Society of Hospital Pharmacists, Vol. II, 72:00, 1974.
Faulkner, S. H.: Ocular paralysis following spinal anaesthesia. Trans. Ophthalmol. Soc. U. K. 64:234, 1944.
Grant, W. M.: Toxicology of the Eye. 2nd Ed., Springfield, Charles C Thomas, 1974, pp. 140–142.

Phillips, O. C., et al.: Neurologic complications following spinal anesthesia with lidocaine: A
prospective review of 10,440 cases. Anesthesiology *30*:284, 1969.
Physicians' Desk Reference. 28th Ed., Oradell, N. J., Medical Economics Co., 1974, pp. 565,
567, 1130, 1565, 1581, 1587.

* * * * * * * * * * * * *

Class: Therapeutic Gases

Generic Name: Carbon Dioxide

Proprietary Name: Carbon Dioxide

Primary Use: This odorless, colorless gas is used as a respiratory stimulant to increase cerebral blood flow and in the maintenance of acid-base balance.

Ocular Side Effects

A. Systemic Administration
1. Blindness
2. Decreased convergence
3. Paralysis of accommodation
4. Decreased dark adaptation
5. Photophobia
6. Visual fields
    a. Constriction
    b. Enlarged blind spot
7. Problems with color vision
    a. Dyschromatopsia
    b. Objects have yellow tinge
8. Retinal vascular engorgement
9. Pupils
    a. Mydriasis
    b. Absence of reaction to light
10. Visual hallucinations
11. Diplopia
12. Decreased vision
13. Abnormal conjugate deviations
14. Papilledema
15. Increased intraocular pressure
16. Ptosis
17. Decreased corneal reflex
18. Proptosis

Clinical Significance: Ocular side effects due to carbon dioxide are not uncommon. While most of them are reversible, some are permanent and have major clinical significance. Carbon dioxide may have a specific toxicity for the retinal ganglion cells which accounts for severe visual defects due to this agent. Nonreactive dilated pupils only occur in severe toxic states.

References

Duke-Elder, S.: Systems of Ophthalmology. St. Louis, C. V. Mosby, Vol. XIV, Part 2, 1972, pp. 1350–1351.

Freedman, A., and Sevel, D.: The cerebro-ocular effects of carbon dioxide poisoning. Arch. Ophthalmol. 76:59, 1966.

Sevel, D., and Freedman, A.: Cerebro-retinal degeneration due to carbon dioxide poisoning. Br. J. Ophthalmol. 51:475, 1967.

Sieker, H. O., and Hickam, J. B.: Carbon dioxide intoxication: The clinical syndrome, its etiology and management, with particular reference to the use of mechanical respirators. Medicine 35:389, 1956.

Walsh, F. B., and Hoyt, W. F.: Clinical Neuro-Ophthalmology. 3rd Ed., Baltimore, Williams & Wilkins, Vol. III, 1969, pp. 2601–2602.

* * * * * * * * * * * *

Generic Name: Oxygen

Proprietary Name: Oxygen

Primary Use: This colorless, odorless, tasteless gas is used in inhalation anesthesia and in hypoxia.

Ocular Side Effects

A. Systemic Administration
1. Retinal vasoconstriction
2. Decreased vision
3. Visual fields
a. Scotomas – paracentral
b. Constriction
4. Retrolental fibroplasia – in newborns or young infants
5. Retinal vasospasms
6. Mydriasis
7. Heightened color perception
8. Retinal detachment
9. Blindness

Clinical Significance: The toxic ocular effects due to oxygen are most prominent in premature infants but may be found in any age group under hyperbaric conditions. Ocular side effects secondary to oxygen therapy are otherwise uncommon. While the ocular changes due to retrolental fibroplasia are irreversible, nearly all other side effects are transient after use of oxygen is discontinued. A report of permanent bilateral blindness probably due to 80 percent oxygen during general anesthesia has been reported. It has been suggested that in some susceptible people severe retinal vasoconstriction or even direct retinal toxicity may occur from oxygen therapy.

References

Goodman, L. S., and Gilman, A. (Eds.): The Pharmacological Basis of Therapeutics. 4th Ed., New York, Macmillan, 1970, pp. 908–921.

Havener, W. H.: Ocular Pharmacology. 2nd Ed., St. Louis, C. V. Mosby, 1970, pp. 366–368.

Kinsey, V. E.: Retrolental fibroplasia. Arch. Ophthalmol. *56*:481, 1956.

Kobayashi, T., and Murakami, S.: Blindness of an adult caused by oxygen. JAMA *219*:741, 1972.

Nichols, C. W., Lambertsen, C. J., and Clark, J. M.: Transient unilateral loss of vision associated with oxygen at high pressure. Arch. Ophthalmol. *81*:548, 1969.

* * * * * * * * * * * *

V. Gastrointestinal Agents

Class: Antacids

Generic Name: 1. Acid Bismuth Sodium Tartrate; 2. Bismuth Carbonate (Bismuth Subcarbonate); 3. Bismuth Oxychloride; 4. Bismuth Salicylate (Bismuth Subsalicylate); 5. Bismuth Sodium Tartrate; 6. Bismuth Sodium Thioglycollate; 7. Bismuth Sodium Triglycollamate

Proprietary Name: 1. Acid Bismuth Solution (G.B.); 2. Lac Bismuth (G.B.); 3. Bismuth Oxychloride Injection (G.B.); 4. Tablettae Bismuthi (Scand.); 5. Bismuth Sodium Tartrate Injection (G.B., Ind.); 6. Thio-Bismol; 7. Bistrimate

Primary Use: Bismuth salts are primarily used as antacids and in the treatment of syphilis and yaws.

Ocular Side Effects

A. Systemic Administration
  1. Eyelids or conjunctiva
     a. Exfoliative dermatitis
     b. Blue discoloration (?)
  2. Subconjunctival hemorrhages
  3. Corneal deposits
  4. Decreased vision (?)

Clinical Significance: Adverse ocular reactions to bismuth preparations are quite rare and seldom of clinical significance. Bismuth-containing corneal deposits have been documented. Only one case of decreased vision has been reported after an overdose of bismuth.

Interactions with Other Drugs

A. Effect of Bismuth Salts on Activity of Other Drugs
  1. Tetracyclines ↓

References

AMA Drug Evaluations. 2nd Ed., Acton, Mass., Publishing Sciences Group, 1973, p. 794.
Cohen, E. L.: Conjunctival haemorrhage after bismuth injection. Lancet *1*:627, 1945.
Fischer, F. P.: Bismuthiase secondaire de la cornee. Ann. Oculist (Paris) *183*:615, 1950.
Grant, W. M.: Toxicology of the Eye. 2nd Ed., Springfield, Charles C Thomas, 1974, pp. 191–192.

Walsh, F. B., and Hoyt, W. F.: Clinical Neuro-Ophthalmology. 3rd Ed., Baltimore, Williams
& Wilkins, Vol. III, 1969, p. 2686.

* * * * * * * * * * * *

Class: Antiemetics

Generic Name: Cyclizine

Proprietary Name: Marezine, Valoid (G.B.)

Primary Use: This piperazine antihistaminic derivative is effective in the management of nausea and vomiting.

Ocular Side Effects

A. Systemic Administration
  1. Decreased vision
  2. Pupils
      a. Mydriasis — may precipitate narrow-angle glaucoma
      b. Decreased reaction to light
  3. Decreased tolerance to contact lenses
  4. Diplopia
  5. Visual hallucinations
  6. Ocular teratogenic effects (?)
      a. Congenital cataracts
      b. Tapetoretinal degeneration

Clinical Significance: Ocular side effects due to cyclizine are rare, reversible, and usually of little clinical significance. Pupillary changes and visual hallucinations primarily occur in overdose situations. A few reports of ocular teratogenic abnormalities have been reported with cyclizine therapy; however, these findings may be coincidental since this drug is used as an antiemetic during pregnancy.

References

Goodman, L. S., and Gilman, A. (Eds.): The Pharmacological Basis of Therapeutics. 4th Ed., New York, Macmillan, 1970, pp. 635–645.
Gott, P. H.: Cyclizine toxicity. Intentional drug abuse of a proprietary antihistamine. N. Engl. J. Med. 279:596, 1968.
Grant, W. M.: Toxicology of the Eye. 2nd Ed., Springfield, Charles C Thomas, 1974, pp. 341–342.
McBride, W.: Cyclizine and congenital abnormalities. Br. Med. J. 1:1157, 1963.
Physicians' Desk Reference. 28th Ed., Oradell, N. J., Medical Economics Co., 1974, p. 654.

* * * * * * * * * * * *

Class: Antispasmodics

Generic Name: 1. Adiphenine; 2. Anisotropine; 3. Atropine Methylnitrate (Atropine Methonitrate); 4. Dicyclomine; 5. Diphemanil; 6. Glycopyrrolate; 7. Hexocyclium; 8. Isopropamide; 9. Mepenzolate; 10. Methantheline; 11. Methixene; 12. Oxyphencyclimine; 13. Oxyphenonium; 14. Pipenzolate; 15. Piperidolate; 16. Poldine; 17. Propantheline; 18. Tridihexethyl

Proprietary Name: *Systemic:* 1. Trasentine; 2. Valpin; 3. Eumydrin, Metropine; 4. Bentyl, Dicycol (Austral.), Dyspas, Merbentyl (G.B.), Procyclomine (Austral.), Wyovin (G.B.); 5. Demotil (Swed.), Prantal; 6. Robinul; 7. Tral, Traline (Fr.); 8. Darbid, Priamide (Belg., Fr.), Tyrimide (G.B.); 9. Cantil; 10. Banthine; 11. Tremaril (Switz.), Tremonil (G.B.), Trest; 12. Daricon, Vio-Thene; 13. Antrenyl, Oxyphenon (Cz.), Spastrex (Austral.); 14. Piptal; 15. Dactil; 16. Nacton; 17. Aclobrom (G.B.), Pantheline (Austral.), Pro-Banthine; 18. Pathilon *Ophthalmic:* 3. Atropine Methylnitrate; 10. Methantheline; 13. Oxyphenonium; 17. Propantheline

Primary Use: *Systemic:* These anticholinergic agents are effective in the management of gastrointestinal tract spasticity and peptic ulcers. *Ophthalmic:* These topical anticholinergic mydriatic and cycloplegic agents are used in refractions and fundus examinations.

Ocular Side Effects

A. Systemic Administration
 1. Decreased vision
 2. Mydriasis — may precipitate narrow-angle glaucoma
 3. Paralysis of accommodation
 4. Photophobia
 5. Problems with color vision
 a. Dyschromatopsia (piperidolate)
 b. Colored flashing lights (propantheline)
 6. Flashing lights (piperidolate)
 7. Eyelids or conjunctiva
 a. Allergic reactions
 b. Exfoliative dermatitis
 8. Loss of eyelashes or eyebrows (?) (glycopyrrolate)
B. Local Ophthalmic Use or Exposure
 1. Mydriasis — may precipitate narrow-angle glaucoma
 2. Photophobia
 3. Paralysis of accommodation
 4. Eyelids or conjunctiva (oxyphenonium)
 a. Allergic reactions
 b. Conjunctivitis — nonspecific
 5. Increased intraocular pressure (oxyphenonium)

Clinical Significance: Ocular side effects due to these anticholinergic agents vary, depending on the drug; however, adverse ocular reactions are seldom significant and are reversible. None of the preceding drugs have little more than 10 to 15 percent of the anticholinergic activity of atropine. The most frequent ocular side effects are decreased vision, mydriasis, decreased accommodation, and photophobia. While these effects are not uncommon with some of these agents, rarely are they severe enough to cause a change in the medication. The weak anticholinergic effect of these agents seldom aggravates open-angle glaucoma; however, it has the potential to precipitate narrow-angle glaucoma attacks.

Interactions with Other Drugs

A. Effect of Anticholinergics on Activity of Other Drugs
  1. Barbiturates ↑ (adiphenine)
B. Effect of Other Drugs on Activity of Anticholinergics
  1. Antihistamines ↑
  2. Monoamine oxidase inhibitors ↑
  3. Phenothiazines ↑
  4. Tricyclic antidepressants ↑

References

AMA Drug Evaluations. 2nd Ed., Acton, Mass., Publishing Sciences Group, 1973, pp. 773–783.
Goodman, L. S., and Gilman, A. (Eds.): The Pharmacological Basis of Therapeutics. 4th Ed., New York, Macmillan, 1970, pp. 536–546.
Havener, W. H.: Ocular Pharmacology. 2nd Ed., St. Louis, C. V. Mosby, 1970, pp. 192, 201.
Leopold, I. H. (Ed.): Glaucoma Drug Therapy: Monograph I Parasympathetic Agents. Irvine, Calif., Allergan Pharmaceuticals, 1975, pp. 19–21.
Meyler, L., and Herxheimer, A. (Eds.): Side Effects of Drugs. Amsterdam, Excerpta Medica, Vol. VII, 1972, pp. 246–249.
Physicians' Desk Reference. 28th Ed., Oradell, N. J., Medical Economics Co., 1974, pp. 538, 604, 669, 702, 728, 756, 817, 825, 869, 1041, 1209, 1280, 1320, 1343, 1355.
Stecher, P. G. (Ed.): The Merck Index: An Encyclopedia of Chemicals and Drugs. 8th Ed., Rahway, N. J., Merck and Co., Inc., 1968.

* * * * * * * * * * * * *

Generic Name: 1. Atropine; 2. Belladonna; 3. Homatropine

Proprietary Name: *Systemic:* 1. Cystospaz, Levsin, Levsinex; 2. Belladonna Extract, Leaf, or Tincture; 3. Malcotran, Mesopin, Novatrin. *Ophthalmic:* 1. Atropisol, Atropt (Austral.), Atroptol (Austral.), BufOpto Atropine, Isopto Atropine, Opulets Atropine (G.B.), SMP Atropine (G.B.); 3. Homatrocel, Isopto Homatropine, SMP Homatropine (G.B.)

Primary Use: *Systemic:* These anticholinergic agents are used in the management of gastrointestinal tract spasticity and peptic ulcers, and to decrease secretions of the respiratory tract. Atropine is also used in the treatment of hyperactive carotid sinus reflex and Parkinson's disease. Homatropine is also used in the treatment of dysmenorrhea. *Ophthalmic:* These topical anticholinergic mydriatic and cycloplegic agents are used in refractions, semiocclusive therapy, accommodative spasms, and uveitis.

Ocular Side Effects

   A. Systemic Administration
- 1. Decreased vision
- 2. Mydriasis — may precipitate narrow-angle glaucoma
- 3. Decrease or paralysis of accommodation
- 4. Photophobia
- 5. Micropsia
- 6. Decreased lacrimation
- 7. Visual hallucinations
- 8. Problems with color vision
  - a. Dyschromatopsia
  - b. Objects have red tinge

   B. Local Ophthalmic Use or Exposure — Topical Application
- 1. Decreased vision
- 2. Decrease or paralysis of accommodation
- 3. Mydriasis — may precipitate narrow-angle glaucoma
- 4. Irritation
  - a. Hyperemia
  - b. Photophobia
  - c. Edema
- 5. Increased intraocular pressure
- 6. Eyelids or conjunctiva
  - a. Allergic reactions
  - b. Conjunctivitis — follicular
- 7. Micropsia
- 8. Decreased lacrimation

   C. Local Ophthalmic Use or Exposure — Subconjunctival Injection
- 1. Brawny scleritis

Clinical Significance: Atropine and homatropine have essentially the same ocular side effects whether they are administered systemically or by topical ocular application. Systemic administration causes fewer and less severe ocular side effects since significantly smaller amounts of the drugs reach the eye. Topical ocular atropine and homatropine may elevate the intraocular pressure in eyes with open-angle glaucoma, but not in normal eyes. Probably the most common side effect which requires the discontinuation of these agents is contact dermatitis. Conjunctival papillary hypertrophy usually suggests a hypersensitivity reaction, while a follicular response suggests a toxic or irritative reaction. These drugs are said to produce a greater pupillary response in patients with Down's syndrome.

Interactions with Other Drugs

   A. Effect of Anticholinergics on Activity of Other Drugs
- 1. Phenothiazines ↑
- 2. Analgesics ↑↓
- 3. Anticholinesterases ↓

   B. Effect of Other Drugs on Activity of Anticholinergics
- 1. Analgesics ↑

2. Antihistamines ↑
3. Monoamine oxidase inhibitors ↑
4. Phenothiazines ↑
5. Tricyclic antidepressants ↑

References

Garin, P.: Les medicaments en rapport avec le systeme digestif. Bull. Soc. Belge Ophtalmol. *160*:267, 1972.
Gleason, M. N., et al.: Clinical Toxicology of Commercial Products. 3rd Ed., Baltimore, Williams & Wilkins, 1969.
Goodman, L. S., and Gilman, A. (Eds.): The Pharmacological Basis of Therapeutics. 4th Ed., New York, Macmillan, 1970, pp. 524–548.
Havener, W. H.: Ocular Pharmacology. 2nd Ed., St. Louis, C. V. Mosby, 1970, pp. 188–195.
Lazenby, G. W., Reed, J. W., and Grant, W. M.: Short-term tests of anticholinergic medication in open-angle glaucoma. Arch. Ophthalmol. *80*:443, 1968.
Lazenby, G. W., Reed, J. W., and Grant, W. M.: Anticholinergic medication in open-angle glaucoma. Long-term tests. Arch. Ophthalmol. *84*:719, 1970.
Leopold, I. H., and Comroe, J. H., Jr.: Effect of intramuscular administration of morphine, atropine, scopolamine and neostigmine on the human eye. Arch. Ophthalmol. *40*:285, 1948.

* * * * * * * * * * * *

Class: Stimulants of the Gastrointestinal

and Urinary Tracts

Generic Name: Bethanechol

Proprietary Name: Mechothane (G.B.), Myotonachol, Myotonine (G.B.), Urecholine

Primary Use: This quaternary ammonium parasympathomimetic agent is effective in the management of postoperative abdominal distention and nonobstructive urinary retention.

Ocular Side Effects

A. Systemic Administration
    1. Nonspecific ocular irritation
        a. Lacrimation
        b. Hyperemia
        c. Burning sensation
    2. Decreased accommodation

Clinical Significance: Adverse ocular reactions due to bethanechol are unusual, but they may continue long after use of the drug is discontinued.

Interactions with Other Drugs
  A. Effect of Other Drugs on Activity of Bethanechol
     1. Anticholinergics ↓
     2. Sympathomimetics ↓

References

Blacow, N. W. (Ed.): Martindale: The Extra Pharmacopoeia. 26th Ed., London, Pharmaceutical Press, 1972, p. 1147.
Goodman, L. S., and Gilman, A. (Eds.): The Pharmacological Basis of Therapeutics. 4th Ed., New York, Macmillan, 1970, pp. 466–472.
Grant, W. M.: Toxicology of the Eye. 2nd Ed., Springfield, Charles C Thomas, 1974, p. 188.
Perritt, R. A.: Eye complications resulting from systemic medications. Ill. Med. J. *117*:423, 1960.

* * * * * * * * * * * *

Generic Name: Carbachol

Proprietary Name: *Systemic:* Carbacholine (Scand.), Carcholin. *Ophthalmic:* Carbacel, Isopto Carbachol, Miostat, P. V. Carbachol

Primary Use: *Systemic:* This quaternary ammonium parasympathomimetic agent is effective in the management of postoperative intestinal atony and urinary retention. *Ophthalmic:* This topical or intraocular agent is used in open-angle glaucoma.

Ocular Side Effects
  A. Systemic Administration
     1. Decreased accommodation
  B. Local Ophthalmic Use or Exposure — Topical Application
     1. Miosis
     2. Decreased vision
     3. Decreased intraocular pressure
     4. Accommodative spasm
     5. Eyelids or conjunctiva
        a. Allergic reactions
        b. Hyperemia
        c. Conjunctivitis — follicular
     6. Ocular pain
     7. Blepharoclonus
     8. Myopia
  C. Local Ophthalmic Use or Exposure — Intracameral Injection
     1. Miosis

Clinical Significance: Probably the most frequent ocular side effect due to carbachol is a decrease in vision secondary to miosis or accommodative spasms. In the younger age groups, transient drug-induced myopia may be quite bothersome. Follicular conjunctivitis is common after long-term therapy, but this in general has minimal clinical significance. If there are significant breaks in the conjunctiva or corneal epithelium, care must be taken not to apply topical ocular carbachol since major systemic side effects may occur.

Interactions with Other Drugs

A.   Effect of Other Drugs on Activity of Carbachol
   1.   Anticholinergics ↓
   2.   Sympathomimetics ↓

References

Beasley, H., et al.: Carbachol in cataract surgery. Arch. Ophthalmol. *80*:39, 1968.

Ellis, P. P., and Smith, D. L.: Handbook of Ocular Therapeutics and Pharmacology. 4th Ed., St. Louis, C. V. Mosby, 1973, pp. 45–46.

Goodman, L. S., and Gilman, A. (Eds.): The Pharmacological Basis of Therapeutics. 4th Ed., New York, Macmillan, 1970, pp. 466–472.

Grant, W. M.: Toxicology of the Eye. 2nd Ed., Springfield, Charles C Thomas, 1974, pp. 228, 706–718.

Physicians' Desk Reference for Ophthalmology. 3rd Ed., Oradell, N. J., Medical Economics Co., 1974/75, p. 239.

* * * * * * * * * * * *

VI. Cardiac, Vascular, and Renal Agents

Class: Agents Used to Treat Migraine

Generic Name: 1. Ergonovine (Ergometrine); 2. Ergotamine; 3. Methylergono-vine; 4. Methysergide

Proprietary Name: 1. Ergomine (Austral.), Ergotrate, Ermalate (Austral.); 2. Ergomar, Ergotart (Austral.), Etin (Austral.), Femergin (G.B.), Gynergen, Lingraine (G.B.); 3. Methergin (G.B.), Methergine, Methylergometrine (G.B.); 4. Deseril (G.B.), Desernil (Fr.), Sansert

Primary Use: These ergot alkaloids and derivatives are effective in the management of migraine or other vascular types of headaches and as oxytocic agents.

Ocular Side Effects

A. Systemic Administration
   1. Decreased vision
   2. Retinal vascular disorders
      a. Spasms
      b. Constriction
      c. Stasis
      d. Thrombosis
      e. Occlusion
   3. Miosis (ergotamine)
   4. Decreased intraocular pressure — minimal
   5. Visual fields
      a. Scotomas (methysergide)
      b. Hemianopsia (ergonovine)
   6. Decreased accommodation (methysergide)
   7. Problems with color vision
      a. Dyschromatopsia
      b. Objects have red tinge
   8. Eyelids or conjunctiva — edema
   9. Loss of eyelashes or eyebrows (?)

Clinical Significance: Ocular side effects due to these ergot alkaloids are rare; however, patients on standard therapeutic dosages may develop significant adverse ocular effects. This is probably due to an unusual susceptibility, sensitivity, or a preexisting disease which is exacerbated by the ergot

137

preparations. Increased ocular vascular complications have been seen in patients with a preexisting occlusive peripheral vascular disease. The course of patients with retinal vascular disease should be followed closely if ergot preparations are necessary for the management of their nonophthalmic disease. Even in a healthy 19-year-old, a standard therapeutic injection of ergotamine apparently precipitated a central retinal artery occlusion.

Interactions with Other Drugs

A. Effect of Ergot Alkaloids on Activity of Other Drugs
    1. Analgesics ↓ (methysergide)
B. Synergistic Activity
    1. Sympathomimetics

References

Christensen, L., and Swan, K. C.: Adrenergic blocking agents in the treatment of glaucoma. Trans. Am. Acad. Ophthalmol. Otolaryngol. 53:489, 1949.

Crews, S. J.: Toxic effects on the eye and visual apparatus resulting from the systemic absorption of recently introduced chemical agents. Trans. Ophthalmol. Soc. U. K. 82:387, 1962.

Goodman, L. S., and Gilman, A. (Eds.): The Pharmacological Basis of Therapeutics. 4th Ed., New York, Macmillan, 1970, pp. 897–907.

Grant, W. M.: Toxicology of the Eye. 2nd Ed., Springfield, Charles C Thomas, 1974, pp. 456–457, 705–706.

Peters, G. S., and Horton, B. T.: Headache: With special reference to the excessive use of ergotamine preparations and withdrawal effects. Proc. Staff Meet. Mayo Clin. 26:153, 1951.

* * * * * * * * * * * * *

Class: Antianginal Agents

Generic Name: Amiodarone

Proprietary Name: Cordarone (Belg., Fr.)

Primary Use: This benzofuran derivative is effective in the treatment of angina pectoris.

Ocular Side Effects

A. Systemic Administration
    1. Yellow-brown corneal deposits
    2. Decreased vision
    3. Problems with color vision — colored haloes around lights
    4. Corneal ulceration
    5. Photosensitivity
    6. Retinal changes (?)

Clinical Significance: Ocular side effects due to amiodarone are probably seen in nearly all patients on long-term usage. The only significant ocular side effect is a whorl-like corneal epithelial pattern indistinguishable from that due to chloroquine. These deposits are dose- and time-related; however, they appear to reach a steady state with no progression even with continued drug use. They are completely reversible, but may take as long as one year to clear. Visual changes are unusual and most often consist of complaints of hazy vision. Slate gray periocular skin pigmentation has been seen secondary to photosensitivity reactions. Although no retinal changes have been directly attributed to this drug, depigmentation of the macula has been suggested in one uncontrolled series.

References

Babel, J., and Stangos, N.: Lesions oculaires iatrogenes; l'action d'un nouveau medicament contre l'angor pectoris. Arch. Ophtalmol. (Paris) 30:197, 1970.
Darleguy, P., et al.: Le retentissement oculaire au cours du traitement par la cordarone. Bull. Soc. Ophtalmol. Fr. 71:82, 1971.
Moreau, P. G., and Pichon, P.: Lesions corneennes par amidarone. Bull. Soc. Ophtalmol. Fr. 70:538, 1970.
Thilges, V.: Le cordarone, cause de micro-depots de l'epithelium corneen semblables à ceux de l'intoxication chloroquinique. Ann. Oculist (Paris) 203:151, 1970.
Watillon, M., Lavergne, G., and Weekers, J. F.: Lesions corneennes au cours du traitement par le cordarone (chlorhydrate d'amiodarone). Bull. Soc. Belge Ophtalmol. 150:715, 1968.

* * * * * * * * * * * *

Generic Name: Amyl Nitrite

Proprietary Name: Vaporole

Primary Use: This short-acting nitrite antianginal agent is effective in the treatment of acute attacks of angina pectoris.

Ocular Side Effects

A. Inhalation Administration
   1. Mydriasis
   2. Decreased vision
   3. Problems with color vision
      a. Dyschromatopsia
      b. Objects have yellow tinge
      c. Colored haloes around objects — mainly blue or yellow
   4. Increased or decreased intraocular pressure
   5. Color hallucinations
   6. Eyelids or conjunctiva — allergic reactions
   7. Retinal vasodilatation

Clinical Significance: Ocular side effects due to amyl nitrite are transient and reversible. Adverse ocular reactions are not uncommon but seldom of clinical significance. There is no evidence that this drug has precipitated narrow-angle glaucoma.

Interactions with Other Drugs

A. Effect of Amyl Nitrite on Activity of Other Drugs
   1. Analgesics ↑
   2. Anticholinergics ↑
   3. Antihistamines ↑
   4. Sympathomimetics ↑
   5. Tricyclic antidepressants ↑
   6. Anticholinesterases ↓
B. Effect of Other Drugs on Activity of Amyl Nitrite
   1. Adrenergic blockers ↑
   2. Anticholinesterases ↓

References

Cristini, G., and Pagliarani, N.: Amyl nitrite test in primary glaucoma. Br. J. Ophthalmol. 37:741, 1953.
Cristini, G., and Pagliarani, N.: Slitlamp study of the aqueous veins in simple glaucoma during the amyl nitrite test. Br. J. Ophthalmol. 39:685, 1955.
Grant, W. M.: Physiological and pharmacological influences upon intraocular pressure. Pharmacol. Rev. 7:143, 1955.
Grant, W. M.: Toxicology of the Eye. 2nd Ed., Springfield, Charles C Thomas, 1974, pp. 134–135.

* * * * * * * * * * * *

Generic Name: 1. Erythrityl Tetranitrate; 2. Isosorbide Dinitrate; 3. Mannitol Hexanitrate; 4. Pentaerythritol Tetranitrate; 5. Trolnitrate

Proprietary Name: 1. Cardilate, Cardiloid, Dolorin (G.B.), Trituratio Erythryli Nitratis (Scand.); 2. Carvasin (Canad.), Cedocard (G.B.), Isoket (Germ.), Isordil, Risordan (Fr.), Sorbangil (Swed.), Sorbitrate, Vascardin (G.B.); 3. Maxitrate, Moloid (Germ.), Nitranitol; 4. Antora, Cardiacap (G.B.), Dilac 80, Duotrate, El-Petn, Equanitrate, Metranil, Mycardol (G.B.), Neo-Corovas, Nitrin, Nitropent (Swed.), Penritol (Austral.), Pentafin, Pentathryn (Austral.), Pentral (G.B.), Pentritol, Pentryate, Pentytrit (Denm.), Perispan, Peritrate, Petn, Quintrate, SK-Petn, Tetrasule, Tranite, Vasitol, Vaso-30/80, Vasodiatol; 5. Angitrit (Norw.), Duronitrin (Austral.), Metamine, Ortin (Switz.), Praenitron (Austral.)

Primary Use: These long-acting vasodilators are used in the treatment of chronic angina pectoris.

Ocular Side Effects

A. Systemic Administration
   1. Decreased vision
   2. Decreased intraocular pressure
   3. Eyelids or conjunctiva — exfoliative dermatitis
   4. Increased intraocular pressure (?)

Clinical Significance: Ocular side effects due to the nitrate vasodilators are uncommon, transitory, and reversible. The primary adverse ocular reaction is transitory blurred vision. Use of these vasodilators is probably not contra-indicated in glaucomatous patients; however, there have been a few reports to the contrary.

Interactions with Other Drugs

A. Effect of Nitrates on Activity of Other Drugs
    1. Analgesics ↑
    2. Anticholinergics ↑
    3. Antihistamines ↑
    4. Sympathomimetics ↑
    5. Tricyclic antidepressants ↑
    6. Anticholinesterases ↓
B. Effect of Other Drugs on Activity of Nitrates
    1. Adrenergic blockers ↑
    2. Anticholinesterases ↓

References

American Hospital Formulary Service. Washington, D. C., American Society of Hospital Pharmacists, Vol. 1, *24*:12, 1959–1963.
Grant, W. M.: Toxicology of the Eye. 2nd Ed., Springfield, Charles C Thomas, 1974, pp. 611–612, 795–796.
Havener, W. H.: Ocular Pharmacology. 2nd Ed., St. Louis, C. V. Mosby, 1970, p. 460.
Whitworth, C. G., and Grant, W. M.: Use of nitrate and nitrite vasodilators by glaucomatous patients. Arch. Ophthalmol. *71*:492, 1964.

* * * * * * * * * * * *

Generic Name: Nitroglycerin (Glyceryl Trinitrate)

Proprietary Name: Anginine (Austral.), Angised (G.B.), Cardabid, Nitora, Nitro-Bid, Nitrocine (G.B.), Nitroglyn, Nitrol, Nitrolan (G.B.), Nitrong, Nitro-SA, Nitrospan, Nitrostat, Nitro-TD, Sustac (G.B.), Trates, Triagin (Austral.), Vasitrin (Austral.)

Primary Use: This short-acting trinitrate vasodilator is effective in the treat-ment of acute attacks of angina pectoris.

Ocular Side Effects

A. Systemic Administration
    1. Decreased vision
    2. Increased or decreased intraocular pressure
    3. Blindness
    4. Retinal vasodilatation
    5. Problems with color vision — colored haloes around lights, mainly yellow or blue
    6. Subconjunctival or retinal hemorrhages secondary to drug-induced anemia

7. Eyelids — exfoliative dermatitis
8. Visual hallucinations (?)
9. Optic atrophy (?)

Clinical Significance: Ocular side effects due to nitroglycerin are uncommon, transient, and reversible. No evidence of significant ocular pressure elevation due to nitroglycerin usage exists in patients with open- or narrow-angle glaucoma. Theoretically, however, the drug does have the potential to precipitate narrow-angle glaucoma, and patients with narrow angles taking this drug should be closely followed. Transitory and reversible blindness due to ingestion of nitroglycerin have been seen, and in one instance, optic atrophy was reported.

Interactions with Other Drugs

A. Effect of Nitroglycerin on Activity of Other Drugs
    1. Analgesics ↑
    2. Anticholinergics ↑
    3. Antihistamines ↑
    4. Sympathomimetics ↑
    5. Tricyclic antidepressants ↑
    6. Anticholinesterases ↓
B. Effect of Other Drugs on Activity of Nitroglycerin
    1. Adrenergic blockers ↑
    2. Anticholinesterases ↓

References

Laws, C. E.: Nitroglycerine head. JAMA *54*:793, 1910.
Resnick, L.: Eye Hazards in Industry. Extent, Cause and Means of Prevention. New York, Columbia University Press, 1941, p. 266.
Stecher, P. G. (Ed.): The Merck Index: An Encyclopedia of Chemicals and Drugs. 8th Ed., Rahway, N. J., Merck and Co., Inc., 1968, pp. 75, 727–728.
Whitworth, C. G., and Grant, W. M.: Use of nitrate and nitrite vasodilators by glaucomatous patients. Arch. Ophthalmol. *71*:492, 1964.
Zahn, K. I.: The effect of nitroglycerine on the retinal circulation. Cesk. Oftalmol. *13*:146, 1957.

* * * * * * * * * * * *

Class: Antiarrhythmic Agents

Generic Name: Methacholine

Proprietary Name: Mecholyl

Primary Use: *Systemic:* This quaternary ammonium parasympathomimetic agent is primarily used in the management of paroxysmal tachycardia, Raynaud's syndrome, and scleroderma. *Ophthalmic:* This topical agent is used in the management of narrow-angle glaucoma and in the diagnosis of Adie's pupil.

Ocular Side Effects

A. Systemic Administration
   1. Decreased accommodation
B. Local Ophthalmic Use or Exposure
   1. Pupils
      a. No effect — normal pupil
      b. Miosis — Adie's pupil
   2. Decreased intraocular pressure
   3. Eyelids or conjunctiva
      a. Allergic reactions
      b. Hyperemia
   4. Myopia
   5. Bloody tears
   6. Blepharoclonus
   7. Lacrimation

Clinical Significance: Topical ocular application of methacholine causes a number of ocular side effects; however, all are reversible and of minimal clinical importance. While miosis normally occurs with topical ocular 10 percent methacholine solutions, no effect is seen with 2.5 percent solutions except in patients with Adie's pupil or familial dysautonomia.

Interactions with Other Drugs

A. Effect of Other Drugs on Activity of Methacholine
   1. Anticholinergics ↓
   2. Sympathomimetics ↓

References

Blacow, N. W. (Ed.): Martindale: The Extra Pharmacopoeia. 26th Ed., London, Pharmaceutical Press, 1972, pp. 1153–1154.

Ellis, P. P., and Smith, D. L.: Handbook of Ocular Therapeutics and Pharmacology. 4th Ed., St. Louis, C. V. Mosby, 1973, pp. 45–46.

Goodman, L. S., and Gilman, A. (Eds.): The Pharmacological Basis of Therapeutics. 4th Ed., New York, Macmillan, 1970, pp. 466–472.

Grant, W. M.: Toxicology of the Eye. 2nd Ed., Springfield, Charles C Thomas, 1974, pp. 706–718.

Havener, W. H.: Ocular Pharmacology. 2nd Ed., St. Louis, C. V. Mosby, 1970, pp. 204–205.

* * * * * * * * * * * *

Generic Name: Oxprenolol

Proprietary Name: Trasicor (G.B.)

Primary Use: This beta-adrenergic blocking agent is effective in the management of cardiac arrhythmias, angina pectoris, and hypertension.

Ocular Side Effects

A. Systemic Administration
1. Decreased vision
2. Eyelids or conjunctiva
a. Allergic reactions
b. Erythema
c. Conjunctivitis — nonspecific
3. Visual hallucinations
4. Decreased lacrimation (?)
5. Oculomucocutaneous syndrome (?)

Clinical Significance: This beta blocker only occasionally causes ocular side effects, and they are usually transitory and insignificant. There is a suspicion, but no conclusive data, that oxprenolol has the potential to cause an oculomucocutaneous syndrome similar to that seen with practolol. At present, one can only closely follow the course of patients on this drug for ocular changes, especially signs of irritation and keratoconjunctivitis sicca.

Interactions with Other Drugs

A. Effect of Oxprenolol on Activity of Other Drugs
1. Phenothiazines ↑
2. Sympathomimetics ↑
3. Tricyclic antidepressants ↑
4. Antihistamines ↓

References

Blacow, N. W. (Ed.): Martindale: The Extra Pharmacopoeia. 26th Ed., London, Pharmaceutical Press, 1972, pp. 1571–1573.

Holt, P. J. A., and Waddington, E.: Oculocutaneous reaction to oxprenolol. Br. Med. J. 2:539, 1975.

Hudson, W. A., and Finnis, W. A.: Oxprenolol and psoriasis-like eruptions. Lancet 1:932, 1975.

Wright, P., and Fraunfelder, F. T.: Practolol induced oculomucocutaneous syndrome. In Leopold, I. H., and Burns, R. P. (Eds.): Symposium on Ocular Therapy. New York, John Wiley & Sons, Inc., Vol. IX. To be published.

* * * * * * * * * * * *

Generic Name: Practolol

Proprietary Name: Eraldin (G.B.)

Primary Use: This beta-adrenergic blocking agent is effective in the management of angina pectoris, certain arrhythmias, and hypertension. It is also used as an adjunct to anesthesia and as a bronchodilator.

Ocular Side Effects

A. Systemic Administration
1. Keratoconjunctivitis
2. Foreign body sensation
3. Photophobia
4. Decreased lacrimation
5. Decreased vision
6. Conjunctiva
   a. Hyperemia
   b. Prominence of papillary tufts
   c. Areas of increased or decreased vascularity
   d. Scarring
   e. Keratinization
   f. Shrinkage — with obliteration of fornix
7. Cornea
   a. Dense yellow or white stromal opacities
   b. Loss of stroma
   c. Perforation
8. Eyelids
   a. Thickening
   b. Hyperemia
   c. "Cafe au lait" pigmentation
   d. Lupoid syndrome
B. Local Ophthalmic Use or Exposure
1. Decreased intraocular pressure

Clinical Significance: Ocular side effects due to practolol occur in approximately 0.2 percent of patients. The severity of the practolol-induced ocular changes is directly proportional to the length of time the patient has been taking the drug. If at the first signs of ocular involvement the drug is discontinued, all the ocular changes are reversible. However, if it remains unrecognized, this may lead to severe irreversible ocular changes including blindness. The most frequent adverse ocular reaction includes various degrees of keratoconjunctivitis sicca. This may progress to severe keratinization, scarring, and loss of conjunctival fornices. Sudden onset of corneal opacities with loss of stromal thickness leading to perforation has been seen. Adverse ocular reactions due to practolol may be unique since a serum intercellular antibody has been found in several patients. This antibody has also been found in the epithelium of eyes with practolol-induced disease. While it is too early to claim an immunologic cause and effect secondary to this drug, it is highly suggestive. While many of the signs and symptoms improve on withdrawal of the drug, reduction of tear secretion persists in most patients.

Interactions with Other Drugs

A. Effect of Practolol on Activity of Other Drugs
1. Alcohol ↑
2. Analgesics ↑
3. Barbiturates ↑

      4. General anesthetics ↑
      5. Phenothiazines ↑
      6. Sympathomimetics ↑↓
  B. Effect of Other Drugs on Activity of Practolol
      1. Alcohol ↑
      2. Analgesics ↑
      3. Barbiturates ↑
      4. General anesthetics ↑
      5. Phenothiazines ↑
      6. Anticholinergics ↓

References

Amos, H. E., Brigden, W. D., and McKerron, R. A.: Untoward effects associated with practolol: Demonstration of antibody binding to epithelial tissue. Br. Med. J. 1:598, 1975.

Blacow, N. W. (Ed.): Martindale. The Extra Pharmacopoeia. 26th Ed., London, Pharmaceutical Press, 1972, pp. 1573–1574.

Felix, R. H., Ive, F. A., and Dahl, M. G. C.: Cutaneous and ocular reactions to practolol. Br. Med. J. 4:321, 1974.

Raftery, E. B., and Denman, A. M.: Systemic lupus erythematosus syndrome induced by practolol. Br. Med. J. 2:452, 1973.

Wright, P., and Fraunfelder, F. T.: Practolol induced oculomucocutaneous syndrome. In Leopold, I. H., and Burns, R. P. (Eds.): Symposium on Ocular Therapy. New York, John Wiley & Sons, Inc., Vol. IX. To be published.

Wright, P.: Untoward effects associated with practolol administration: Oculomucocutaneous syndrome. Br. Med. J. 1:595, 1975.

* * * * * * * * * * * * *

Generic Name: Propranolol

Proprietary Name: Dociton (Germ.), Inderal

Primary Use: This beta-adrenergic blocking agent is effective in the management of angina pectoris, certain arrhythmias, hypertrophic subaortic stenosis, pheochromocytoma, and certain hypertensive states.

Ocular Side Effects

  A. Systemic Administration
      1. Diplopia
      2. Decreased vision
      3. Eyelids or conjunctiva
         a. Allergic reactions
         b. Erythema
         c. Conjunctivitis — nonspecific
         d. Purpura
         e. Stevens-Johnson syndrome
      4. Decreased intraocular pressure
      5. Visual hallucinations
      6. Decreased lacrimation (?)

B. Local Ophthalmic Use or Exposure
   1. Anesthetic
   2. Conjunctival hyperemia
   3. Irritation
   4. Decreased intraocular pressure
   5. Miosis
   6. Decreased lacrimation (?)

Clinical Significance: Adverse ocular side effects due to propranolol are usually insignificant and transient. As with all beta-adrenergic blocking agents, one needs to be aware of the possibility of sicca-like syndrome. Topical ocular use has little clinical application although it has been advocated for thyrotoxic lid retraction and glaucoma therapy.

Interactions with Other Drugs

A. Effect of Propranolol on Activity of Other Drugs
   1. Alcohol ↑
   2. Analgesics ↑
   3. Barbiturates ↑
   4. General anesthetics ↑
   5. Phenothiazines ↑
   6. Sympathomimetics ↑↓
B. Effect of Other Drugs on Activity of Propranolol
   1. Alcohol ↑
   2. Analgesics ↑
   3. Barbiturates ↑
   4. General anesthetics ↑
   5. Phenothiazines ↑
   6. Anticholinergics ↓

References

Cote, G., and Drance, S. M.: The effect of propranolol on human intraocular pressure. Can. J. Ophthalmol. 3:207, 1968.
Crombie, A. L., and Lawson, A. A. H.: Adrenergic blocking agents. Br. J. Ophthalmol. 52:616, 1968.
Davidson, S. I.: Report of ocular adverse reactions. Trans. Ophthalmol. Soc. U. K. 93:495, 1973.
Ginn, W. M., Jr., and Orgain, E. S.: Propranolol hydrochloride in the treatment of angina pectoris. JAMA 198:1214, 1966.
Phillips, C. I., Howitt, G., and Rowlands, D. J.: Propranolol as ocular hypotensive agent. Br. J. Ophthalmol. 51:222, 1967.
Sneddon, J. M., and Turner, P.: Adrenergic blockade and the eye signs of thyrotoxicosis. Lancet 2:525, 1966.

* * * * * * * * * * * *

Generic Name: Quinidine

Proprietary Name: Auriquin (G.B.), Cardioquin, Cin-Quin, Kinidin (G.B.), Quinaglute, Quinicardine (G.B.), Quinidex, Quinidoxin (Austral.), Quinora

Primary Use: This isomer of quinine is effective in the treatment and prevention of atrial, nodal, and ventricular arrhythmias.

Ocular Side Effects

A. Systemic Administration
   1. Decreased vision
   2. Problems with color vision — dyschromatopsia
   3. Mydriasis
   4. Visual fields
      a. Scotomas
      b. Constriction
   5. Photophobia
   6. Diplopia
   7. Night blindness
   8. Eyelids or conjunctiva
      a. Allergic reactions
      b. Angioneurotic edema
      c. Exfoliative dermatitis
   9. Subconjunctival or retinal hemorrhages secondary to drug-induced anemia
   10. Blindness (?)

Clinical Significance: Ocular side effects due to quinidine are rare, and nearly all are transitory and reversible with discontinued use of the drug. Adverse ocular reactions are primarily dose-dependent and are cumulative.

Interactions with Other Drugs

A. Effect of Quinidine on Activity of Other Drugs
   1. Adrenergic blockers ↑
   2. Antibiotics (apnea) ↑
   3. Anticholinergics ↑
   4. Phenothiazines ↑
   5. Anticholinesterases ↓
B. Effect of Other Drugs on Activity of Quinidine
   1. Antacids ↑
   2. Anticholinergics ↑
   3. Carbonic anhydrase inhibitors ↑
   4. Phenothiazines ↑

References

AMA Drug Evaluations. 2nd Ed., Acton, Mass., Publishing Sciences Group, 1973, pp. 14–15.
Is quinidine outdated?: Br. Med. J. *1*:331, 1969.
Monninger, R., and Platt, D.: Toxic amblyopia due to quinidine. Am. J. Ophthalmol. *43*:107, 1957.
Physicians' Desk Reference. 28th Ed., Oradell, N. J., Medical Economics Co., 1974, pp. 707, 826, 1205.
Taylor, D. R., and Potashnick, R.: Quinidine-induced exfoliative dermatitis. JAMA *145*:641, 1951.

* * * * * * * * * * * * *

Class: Antihypertensive Agents

Generic Name: 1. Alkavervir; 2. Cryptenamine; 3. Protoveratrines A and B; 4. Veratrum

Proprietary Name: 1. Veriloid (G.B.); 2. Unitensen; 3. Protalba-R, Puroverine (G.B.); 4. Danbar (G.B.), Vertavis

Primary Use: These veratrum alkaloids are used in the management of mild to moderate hypertension and various forms of renal dysfunction.

Ocular Side Effects

A. Systemic Administration
   1. Decreased vision
   2. Mydriasis — may precipitate narrow-angle glaucoma
   3. Extraocular myotonia

Clinical Significance: Few ocular side effects have been reported for these drugs. All adverse ocular effects are reversible and seldom of clinical significance.

Interactions with Other Drugs

A. Effect of Veratrum Alkaloids on Activity of Other Drugs
   1. Adrenergic blockers ↑
   2. General anesthetics ↑
   3. Monoamine oxidase inhibitors ↑
   4. Sympathomimetics ↑↓
   5. Tricyclic antidepressants ↓
B. Effect of Other Drugs on Activity of Veratrum Alkaloids
   1. Adrenergic blockers ↑
   2. Alcohol ↑
   3. Analgesics ↑
   4. General anesthetics ↑
   5. Monoamine oxidase inhibitors ↑
   6. Local anesthetics ↓
   7. Sympathomimetics ↓
   8. Tricyclic antidepressants ↓

References

AMA Drug Evaluations. 2nd Ed., Acton, Mass., Publishing Sciences Group, 1973, pp. 60–61.

Beasley, J., and Robinson, K.: Intolerance to "verloid." Br. Med. J. *1*:316, 1954.

Kolb, E. J., and Korein, J.: Neuromuscular toxicity of veratrum alkaloids. Neurology *11*:159, 1961.

Meyler, L., and Herxheimer, A. (Eds.): Side Effects of Drugs. Amsterdam, Excerpta Medica, Vol. VII, 1972, p. 304.

Walsh, F. B., and Hoyt, W. F.: Clinical Neuro-Ophthalmology. 3rd Ed., Baltimore, Williams & Wilkins, Vol. III, 1969, p. 2655.

* * * * * * * * * * * * *

Generic Name: 1. Alseroxylon;   2. Deserpidine;   3. Rauwolfia   Serpentina; 4. Rescinnamine; 5. Reserpine; 6. Syrosingopine

Proprietary Name: 1. Rautensin, Rauwiloid; 2. Harmonyl; 3. Hyperloid, Hypertane (G.B.), Hypertensan (G.B.), Raudixin, Rauval, Rauwoldin, Serenol (Austral.), Serfolia, Wolfina; 4. Anaprel 500 (G.B.), Moderil; 5. Lemiserp, Raurine, Rau-Sed, Reserdrex (Austral.), Reserpoid, Ryser (Austral.), Sandril, Serfin, Serpanray, Serpasil, Serpate, Serpiloid (Austral.), Sertina, Tenserp (Austral.), Vio-Serpine; 6. Singoserp

Primary Use: These rauwolfia alkaloids are used in the management of hypertension and agitated psychotic states.

Ocular Side Effects

- A. Systemic Administration
    1. Conjunctival hyperemia
    2. Horner's syndrome
        - a. Miosis
        - b. Ptosis
        - c. Increased sensitivity to topical ocular epinephrine preparations
    3. Nonspecific ocular irritation
        - a. Lacrimation
        - b. Hyperemia
    4. Extraocular muscles
        - a. Oculogyric crises
        - b. Decreased spontaneous movements
        - c. Abnormal conjugate deviations
        - d. Jerky pursuit movements
    5. Decreased vision
    6. Retinal hemorrhages
    7. Decreased intraocular pressure
    8. Mydriasis — may precipitate narrow-angle glaucoma
    9. Problems with color vision
        - a. Dyschromatopsia
        - b. Objects have yellow tinge
    10. Optic atrophy (?)
    11. Uveitis (?)

Clinical Significance: Most of the preceding ocular side effects have been primarily due to reserpine instead of the other rauwolfia alkaloids. However, the general toxicity of deserpidine and rescinnamine is said to be about the same as that of reserpine. The other drugs listed are probably less toxic. Ocular side effects are not uncommon, but nearly all are reversible.

Interactions with Other Drugs

A.   Effect of Rauwolfia Alkaloids on Activity of Other Drugs
1.   Alcohol ↑
2.   Barbiturates ↑
3.   General anesthetics ↑
4.   Monoamine oxidase inhibitors ↑
5.   Sympathomimetics ↑↓
6.   Analgesics ↓
7.   Anticholinergics ↓
8.   Salicylates ↓
B.   Effect of Other Drugs on Activity of Rauwolfia Alkaloids
1.   Adrenergic blockers ↑
2.   Alcohol ↑
3.   Antihistamines ↑
4.   General anesthetics ↑
5.   Phenothiazines ↑
6.   Monoamine oxidase inhibitors ↑↓
7.   Sympathomimetics ↓
8.   Tricyclic antidepressants ↓

References

Freedman, D. X., and Benton, A. J.: Persisting effects of reserpine in man. N. Engl. J. Med. *264*:529, 1961.
Kaplan, M. R., and Pilger, I. S.: The effect of rauwolfia serpentina derivatives on intraocular pressure. Am. J. Ophthalmol. *43*:550, 1957.
Kline, N. S., Barsa, J., and Gosline, E.: Management of side effects of reserpine and combined reserpine-chlorpromazine treatment. Dis. Nerv. Syst. *17*:352, 1956.
Raymond, L. F.: Ocular pathology in reserpine sensitivity: Report of two cases. J. Med. Soc. N. J. *60*:417, 1963.
Walsh, F. B., and Hoyt, W. F.: Clinical Neuro-Ophthalmology. 3rd Ed., Baltimore, Williams & Wilkins, Vol. I and Vol. III, 1969, pp. 447, 2638, 2668.

* * * * * * * * * * * *

Generic Name: 1. Chlorisondamine;   2. Mecamylamine;   3. Pentolinium; 4. Tetraethylammonium; 5. Trimethaphan (Trimetaphan); 6. Trimethidinium

Proprietary Name: 1. Ecolid; 2. Inversine, Mevasine, (Austral.); 3. Ansolysen; 4. Etamon; 5. Arfonad; 6. Trimethidinium

Primary Use: These ganglionic blocking agents are used in the management of moderate to severe hypertension and are used to produce controlled hypotension for the reduction of surgical hemorrhage.

Ocular Side Effects

A.   Systemic Administration
1.   Decreased vision
2.   Mydriasis
3.   Paralysis of accommodation

4. Conjunctival edema
5. Decreased intraocular pressure
6. Ptosis (tetraethylammonium)
7. Colored flashing lights (mecamylamine)
8. Decreased lacrimation (chlorisondamine)
9. Blindness (chlorisondamine)

Clinical Significance: Although ocular side effects due to the ganglionic blocking agents are common, they are transitory, reversible, and seldom of major significance. Since these drugs can cause profound hypotensive episodes, visual complaints probably occur on a cerebral basis. Mydriasis and cycloplegic effects are probably due to the parasympatholytic effect of these drugs. Side effects tend to become less pronounced as administration of the drug is continued.

Interaction with Other Drugs

A. Effect of Ganglionic Blocking Agents on Activity of Other Drugs
1. Carbonic anhydrase inhibitors ↑
2. Diuretics ↑
3. General anesthetics ↑
4. Monoamine oxidase inhibitors ↑
5. Sympathomimetics ↑↓
6. Anticholinesterases ↓
B. Effect of Other Drugs on Activity of Ganglionic Blocking Agents
1. Adrenergic blockers ↑
2. Alcohol ↑
3. Carbonic anhydrase inhibitors ↑
4. Diuretics ↑
5. General anesthetics ↑
6. Monoamine oxidase inhibitors ↑
7. Phenothiazines ↑
8. Sympathomimetics ↑↓
9. Anticholinesterases ↓
10. Tricyclic antidepressants ↓

References

Drucker, A. P., Sadove, M. S., and Unna, K.: Ocular manifestations of intravenous tetraethylammonium chloride in man. Am. J. Ophthalmol. *33*:1564, 1950.

Grant, W. M.: Toxicology of the Eye. 2nd Ed., Springfield, Charles C Thomas, 1974, pp. 260, 643, 985.

Stecher, P. G. (Ed.): The Merck Index: An Encyclopedia of Chemicals and Drugs. 8th Ed., Rahway, N. J., Merck and Co., Inc., 1968.

von Oettingen, W. F.: Poisoning: A Guide to Clinical Diagnosis and Treatment. 2nd Ed., Philadelphia, W. B. Saunders, 1958.

Walsh, F. B., and Hoyt, W. F.: Clinical Neuro-Ophthalmology. 3rd Ed., Baltimore, Williams & Wilkins, Vol. III, 1969, p. 2668.

* * * * * * * * * * * *

Generic Name: Diazoxide

Proprietary Name: Eudemine (G.B.), Hyperstat

Primary Use: This nondiuretic benzothiadiazine derivative is used in the emergency treatment of malignant hypertension.

Ocular Side Effects

A. Systemic Administration
  1. Lacrimation
  2. Eyelids or conjunctiva
    a. Allergic reactions
    b. Erythema
  3. Decreased vision
  4. Cataracts

Clinical Significance: Ocular side effects due to diazoxide are uncommon except for increased lacrimation, which occurs in up to 20 percent of patients taking this agent. In some instances, the lacrimation continued long after discontinued use of diazoxide. The cause of this unusual phenomenon is unknown. Acute reversible cataracts are extremely rare and are seen primarily in infants as a result of osmotic imbalance in hyperglycemia and hyperosmolar coma.

Interactions with Other Drugs

A. Effect of Diazoxide on Activity of Other Drugs
  1. Tricyclic antidepressants ↑
B. Effect of Other Drugs on Activity of Diazoxide
  1. Adrenergic blockers ↑
  2. Alcohol ↑
  3. Analgesics ↑
  4. Monoamine oxidase inhibitors ↑
  5. Tricyclic antidepressants ↑

References

AMA Drug Evaluations. 2nd Ed., Acton, Mass., Publishing Sciences Group, 1973, pp. 57–58.
Blacow, N. W. (Ed.): Martindale: The Extra Pharmacopoeia. 26th Ed., London, Pharmaceutical Press, 1972, pp. 736–737.
Grant, W. M.: Toxicology of the Eye. 2nd Ed., Springfield, Charles C Thomas, 1974, p. 360.
Physicians' Desk Reference. 28th Ed., Oradell, N. J., Medical Economics Co., 1974, p. 1304.
Thomson, A., et al.: Clinical observations on an antihypertensive chlorothiazide analogue devoid of diuretic activity. Can. Med. Assoc. J. 87:1306, 1962.

* * * * * * * * * * * * *

Generic Name: Furosemide. See under *Diuretics.*

* * * * * * * * * * * * *

Generic Name: Guanethidine

Proprietary Name: *Systemic:* Abapressine (Pol.), Ismelin. *Ophthalmic:* Ismelin (G.B.)

Primary Use: *Systemic:* This adrenergic blocker is effective in the treatment of moderate to severe hypertension. *Ophthalmic:* This topical adrenergic blocker is used in the management of open-angle glaucoma and lid retraction due to thyroid disorders.

Ocular Side Effects

- A.   Systemic Administration
    1.   Decreased vision
    2.   Nonspecific ocular irritation
        a.   Hyperemia
        b.   Photophobia
        c.   Edema
    3.   Horner's syndrome
        a.   Miosis
        b.   Ptosis
        c.   Enophthalmos (?)
    4.   Diplopia
    5.   Decreased intraocular pressure
    6.   Accommodative spasm
    7.   Flashing lights
    8.   Subconjunctival or retinal hemorrhages secondary to drug-induced anemia
    9.   Retinal vasospasms (?)
- B.   Local Ophthalmic Use or Exposure
    1.   Irritation
        a.   Hyperemia
        b.   Photophobia
        c.   Ocular pain
        d.   Edema
        e.   Burning sensation
    2.   Horner's syndrome
        a.   Miosis
        b.   Ptosis
        c.   Enophthalmos
    3.   Decreased intraocular pressure
    4.   Mydriasis
    5.   Punctate keratitis
    6.   Exacerbation of viral keratoconjunctivitis (?)

Clinical Significance: Topical ocular application or systemic administration of guanethidine frequently causes ocular side effects. These adverse ocular reactions are reversible and transitory with discontinued use of the drug.

Interactions with Other Drugs

  A. Effect of Guanethidine on Activity of Other Drugs
    1. General anesthetics ↑
    2. Monoamine oxidase inhibitors ↑
    3. Sympathomimetics ↑↓
    4. Anticholinergics ↓
  B. Effect of Other Drugs on Activity of Guanethidine
    1. Alcohol ↑
    2. General anesthetics ↑
    3. Phenothiazines ↑↓
    4. Antihistamines ↓
    5. Local anesthetics ↓
    6. Monoamine oxidase inhibitors ↓
    7. Sympathomimetics ↓
    8. Tricyclic antidepressants ↓

References

Bonomi, L., and Di Comite, P.: Outflow facility after guanethidine sulfate administration. Arch. Ophthalmol. 78:337, 1967.
Cant, J. S., and Lewis, D. R. H.: Unwanted pharmacological effects of local guanethidine in the treatment of dysthyroid upper lid retraction. Br. J. Ophthalmol. 53:239, 1969.
Crombie, A. L., and Lawson, A. A. H.: Long-term trial of local guanethidine in treatment of eye signs of thyroid dysfunction and idiopathic lid retraction. Br. Med. J. 4:592, 1967.
Davidson, S. I.: Reports of ocular adverse reactions. Trans. Ophthalmol. Soc. U. K. 93:495, 1973.
Gay, A. J., and Wolkstein, M. A.: Topical guanethidine therapy for endocrine lid retraction. Arch. Ophthalmol. 76:364, 1966.
Gloster, J.: Guanethidine and glaucoma. Trans. Ophthalmol. Soc. U. K. 94:573, 1974.
Stirpe, M., and Bucci, M.: Guanethidine and pupillary reaction. Surv. Ophthalmol. 9:227, 1964.

* * * * * * * * * * * * *

Generic Name: Hexamethonium

Proprietary Name: Vegolysen (G.B.)

Primary Use: This ganglionic blocking agent is used primarily in emergency hypertensive crises.

Ocular Side Effects

  A. Systemic Administration
    1. Decreased vision
    2. Mydriasis — may precipitate narrow-angle glaucoma
    3. Paralysis of accommodation
    4. Macular edema
    5. Decreased lacrimation
    6. Decreased intraocular pressure
    7. Visual fields
      a. Constriction

        b. Hemianopsia
    8. Conjunctival edema
    9. Retinal vasodilatation
  10. Optic atrophy
  11. Blindness
  12. Periorbital edema (?)

Clinical Significance: Hexamethonium frequently causes adverse ocular reactions, but the drug itself is rarely used except in severe end-stage hypertension or in a hypertensive crisis. While decreased vision, mydriasis, and paralysis of accommodation are common and reversible, most other ocular side effects are infrequent. Many of the drug-induced ocular side effects can be explained by a rapid change in the blood pressure.

Interactions with Other Drugs

  A. Effect of Hexamethonium on Activity of Other Drugs
    1. Carbonic anhydrase inhibitors ↑
    2. Sympathomimetics ↑
    3. Anticholinesterases ↓
  B. Effect of Other Drugs on Activity of Hexamethonium
    1. Alcohol ↑
    2. Monoamine oxidase inhibitors ↑

References

Barnett, A. J.: Ocular effects of methonium compounds, Br. J. Ophthalmol. 36:593, 1952.
Bruce, G. M.: Permanent bilateral blindness following use of hexamethonium chloride. Arch. Ophthalmol. 54:422, 1955.
Cameron, A. J., and Burn, R. A.: Hexamethonium and glaucoma. Br. J. Ophthalmol. 36:482, 1952.
Goldsmith, A. J., and Hewer, A. J.: Unilateral amaurosis with partial recovery after using hexamethonium iodide. Br. Med. J. 2:759, 1952.
Walsh, F. B., and Hoyt, W. F.: Clinical Neuro-Ophthalmology. 3rd Ed., Baltimore, Williams & Wilkins, Vol. III, 1969, pp. 2667–2668.

* * * * * * * * * * * *

Generic Name: Hydralazine

Proprietary Name: Apresoline, Dralzine, Hydrallazine (G.B.), Lopress

Primary Use: This phthalazine derivative is effective in the management of essential or malignant hypertension, hypertensive complications of pregnancy, and hypertension associated with acute glomerulonephritis.

Ocular Side Effects

  A. Systemic Administration
    1. Decreased vision
    2. Nonspecific ocular irritation
      a. Lacrimation
      b. Photophobia

3. Eyelids or conjunctiva
   a. Allergic reactions
   b. Erythema
   c. Conjunctivitis — nonspecific
   d. Edema
   e. Urticaria
   f. Lupoid syndrome
4. Periorbital edema
5. Colored flashing lights
6. Subconjunctival or retinal hemorrhages secondary to drug-induced anemia

Clinical Significance: All ocular side effects due to hydralazine are reversible, transient, and seldom of clinical significance.

Interactions with Other Drugs

A. Effect of Hydralazine on Activity of Other Drugs
   1. General anesthetics ↑
   2. Monoamine oxidase inhibitors ↑
   3. Sympathomimetics ↑↓
B. Effect of Other Drugs on Activity of Hydralazine
   1. Alcohol ↑
   2. Diuretics ↑
   3. General anesthetics ↑
   4. Monoamine oxidase inhibitors ↑↓
   5. Sympathomimetics ↓
   6. Tricyclic antidepressants ↓

References

Blacow, N. W. (Ed.): Martindale: The Extra Pharmacopoeia. 26th Ed., London, Pharmaceutical Press, 1972, pp. 797–798.
Grant, W. M.: Toxicology of the Eye. 2nd Ed., Springfield, Charles C Thomas, 1974, p. 553.
Grob, D., Langford, H. G., and Ziegler, B.: Further observations on the effects of autonomic blocking agents in patients with hypertension. 1. General systemic effects of Hexamethonine, Pentamethonium and Hydrazinophthalazine. Circulation 8:205, 1953.
von Oettingen, W. F.: Poisoning: A Guide to Clinical Diagnosis and Treatment. 2nd Ed., Philadelphia, W. B. Saunders, 1958.
Walsh, F. B., and Hoyt, W. F.: Clinical Neuro-Ophthalmology. 3rd Ed., Baltimore, Williams & Wilkins, Vol. III, 1969, p. 2668.

* * * * * * * * * * * *

Generic Name: Methyldopa

Proprietary Name: Aldomet

Primary Use: This adrenergic blocker is effective in the management of acute or severe hypertension.

Ocular Side Effects

A.   Systemic Administration
1.   Decreased vision
2.   Decreased intraocular pressure — minimal
3.   Eyelids or conjunctiva
a.   Allergic reactions
b.   Conjunctivitis — nonspecific
c.   Edema
4.   Subconjunctival or retinal hemorrhages secondary to drug-induced anemia
5.   Paralysis of extraocular muscles (?)

Clinical Significance: Adverse ocular side effects due to methyldopa are rare and insignificant. Lowering of intraocular pressure due to this drug has been documented; however, this decrease is only minimal. Only one case of Bell's palsy has been reported, and this may well have been coincidental.

Interactions with Other Drugs

A.   Effect of Methyldopa on Activity of Other Drugs
1.   General anesthetics ↑
2.   Monoamine oxidase inhibitors ↑
3.   Sympathomimetics ↑↓
4.   Tricyclic antidepressants ↓
B.   Effect of Other Drugs on Activity of Methyldopa
1.   Adrenergic blockers ↑
2.   Alcohol ↑
3.   General anesthetics ↑
4.   Phenothiazines ↑
5.   Monoamine oxidase inhibitors ↑↓
6.   Barbiturates ↓
7.   Sympathomimetics ↓
8.   Tricyclic antidepressants ↓

References

AMA Drug Evaluations. 2nd Ed., Acton, Mass., Publishing Sciences Group, 1973, pp. 54–55.

Davidson, S. I.: Reports of ocular adverse reactions: Trans. Ophthalmol. Soc. U. K. 93:495, 1973.

Kastrup, E. K., and Schwach, G. H. (Eds.): Facts and Comparisons. St. Louis, Facts and Comparisons, Inc., 1974, pp. 167h–168a.

Okun, R., et al.: Long-term effectiveness of methyldopa in hypertension. Calif. Med. 104:46, 1966.

Peczon, J. D.: Effect of methyldopa on intraocular pressure in human eyes. Am. J. Ophthalmol. 60:82, 1965.

Suda, K., et al.: On the hypotensive effect of Aldomet. J. Clin. Ophthalmol. 18:191, 1964.

* * * * * * * * * * * *

Generic Name: Pargyline

Proprietary Name: Eutonyl

Primary Use: This nonhydrazine monoamine oxidase inhibitor is used in the treatment of moderate to severe hypertension.

Ocular Side Effects

A. Systemic Administration
  1. Pupils
    a. Mydriasis
    b. Decreased reaction to light
  2. Decreased accommodation
  3. Visual hallucinations
  4. Hyperactive eye movements
  5. Problems with color vision
    a. Dyschromatopsia
    b. Achromatopsia, red-green defect
B. Local Ophthalmic Use or Exposure
  1. Decreased intraocular pressure

Clinical Significance: Significant ocular side effects due to pargyline are rare, and those reported are primarily in overdose situations. Optic nerve damage has not been found as a side effect of this drug, although it has been seen with other monoamine oxidase inhibitors. A well-documented study has reported a significant decrease in intraocular pressure in patients with chronic simple or absolute glaucoma following application of topical ocular pargyline.

Interactions with Other Drugs

A. Effect of Pargyline on Activity of Other Drugs
  1. Alcohol ↑
  2. Analgesics ↑
  3. Anticholinergics ↑
  4. Antihistamines ↑
  5. Barbiturates ↑
  6. Carbonic anhydrase inhibitors ↑
  7. General anesthetics ↑
  8. Monoamine oxidase inhibitors ↑
  9. Sedatives and hypnotics ↑
  10. Sympathomimetics ↑
  11. Tricyclic antidepressants ↑
  12. Local anesthetics ↑↓
  13. Phenothiazines ↑↓
  14. Adrenergic blockers ↓
B. Effect of Other Drugs on Activity of Pargyline
  1. Adrenergic blockers ↑
  2. Diuretics ↑
  3. General anesthetics ↑

4. Monoamine oxidase inhibitors ↑
5. Tricyclic antidepressants ↑
6. Analgesics ↑↓
7. Phenothiazines ↑↓
8. Alcohol ↓
9. Barbiturates ↓

References

Grant, W. M.: Toxicology of the Eye. 2nd Ed., Springfield, Charles C Thomas, 1974, pp. 788–789.

Lipkin, D., and Kushnick, T.: Pargyline hydrochloride poisoning in a child. JAMA *201*:135, 1967.

Mehra, K. S., Roy, P. N., and Singh, R.: Pargyline drops in glaucoma. Arch. Ophthalmol. *92*:453, 1974.

Sutnick, A. I., et al.: Psychotic reactions during therapy with pargyline. JAMA *188*:610, 1964.

Walsh, F. B., and Hoyt, W. F.: Clinical Neuro-Ophthalmology. 3rd Ed., Baltimore, Williams & Wilkins, Vol. III, 1969, p. 2628.

* * * * * * * * * * * * *

Class: Digitalis Glycosides

Generic Name: 1. Acetyldigitoxin; 2. Deslanoside; 3. Digitoxin; 4. Digoxin; 5. Gitalin; 6. Lanatoside C; 7. Ouabain

Proprietary Name: 1. Acylanid, Acylanide (Fr.), Lanacetyl (Pol.); 2. Cediland-D, Lanacard C (Pol.); 3. Crystodigin, Digimerck (Germ.), Digitaline, Digitox (Austral.), Digix (Austral.), Purodigin, Purpurid (Germ.); 4. Cardiox (Austral.), Cardoxin (Austral.), Coragoxine (Fr.), Davoxin, Dialoxin (Austral.), Digolan (Austral.), Fibroxin (Austral.), Lanicor (Germ.), Lanoxin, Prodigox (Austral.), Saroxin; 5. Cordigitum (U.S.S.R.), Gitalen (U.S.S.R.), Gitaligin; 6. Cedilanid, Lanocide (Austral.); 7. Cardibaine (Fr.), Ouabaine (G.B.), Purostrophan (Germ.), Strophoperm (Germ.)

Primary Use: Digitalis glycosides are effective in the control of congestive heart failure and certain arrhythmias.

Ocular Side Effects

A. Systemic Administration
    1. Problems with color vision
        a. Dyschromatopsia
        b. Objects have yellow, green, blue, or red tinge
        c. Achromatopsia, blue-yellow defect
        d. Colored haloes around lights — mainly blue

2. Visual sensations
   a. Flickering vision — often yellow or green
   b. Colored borders to objects
   c. Glare phenomenon — objects appear covered with brown, orange, or white snow
   d. Light flashes
   e. Scintillating scotomas
   f. Frosted appearance of objects
3. Scotomas — central or paracentral
4. Decreased vision
5. Diplopia
6. Decreased intraocular pressure
7. Retrobulbar neuritis
8. Eyelids or conjunctiva
   a. Allergic reactions
   b. Angioneurotic edema
9. Mydriasis (digoxin)
10. Visual hallucinations (digoxin)
11. Paresis of extraocular muscles (digitoxin)
12. Photophobia (digitoxin)

Clinical Significance: Nearly all of the ocular side effects due to the digitalis glycosides are reversible. They are most frequently seen with the long-acting agents such as digoxin or digitoxin, and least often with short-acting agents such as ouabain. The most unique adverse ocular reaction to this group of drugs is the glare phenomenon or the snowy appearance of objects. While common to all the drugs in this group, it is severest and most frequent with acetyldigitoxin. Intraocular pressure is decreased by deslanoside, digitoxin, digoxin, gitalin, and lanatoside C. Clinical use of these drugs for the treatment of glaucoma is not practical since the required therapeutic systemic dose is very near toxic levels. Topical ocular application of these agents causes keratopathy.

Interactions with Other Drugs

A. Effect of Digitalis Glycosides on Activity of Other Drugs
   1. Adrenergic blockers ↑
   2. Sympathomimetics ↑
B. Effect of Other Drugs on Activity of Digitalis Glycosides
   1. Adrenergic blockers ↑
   2. Sympathomimetics ↑
   3. Antacids ↓
   4. Barbiturates ↓
   5. Phenylbutazone ↓

References

AMA Drug Evaluations. 2nd Ed., Acton, Mass., Publishing Sciences Group, 1973, pp. 1–8.
Grant, W. M.: Toxicology of the Eye. 2nd Ed., Springfield, Charles C Thomas, 1974, p. 244.
Lely, A. H., and Van Enter, C. H. J.: Large scale digitoxin intoxication. Br. Med. J. 3:737, 1970.

Physicians' Desk Reference. 28th Ed., Oradell, N. J., Medical Economics Co., 1974, pp. 895, 1398.
Robertson, D. M., Hollenhorst, R. W., and Callahan, J. A.: Ocular manifestations of digitalis toxicity. Arch. Ophthalmol. 76:640, 1966.

* * * * * * * * * * * * *

Generic Name: Digitalis

Proprietary Name: Digifortis, Pil-Digis

Primary Use: The active constituents of digitalis are the glycosides which are effective in the control of congestive heart failure and certain arrhythmias.

Ocular Side Effects

A. Systemic Administration
   1. Problems with color vision
      a. Dyschromatopsia
      b. Objects have yellow, green, blue, or red tinge
      c. Achromatopsia, blue-yellow defect
      d. Colored haloes around lights — mainly blue
   2. Visual sensations
      a. Flickering vision — often yellow or green
      b. Colored borders to objects
      c. Glare phenomenon — objects appear covered with brown, orange, or white snow
      d. Light flashes
      e. Scintillating scotomas
      f. Frosted appearance of objects
   3. Decreased vision
   4. Visual fields
      a. Scotomas — central or paracentral
      b. Constriction
   5. Mydriasis
   6. Visual hallucinations — especially bright floating spots
   7. Diplopia
   8. Ptosis
   9. Paresis of extraocular muscles
   10. Accommodative spasm
   11. Eyelids or conjunctiva
      a. Allergic reactions
      b. Angioneurotic edema
   12. Blindness
   13. Retrobulbar or optic neuritis
   14. Myopia (?)
   15. Miosis (?)
   16. Nystagmus (?)
   17. Optic atrophy (?)
   18. Exophthalmos (?)

Clinical Significance: Ocular side effects are common with digitalis and are probably seen more frequently with it than with all the other digitalis glycosides combined. Most of the ocular side effects are transitory and reversible. The glare phenomenon and disturbances with color vision are the most striking and the most common adverse ocular reactions seen. Most patients on digitalis therapy are also taking numerous other drugs, and it may be difficult to decide which side effect is due to which medication. A recent report suggests that after long-term digitalis therapy, a reversible red-green color defect occurs in the majority of patients.

Interactions with Other Drugs

A. Effect of Digitalis on Activity of Other Drugs
    1. Adrenergic blockers ↑
    2. Sympathomimetics ↑
B. Effect of Other Drugs on Activity of Digitalis
    1. Adrenergic blockers ↑
    2. Sympathomimetics ↑
    3. Antacids ↓
    4. Barbiturates ↓
    5. Phenylbutazone ↓

References

AMA Drug Evaluations. 2nd Ed., Acton, Mass., Publishing Sciences Group, 1973, pp. 1–8.
American Hospital Formulary Service. Washington, D. C., American Society of Hospital Pharmacists, Vol. 1, 24:04, 1968.
Goodman, L. S., and Gilman, A. (Eds.): The Pharmacologic Basis of Therapeutics. 4th Ed., New York, Macmillan, 1970, pp. 677–708.
Manninen, V.: Impaired colour vision in diagnosis of digitalis intoxication. Br. Med. J. 4:653, 1974.
Peczon, J. D.: Clinical evaluation of digitalization in glaucoma. Arch. Ophthalmol. 71:500, 1964.
White, P. D.: An important toxic effect of digitalis overdosage on the vision. N. Engl. J. Med. 272:904, 1965.

* * * * * * * * * * * *

Class: Diuretics

Generic Name: 1. Bendroflumethiazide; 2. Benzthiazide; 3. Chlorothiazide (Chlorthiazide); 4. Chlorthalidone; 5. Cyclothiazide; 6. Hydrochlorothiazide; 7. Hydroflumethiazide; 8. Methyclothiazide; 9. Polythiazide; 10. Trichlormethiazide

Proprietary Name: 1. Aprinox (G.B.), Aprinox-M (Austral.), Bendrofluazide (G.B.), Benuron, Berkozide (G.B.), Bristuric (Austral.), Centyl (G.B.), Naturetin, Naturine (Fr.), Pluryl (Austral.); 2. Aquatag, Diucen, Exna, Lemazide,

Proaqua; 3. Diuril, Flumen (Ital.), Minzil (Ital.), Salisan (Denm.), Saluren (Ital.), Saluric (G.B.), Yadalan (Span.); 4. Hygroton, Igroton (Ital.); 5. Anhydron, Doburil (Austral.); 6. Aquarius (Canad.), Direma (G.B.), Esidrex (G.B.), Esidrix, Hydrid (Canad.), Hydro-Aquil (Canad.), Hydro-Diuril, Hydro-Saluric (G.B.), Hydrozide (Canad.), Neo-Codema (Canad.), Neo-Flumen (Austral.), Oretic; 7. Bristab (Austral.), Di-Ademil (Austral.), Hydrenox (G.B.), Leodrine (Fr.), NaClex (G.B.), Rontyl (Denm.), Saluron; 8. Aquatensen, Duretic (Canad.), Enduron; 9. Nephril (G.B.), Renese; 10. Metahydrin, Naqua

Primary Use: These benzothiadiazide diuretics are effective in the maintenance therapy of edema associated with chronic congestive heart failure, essential hypertension, renal dysfunction, cirrhosis, pregnancy, premenstrual tension, and hormonal imbalance.

Ocular Side Effects
    A. Systemic Administration
        1. Decreased vision
        2. Myopia
        3. Problems with color vision
            a. Objects have yellow tinge
            b. Large yellow spots on white background
        4. Retinal edema
        5. Eyelids or conjunctiva
            a. Allergic reactions
            b. Photosensitivity
            c. Purpura
            d. Erythema multiforme
            e. Stevens-Johnson syndrome
        6. Decreased intraocular pressure — minimal
        7. Paralysis of accommodation
        8. Subconjunctival or retinal hemorrhages secondary to drug-induced anemia
        9. Cortical blindness (?)

Clinical Significance: Ocular side effects due to these benzothiadiazides occur only occasionally and are usually transitory. Myopia is probably caused by an increase in the anteroposterior diameter of the lens which may be reversible even if use of the drug is continued.

Interactions with Other Drugs
    A. Effect of Thiazides on Activity of Other Drugs
        1. Adrenergic blockers ↑
        2. Monoamine oxidase inhibitors ↑
        3. Phenothiazines ↑
        4. Tricyclic antidepressants ↑
        5. Sympathomimetics ↑↓
    B. Effect of Other Drugs on Activity of Thiazides
        1. Alcohol ↑
        2. Analgesics ↑

3. Barbiturates ↑
4. General anesthetics ↑
5. Monoamine oxidase inhibitors ↑
6. Tricyclic antidepressants ↑↓
7. Sympathomimetics ↓

References

Beasley, F. J.: Transient myopia and retinal edema during hydrochlorothiazide (Hydro-Diuril) therapy. Arch. Ophthalmol. 65:212, 1961.
Ericson, L. A.: Hygroton-induced myopia and retinal edema. Acta Ophthalmol. 41:538, 1963.
Pallin, O., and Ericson, R.: Ultrasound studies in a case of Hygroton-induced myopia. Acta Ophthalmol. 43:692, 1965.
Peczon, J. D., and Grant, W. M.: Diuretic drugs in glaucoma. Am. J. Ophthalmol. 66:680, 1968.
Weinstock, F. J.: Transient severe myopia. JAMA 217:1245, 1971.

* * * * * * * * * * * * *

Generic Name: Ethacrynic Acid

Proprietary Name: Edecril (Austral.), Edecrin

Primary Use: This phenoxyacetic acid derivative is effective as a short-acting diuretic in all types of edema.

Ocular Side Effects

A. Systemic Administration
   1. Decreased vision
   2. Nystagmus
   3. Subconjunctival or retinal hemorrhages secondary to drug-induced anemia.

Clinical Significance: Few ocular side effects have been reported due to ethacrynic acid therapy. Although blurring of vision is not uncommon, it is seldom of major significance. Ethacrynic acid in dust form is highly irritating to the eyes.

Interactions with Other Drugs

A. Effect of Ethacrynic Acid on Activity of Other Drugs
   1. Alcohol ↑
   2. Carbonic anhydrase inhibitors ↑

References

AMA Drug Evaluations. 2nd Ed., Acton, Mass., Publishing Sciences Group, 1973, pp. 73–74.
Peczon, J. D., and Grant, W. M.: Diuretic drugs in glaucoma. Am. J. Ophthalmol. 66:680, 1968.
Pillay, V. K. G., et al.: Transient and permanent deafness following treatment with ethacrynic acid in renal failure. Lancet 1:77, 1969.

Schneider, W. J., and Becker, E. L.: Acute transient hearing loss after ethacrynic acid
    therapy. Arch. Intern. Med. *117*:715, 1966.
Schwartz, F. D., Pillay, V. K. G., and Kark, R. M.: Ethacrynic acid: Its usefulness and
    untoward effects. Am. Heart J. *79*:427, 1970.

* * * * * * * * * * * * *

Generic Name: Furosemide

Proprietary Name: Frusemide (G.B.), Furantral (Pol.), Lasix

Primary Use: This potent sulfonamide diuretic is effective primarily in the
  treatment of hypertension complicated by congestive heart failure or renal
  impairment.

Ocular Side Effects

  A.   Systemic Administration
    1.   Decreased vision
    2.   Problems with color vision — dyschromatopsia
    3.   Eyelids or conjunctiva
        a.   Allergic reactions
        b.   Erythema multiforme
        c.   Exfoliative dermatitis
    4.   Visual hallucinations
    5.   Decreased intraocular pressure — minimal
    6.   Decreased tolerance to contact lenses
    7.   Subconjunctival or retinal hemorrhages secondary to drug-induced
         anemia
    8.   Decreased accommodation (?)
    9.   Photophobia (?)
    10.   Ocular teratogenic effects (?)

Clinical Significance: Furosemide has potent systemic side effects and is not
  commonly used. Ocular side effects are rare and seldom of significance. One
  instance of a baby born blind after the mother took 40 mg of furosemide 3
  times daily during her second trimester has been reported.

Interactions with Other Drugs

  A.   Effect of Furosemide on Activity of Other Drugs
    1.   Adrenergic blockers ↑
    2.   Monoamine oxidase inhibitors ↑
    3.   Phenothiazines ↑
    4.   Tricyclic antidepressants ↑
  B.   Effect of Other Drugs on Activity of Furosemide
    1.   Adrenergic blockers ↑
    2.   Monoamine oxidase inhibitors ↑
    3.   Phenothiazines ↑
    4.   Tricyclic antidepressants ↑

C.   Cross Sensitivity
   1.   Sulfonamides

References

AMA Drug Evaluations. 2nd Ed., Acton, Mass., Publishing Sciences Group, 1973, pp. 50, 74–75.

Davidson, S. I.: Reports of ocular adverse reactions. Trans. Ophthalmol. Soc. U. K. *93*:495, 1973.

Peczon, J. D., and Grant, W. M.: Diuretic drugs in glaucoma. Am. J. Ophthalmol. *66*:680, 1968.

Physicians' Desk Reference. 28th Ed., Oradell, N. J., Medical Economics Co., 1974, p. 793.

* * * * * * * * * * * *

Generic Name: Spironolactone

Proprietary Name: Aldactone

Primary Use: This aldosterone antagonist is effective in the treatment of edema associated with cirrhosis, nephrotic syndrome, congestive heart failure, and essential hypertension. It is also used in the diagnosis of hyperaldosteronism.

Ocular Side Effects

A.   Systemic Administration
   1.   Decreased vision
   2.   Myopia
   3.   Decreased intraocular pressure — minimal

Clinical Significance: Few significant ocular side effects due to spironolactone have been reported, and all are transitory and reversible.

Interactions with Other Drugs

A.   Effect of Other Drugs on Activity of Spironolactone
   1.   General anesthetics ↑
   2.   Monoamine oxidase inhibitors ↑
   3.   Other diuretics ↑
   4.   Salicylates ↓

References

AMA Drug Evaluation. 2nd Ed., Acton, Mass., Publishing Sciences Group, 1973, p. 76.
Belci, C.: Miopia transitoria in corso di terapia con diuretici. Boll. Oculist *47*:24, 1968.
Duke-Elder, S.: Systems of Ophthalmology. St. Louis, C. V. Mosby, Vol. XIV, Part 2, 1972, p. 1343.
Grant, W. M.: Toxicology of the Eye. 2nd Ed., Springfield, Charles C Thomas, 1974, p. 939.
Meyler, L., and Herxheimer, A. (Eds.): Side Effects of Drugs. Amsterdam, Excerpta Medica, Vol. VII, 1972, p. 313.

* * * * * * * * * * * *

Class: Osmotics

Generic Name: Glycerin (Glycerol)

Proprietary Name: *Systemic:* Glyrol. *Ophthalmic:* Ophthalgan

Primary Use: *Systemic:* This trihydric alcohol is a hyperosmotic agent used to decrease intraocular pressure in various acute glaucomas and in preoperative intraocular procedures. *Ophthalmic:* This topical trihydric alcohol is a hyperosmotic used to reduce corneal edema for diagnostic procedures, increased comfort, or improved vision.

Ocular Side Effects

A. Systemic Administration
    1. Decreased intraocular pressure
    2. Subconjunctival or retinal hemorrhages
    3. Visual hallucinations
B. Local Ophthalmic Use or Exposure
    1. Irritation
        a. Lacrimation
        b. Hyperemia
        c. Ocular pain
        d. Burning sensation
    2. Subconjunctival hemorrhages

Clinical Significance: Systemic glycerin causes decreased intraocular pressure, which is an intended ocular response, and has surprisingly few other ocular effects. Visual hallucinations probably occur due to cerebral dehydration. Topical ocular glycerin has caused subconjunctival hemorrhages and with continued use may cause ocular irritation.

Interactions with Other Drugs

A. Effect of Glycerin on Activity of Other Drugs
    1. Ascorbic acid ↑
B. Effect of Other Drugs on Activity of Glycerin
    1. Anticholinesterases ↑
    2. Ascorbic acid ↑
    3. Carbonic anhydrase inhibitors ↑

References

AMA Drug Evaluations. 2nd Ed., Acton, Mass., Publishing Sciences Group, 1973, p. 685.
Cogan, D. G.: Clearing of edematous corneas by glycerine. Am. J. Ophthalmol. *26*:551, 1943.
Havener, W. H.: Ocular Pharmacology. 2nd Ed., St. Louis, C. V. Mosby, 1970, pp. 357–362, 431.

Hovland, K. R.: Effects of drugs on aqueous humor dynamics. Int. Ophthalmol. Clin. 11:(2):99, 1971.

Virno, M., et al.: Oral glycerol in ophthalmology. Am. J. Ophthalmol. 55:1133, 1963.

* * * * * * * * * * * *

Generic Name: 1. Isosorbide; 2. Mannitol

Proprietary Name: 1. Hydronol; 2. Osmitrol

Primary Use: These hyperosmotic agents are used to decrease intraocular pressure in various acute glaucomas and in preoperative intraocular procedures. Mannitol is also used in the management of oliguria and anuria.

Ocular Side Effects

A. Systemic Administration
1. Decreased intraocular pressure
2. Decreased vision
3. Subconjunctival or retinal hemorrhages
4. Visual hallucinations

Clinical Significance: Isosorbide is excreted unchanged in the urine so that both systemic and ocular side effects are rare. Adverse ocular reactions are more frequent with mannitol since it is administered parenterally and is a more potent agent. Probably all ocular side effects listed are secondary to dehydration effects.

References

Barry, K., Khoury, A. H., and Brooks, M. H.: Mannitol and isosorbide. Arch. Ophthalmol. 81:695, 1969.

Becker, B., Kolker, A. E., and Krupin, T.: Isosorbide. An oral hyperosmotic agent. Arch. Ophthalmol. 78:147, 1967.

Havener, W. H.: Ocular Pharmacology. 2nd Ed., St. Louis, C. V. Mosby, 1970, pp. 356–357, 362–364.

Smith, E. W., and Drance, S. M.: Reduction of human intraocular pressure with intravenous mannitol. Arch. Ophthalmol. 68:734, 1962.

Weiss, D., Shaffer, R. N., and Wise, B. L.: Mannitol infusion to reduce intraocular pressure. Arch. Ophthalmol. 68:341, 1962.

* * * * * * * * * * * *

Generic Name: Urea

Proprietary Name: Ureaphil, Urevert (G.B.)

Primary Use: This hyperosmotic agent is used to decrease temporarily intracranial, cerebrospinal, or intraocular pressure.

Ocular Side Effects

    A. Systemic Administration
        1. Decreased intraocular pressure
        2. Rebound glaucoma
        3. Subconjunctival or retinal hemorrhages
        4. Visual hallucinations
        5. Nystagmus (?)

Clinical Significance: Urea rarely causes ocular side effects other than the intended response of decreased intraocular pressure. However, on occasion a "rebound glaucoma" may occur, possibly caused by the following proposed mechanism. Urea lowers intraocular pressure by drawing intraocular fluid into the vascular system. In rare instances, when the urea concentration is higher within the eye than intravascularly, an increased amount of extravascular fluid flows into the eye. The vitreous may then expand, causing the anterior chamber to precipitate a narrow-angle attack.

Interactions with Other Drugs

    A. Effect of Other Drugs on Activity of Urea
        1. Anticholinesterases ↑
        2. Carbonic anhydrase inhibitors ↑

References

American Hospital Formulary Service. Washington, D. C., American Society of Hospital Pharamacists, Vol. II, 40:28, 1967.
Havener, W. H.: Ocular Pharmacology. 2nd Ed., St. Louis, C. V. Mosby, 1970, pp. 345–355.
Hill, K., Whitney, J. B., and Trotter, R. R.: Intravenous hypertonic urea in the management of acute angle-closure glaucoma. Arch. Ophthalmol. 65:497, 1961.
Kwito, M. L., Kronenberg, B., and Galin, M. A.: The effect of intravenous urea on ocular fluid dynamics. Ann. Ottal. 94:1039, 1968.

* * * * * * * * * * * *

Class: Peripheral Vasodilators

Generic Name: 1. Aluminum Nicotinate; 2. Niacinamide (Nicotinamide); 3. Nicotinic Acid; 4. Nicotinyl Alcohol

Proprietary Name: 1. Nicalex; 2. Nicamid (Switz.), Nicobion (Germ.); 3. Efacin, Niacin, Nicangin (Swed.), Nico-400, Nicobid, Nicocap, Nicotinex, Nicyl (Fr.), Vasotherm, Wampocap; 4. Roniacol

Primary Use: Nicotinic acid and its derivatives are used as peripheral vasodilators, as vitamins, and in the treatment of hyperlipidemia.

Ocular Side Effects

A. Systemic Administration
1. Decreased vision
2. Cystoid macular edema
3. Eyelids or conjunctiva
    a. Allergic reactions
    b. Hyperpigmentation
    c. Angioneurotic edema
    d. Urticaria
4. Scotomas — paracentral (?)
5. Proptosis (?)
6. Increased intraocular pressure (?)

Clinical Significance: Massive dosages of these drugs have been shown to cause ocular side effects, all of which have been reversible after use is discontinued. An atypical cystoid macular edema is believed to be attributable to nicotinic acid. The macular disorder improves or disappears completely following discontinuance of nicotinic acid therapy.

Interactions with Other Drugs

A. Effect of Nicotinic Acid Derivatives on Activity of Other Drugs
1. Phenothiazines ↑

References

AMA Drug Evaluations. 2nd Ed., Acton, Mass., Publishing Sciences Group, 1973, pp. 29, 151, 161.
Chazin, B. J.: Effect of nicotinic acid on blood cholesterol. Geriatrics 15:423, 1960.
Gass, J. D.: Nicotinic acid maculopathy. Am. J. Ophthalmol. 76:500, 1973.
Harris, J. L.: Toxic amblyopia associated with administration of nicotinic acid. Am. J. Ophthalmol. 55:133, 1963.
Parsons, W. B., Jr., and Flinn, J. H.: Reduction in elevated blood cholesterol levels by large doses of nicotinic acid. JAMA 165:234, 1957.

* * * * * * * * * * * * *

Generic Name: Phenoxybenzamine

Proprietary Name: Dibenyline (G.B.), Dibenzyline

Primary Use: This alpha-adrenergic blocking agent is used in the management of pheochromocytoma and sometimes in the treatment of vasospastic peripheral vascular disease other than the obstructive types.

Ocular Side Effects

A. Systemic Administration
1. Miosis
2. Ptosis
3. Conjunctival hyperemia
4. Decreased intraocular pressure (?)

Clinical Significance: Ocular side effects such as miosis due to phenoxybenzamine are common, but they are seldom a problem except when associated with posterior subcapsular or central lens changes. Ptosis and conjunctival hyperemia are seldom clinically significant although they are frequently seen. All adverse ocular reactions are reversible and transitory after discontinued drug use.

Interactions with Other Drugs

A. Effect of Phenoxybenzamine on Activity of Other Drugs
  1. Sympathomimetics ↓

References

AMA Drug Evaluations. 2nd Ed., Acton, Mass., Publishing Sciences Group, 1973, p. 30.
Goodman, L. S., and Gilman, A. (Eds.): The Pharmacological Basis of Therapeutics. 4th Ed., New York, Macmillan, 1970, pp. 550–557.
Grant, W. M.: Toxicology of the Eye. 2nd Ed., Springfield, Charles C Thomas, 1974, p. 814.
Walsh, F. B., and Hoyt, W. F.: Clinical Neuro-Ophthalmology. 3rd Ed., Baltimore, Williams & Wilkins, Vol. 1, 1969, p. 447.

* * * * * * * * * * * *

Generic Name: Tolazoline

Proprietary Name: Priscol (G.B.), Priscoline, Toline (Austral.), Vasodil (Swed.), Zoline (G.B.)

Primary Use: This alpha-adrenergic blocking agent is used in the management of spastic peripheral vascular disorders and as a diagnostic test for open-angle glaucoma.

Ocular Side Effects

A. Systemic Administration
  1. Intraocular pressure
    a. Increased
    b. Decreased — especially in hypertensive individuals
B. Local Ophthalmic Use or Exposure — Subconjunctival Injection
  1. Increased intraocular pressure — especially in open-angle glaucoma
  2. Ptosis
  3. Miosis
  4. Conjunctival hyperemia

Clinical Significance: In general, the ocular pressure response from systemic tolazoline is of little clinical significance because of its variability and small amplitude. However, in hypertensive individuals the transient decreased intraocular pressure induced by tolazoline may be significant. Ocular side effects from subconjunctival injections are common but rarely significant. Increased intraocular pressure may be attributable in part to vasodilatation.

Interactions with Other Drugs

A. Effect of Tolazoline on Activity of Other Drugs
1. General anesthetics ↑
2. Monoamine oxidase inhibitors ↑
B. Effect of Other Drugs on Activity of Tolazoline
1. General anesthetics ↑
2. Monoamine oxidase inhibitors ↑

References

Duke-Elder, S.: Systems of Ophthalmology. St. Louis, C. V. Mosby, Vol. XIV, Part 2, 1972, p. 1046.

Newell, F. W., Ridgway, W. L., and Zeller, R. W.: The treatment of glaucoma with dibenamine. Am. J. Ophthalmol. *34*:527, 1951.

Sugar, S., and Santos, R.: The Priscoline provocative test. Am. J. Ophthalmol. *40*:510, 1955.

Walsh, F. B., and Hoyt, W. F.: Clinical Neuro-Ophthalmology. 3rd Ed., Baltimore, Williams & Wilkins, Vol. I, 1969, p. 447.

Zarrabi, M.: Quelques observations sur le Priscol en ophtalmologie. Ophthalmologica *122*:76, 1951.

* * * * * * * * * * * *

Class: Vasopressors

Generic Name: Ephedrine

Proprietary Name: *Systemic:* Ectasule Minus, Slo-Fedrin, Spaneph (G.B.), Zephrol (G.B.) *Ophthalmic:* Ephedrine Hydrochloride Mimims (G.B.)

Primary Use: *Systemic:* This sympathomimetic amine is effective as a vasopressor, a bronchodilator, and a nasal decongestant. *Ophthalmic:* This topical sympathomimetic amine is used as a conjunctival vasoconstrictor.

Ocular Side Effects

A. Systemic Administration
1. Mydriasis — may precipitate narrow-angle glaucoma
2. Visual hallucinations
3. Decreased intraocular pressure
4. Rebound miosis (?)
B. Local Ophthalmic Use or Exposure
1. Conjunctival vasoconstriction
2. Decreased vision
3. Eyelids or conjunctiva
a. Allergic reactions
b. Conjunctivitis — nonspecific

    4.   Irritation
       a.   Lacrimation
       b.   Rebound hyperemia
       c.   Photophobia
    5.   Mydriasis — may precipitate narrow-angle glaucoma
    6.   Aqueous floaters — pigment debris
    7.   Decreased intraocular pressure (?)

Clinical Significance: Ocular side effects from systemic administration of ephedrine are rare and topical ocular ephedrine solutions are seldom used in concentrations sufficient to cause significant side effects other than the intended response of vasoconstriction. Repeated use, however, may cause rebound conjunctival hyperemia or, in some instances, loss of the drug's vasoconstrictive effect.

Interactions with Other Drugs

   A.   Effect of Ephedrine on Activity of Other Drugs
     1.   Sympathomimetics ↑
     2.   Adrenergic blockers ↓
     3.   Local anesthetics ↓
   B.   Effect of Other Drugs on Activity of Ephedrine
     1.   Monoamine oxidase inhibitors ↑
     2.   Sympathomimetics ↑
     3.   Adrenergic blockers ↓
   C.   Contraindications
     1.   Ophthalmic lotions containing polyvinyl alcohol

References

AMA Drug Evaluations. 2nd Ed., Acton, Mass., Publishing Sciences Group, 1973, pp. 40, 460, 470, 726–727.

Hardesty, J. F.: Control of intraocular hypertension by systemic medication. Trans. Am. Ophthalmol. Soc. *32*:497, 1934.

Havener, W. H.: Ocular Pharmacology. 2nd Ed., St. Louis, C. V. Mosby, 1970, p. 188.

Mitchell, D. W. A.: The effect of ephedrine instillations on intraocular pressure. Br. J. Physiol. Opt. NS *14*:38, 1957.

Walsh, F. B., and Hoyt, W. F.: Clinical Neuro-Ophthalmology. 3rd Ed., Baltimore, Williams & Wilkins, Vol. I, 1969, p. 446.

* * * * * * * * * * * *

Generic Name: Epinephrine

Proprietary Name: *Systemic:* Adrenalin, Adrenaline (G.B.), Asmolin, Sus-Phrine *Ophthalmic:* Adrenaline (G.B.), E1, Epifrin, Epinal, Epitrate, Eppy, Glaucon, IOP, Laevo-Glaucosan (Germ.), Lyophrin (G.B.), Mytrate, Oculo-guttae Adrenalini (Denm.)

Primary Use: *Systemic:* This sympathomimetic amine is effective as a vasopressor, a bronchodilator, and a vasoconstrictor in prolonging the action of
anesthetics. *Ophthalmic:* This topical sympathomimetic amine is used in the
management of open-angle glaucoma.

Ocular Side Effects

A. Systemic Administration
1. Mydriasis — may precipitate narrow-angle glaucoma
2. Problems with color vision
a. Dyschromatopsia
b. Objects have green tinge
c. Achromatopsia — red defect
3. Hemianopsia
4. Lacrimation
B. Local Ophthalmic Use or Exposure
1. Decreased intraocular pressure
2. Decreased vision
3. Mydriasis — may precipitate narrow-angle glaucoma
4. Eyelids or conjunctiva
a. Allergic reactions
b. Blepharoconjunctivitis
c. Vasoconstriction
5. Irritation
a. Lacrimation
b. Rebound hyperemia
c. Photophobia
d. Ocular pain
e. Burning sensation
6. Adrenochrome deposits
a. Conjunctiva
b. Cornea
c. Nasolacrimal system
7. Cystoid macular edema
8. Keratitis
9. Corneal edema
10. Subconjunctival or retinal hemorrhages
11. Loss of eyelashes or eyebrows
12. Paradoxical pressure elevation in open-angle glaucoma
13. Scotomas
14. Aqueous floaters — pigment debris
15. Periorbital edema
16. Vitreous floaters (?)

Clinical Significance: Ocular side effects from systemic epinephrine are rare;
however, topical ocular application may commonly cause significant side
effects other than the intended responses of decreased intraocular pressure and
conjunctival vasoconstriction. Not infrequently, the drug must be stopped
after prolonged use because of ocular discomfort and rebound conjunctival

hyperemia. While most epinephrine-induced ocular side effects are reversible, there are some, such as advanced cystoid macular edema, which may be irreversible. Cystoid macular changes secondary to epinephrine occur more frequently in aphakic patients.

Interactions with Other Drugs

A. Effect of Epinephrine on Activity of Other Drugs
  1. Local anesthetics ↑
  2. Urea ↑
  3. Anticholinesterases ↓
B. Effect of Other Drugs on Activity of Epinephrine
  1. Antihistamines ↑
  2. Monoamine oxidase inhibitors ↑
  3. Sympathomimetics ↑
  4. Tricyclic antidepressants ↑
  5. Adrenergic blockers ↓
  6. Alcohol ↓
  7. Phenothiazines ↓

References

Becker, B., and Morton, W. R.: Topical epinephrine in glaucoma suspects. Am. J. Ophthalmol. 62:272, 1966.

Drance, S. M., and Ross, R. A.: The ocular effects of epinephrine. Surv. Ophthalmol. 14:330, 1970.

Obstbaum, S. A., Kolker, A. E., and Phelps, C. D.: Low-dose epinephrine. Arch. Ophthalmol. 92:118, 1974.

Reinecke, R. D., and Kuwabara, T.: Corneal deposits secondary to topical epinephrine. Arch. Ophthalmol. 70:170, 1963.

Spaeth, G. L.: Nasolacrimal duct obstruction caused by topical epinephrine. Arch. Ophthalmol. 77:355, 1967.

* * * * * * * * * * * *

Generic Name: Hydroxyamphetamine

Proprietary Name: Paredrine (*Systemic* and *Ophthalmic*)

Primary Use: *Systemic:* This sympathomimetic amine is effective as a vasopressor and is used in the treatment of heart block and postural hypotension. *Ophthalmic:* This topical sympathomimetic amine is used as a mydriatic.

Ocular Side Effects

A. Local Ophthalmic Use or Exposure
  1. Mydriasis — may precipitate narrow-angle glaucoma
  2. Decreased vision
  3. Irritation
      a. Lacrimation
      b. Photophobia
      c. Ocular pain

4. Paradoxical pressure elevation in open-angle glaucoma
5. Eyelids or conjunctiva — allergic reactions
6. Paralysis of accommodation — minimal
7. Problems with color vision —objects have a blue tinge

Clinical Significance: Other than precipitating narrow-angle glaucoma, ocular side effects from topical ocular administration of hydroxyamphetamine are insignificant and reversible. Some feel this may be the safest mydriatic to use with a shallow anterior chamber since it is slow-acting and possibly more easily counteracted by miotics. Administration of 1 percent hydroxyamphetamine eyedrops causes a more pronounced mydriasis in patients with mongolism or Down's syndrome than in normal patients.

Interactions with Other Drugs

A. Effect of Hydroxyamphetamine on Activity of Other Drugs
  1. Analgesics ↑
  2. Tricyclic antidepressants ↑
  3. Adrenergic blockers ↓
  4. Alcohol ↓
  5. Antihistamines ↓
B. Effect of Other Drugs on Activity of Hydroxyamphetamine
  1. Local anesthetics ↑
  2. Monoamine oxidase inhibitors ↑
  3. Tricyclic antidepressants ↑
  4. Adrenergic blockers ↓
  5. Phenothiazines ↓

References

Gartner, S., and Billet, E.: Mydriatic glaucoma. Am. J. Ophthalmol. 43:975, 1957.
Grant, W. M.: Toxicology of the Eye. 2nd Ed., Springfield, Charles C Thomas, 1974, pp. 567–568.
Kronfeld, P. C., McGarry, H. I., and Smith, H. E.: The effect of mydriatics upon the intraocular pressure in so-called primary wide-angle glaucoma. Am. J. Ophthalmol. 26:245, 1943.
Priest, J. H.: Atropine response of the eyes in mongolism. Am. J. Dis. Child. 100:869, 1960.
Walsh, F. B., and Hoyt, W. F.: Clinical Neuro-Ophthalmology. 3rd Ed., Baltimore, Williams & Wilkins, Vol. I, 1969, p. 446.

* * * * * * * * * * * *

Generic Name: 1. Levarterenol; 2. Mephentermine; 3. Metaraminol; 4. Methoxamine

Proprietary Name: 1. Levophed, Noradrenaline (G.B.); 2. Mephine (G.B.), Wyamine; 3. Aramine; 4. Vasoxine (G.B.), Vasoxyl

Primary Use: These sympathomimetic amines are used in the management of hypotension and shock.

Ocular Side Effects

A. Systemic Administration
1. Mydriasis — may precipitate narrow-angle glaucoma
2. Horizontal nystagmus
3. Photophobia (levarterenol)

Clinical Significance: Ocular side effects due to these sympathomimetic amines are reversible and transitory. Seldom are adverse ocular reactions seen due to these drugs except in overdose situations.

Interactions with Other Drugs

A. Effect of Sympathomimetics on Activity of Other Drugs
1. Monoamine oxidase inhibitors ↑ (levarterenol)
2. Tricyclic antidepressants ↑
3. Adrenergic blockers ↑↓
4. Analgesics ↓
5. Anticholinesterases ↓
6. Phenothiazines ↓ (levarterenol)
B. Effect of Other Drugs on Activity of Sympathomimetics
1. Alcohol ↑
2. Anticholinergics ↑
3. Antihistamines ↑
4. General anesthetics ↑ (levarterenol)
5. Monoamine oxidase inhibitors ↑
6. Tricyclic antidepressants ↑
7. Adrenergic blockers ↑↓
8. Phenothiazines ↑↓
9. Anticholinesterases ↓

References

Goodman, L. S., and Gilman, A. (Eds.): The Pharmacological Basis of Therapeutics. 4th Ed., New York, Macmillan, 1970, p. 497–499, 508–511.

Grant, W. M.: Toxicology of the Eye. 2nd Ed., Springfield, Charles C Thomas, 1974, pp. 664, 677–678.

Horler, A. R., and Wynne, N. A.: Hypertensive crises due to pargyline and metaraminol. Br. Med. J. 2:460, 1965.

Watillon, M., and Robe-Vanwijck, A.: Les medicaments cardiovasculaires. Bull. Soc. Belge Ophtalmol. 160:174, 1972.

* * * * * * * * * * * *

Generic Name: Phenylephrine

Proprietary Name: *Systemic:* Neo-Synephrine *Ophthalmic:* Degest, Efricel, I-Care (Austral.), Neo-Synephrine, Prefrin, Tear-Efrin

Primary Use: *Systemic:* This sympathomimetic amine is effective as a vasopressor and is used in the management of hypotension, shock, and tachycardia. *Ophthalmic:* This topical sympathomimetic amine is used as a vasoconstrictor and a mydriatic.

Ocular Side Effects

A. Local Ophthalmic Use or Exposure
   1. Mydriasis — may precipitate narrow-angle glaucoma
   2. Decreased vision
   3. Conjunctival vasoconstriction
   4. Rebound miosis
   5. Irritation
      a. Lacrimation
      b. Rebound hyperemia
      c. Photophobia
      d. Ocular pain
   6. Punctate keratitis
   7. Eyelids or conjunctiva — allergic reactions
   8. Aqueous floaters — pigment debris
   9. Corneal edema
   10. Paradoxical pressure elevation in open-angle glaucoma
   11. Cystoid macular edema (?)

Clinical Significance: Other than the possibility of precipitating narrow-angle glaucoma, the ocular side effects due to phenylephrine are usually of little significance. A 10 percent concentration of phenylephrine can cause significant adverse ocular reactions; however, the drug is seldom applied at this concentration except in single-dosage situations or for short periods of time.

Interactions with Other Drugs

A. Effect of Phenylephrine on Activity of Other Drugs
   1. Local anesthetics ↑↓
   2. Adrenergic blockers ↓
   3. Phenothiazines ↓
B. Effect of Other Drugs on Activity of Phenylephrine
   1. Adrenergic blockers ↑
   2. Monoamine oxidase inhibitors ↑
   3. Tricyclic antidepressants ↑

References

Grant, W. M.: Toxicology of the Eye. 2nd Ed., Springfield, Charles C Thomas, 1974, pp. 819–820.

Harris, L. S.: Cycloplegic-induced intraocular pressure elevations. Arch. Ophthalmol. 79:242, 1968.

Holtman, H. W., and Meyer, W.: Problems of the side effects of neosynephrine. Albrecht von Graefes Arch. Klin. Ophthalmol. 185:221, 1972.

Lansche, R. K.: Systemic reactions to topical epinephrine and phenylephrine. Am. J. Ophthalmol. 61:95, 1966.

McReynolds, W. U., Havener, W. H., and Henderson, J. W.: Hazards of the use of sympathomimetic drugs in ophthalmology. Arch. Ophthalmol. 56:176, 1956.

* * * * * * * * * * * * *

VII. Hormones and Agents Affecting Hormonal Mechanisms

Class: Adrenal Corticosteroids

Generic Name: 1. Adrenal Cortex Injection; 2. Aldosterone; 3. Betamethasone; 4. Cortisone; 5. Desoxycorticosterone (Desoxycortone); 6. Dexamethasone; 7. Fludrocortisone; 8. Fluorometholone; 9. Fluprednisolone; 10. Hydrocortisone; 11. Medrysone; 12. Methylprednisolone; 13. Paramethasone; 14. Prednisolone; 15. Prednisone; 16. Triamcinolone

Proprietary Name: *Systemic:* 1. Supracort (G.B.); 2. Aldocorten (G.B.); 3. Betasolon (Ital.), Betnelan (G.B.), Celestan (Germ.), Celestene (Fr.), Celestone, Desacort-Beta (Ital.), Minisone (Ital.), Rinderon (Jap.); 4. Adreson (G.B.), Austracort (Austral.), Cortelan (G.B.), Cortic (Austral.), Cortilen (Ital.), Cortistab (G.B.), Cortisyl (G.B.), Cortone, Neosone, Novocort (Canad.); 5. Cortate, Cortiron (Germ.), Doca, Percorten, Surrenon (Ital.), Syncorta (Jap.), Syncortyl (Fr.); 6. Carulon (Jap.), Corson (Jap.), Cortisumman (Germ.), Decadron, Decaesadril (Ital.), Decasterolone (Ital.), Decofluor (Ital.), Dectan (Jap.), Deltafluorene (Austral.), Deronil, Desacort (Ital.), Desacortone (Ital.), Desalark (Ital.), Desameton (Ital.), Deseronil (Ital.), Dexa Cortisyl (G.B.), Dexa-Dabrosan (Germ.), Dexamed (Germ.), Dexameth, Dexapolcort (Pol.), Dexa-Scheroson (Germ.), Dexasone (Austral.), Dexinolon (Germ.), Fluormone (Ital.), Fluorocort (Ital.), Fortecortin (Germ.), Gammacorten, Hexadrol, Hightisone (Jap.), Metasolon (Jap.), Millicorten (Germ.), Oradexon (G.B.), Orgadrone (Jap.); 7. Alflorone, Cortineff (Pol.), F-Cortef, Florinef, Scherofluron (Germ.); 9. Alphadrol, Etadrol (Ital.); 10. Cortef, Cortifan, Cortiment (Canad.), Cortiphate (Canad.), Cortril, Efcortesol (G.B.), Ficortril (Germ.), Hycor (Austral.), Hycortole, Hydrocortistab (G.B.), Hydrocortone, Incortin-H (Germ.), Phiacort (Austral.), Solu-Cortef; 12. Caberdelta M (Ital.), Depo-Medrol, Depo-Medrone (G.B.), Medesone (Ital.), Medrol, Medrone (G.B.), Solu-Medrol, Urbason (Germ.); 13. Alondra (Arg.), Dilar (Fr.), Haldrate (G.B.), Haldrone, Metilar (G.B.), Monocortin (Germ.), Paramesone (Jap.); 14. Adnisone (Austral.), Anpilone (G.B.), Codilcortone (G.B.), Codelsol (G.B.), Cormalone (Canad.), Dacortin (Swed.), Dacortin H (Span.), Decortin-H (Germ.), Delcortol (Denm.), Delta-Cortef, Deltacortenolo (Ital.), Delta-Cortilen (Ital.), Deltacortril (G.B.), Delta-Genacort (G.B.), Deltalone (G.B.), Deltasolone (Austral.), Deltastab (G.B.), Deltidrosol (Ital.), Deltilen (Ital.), Di-Adreson-F (G.B.), Donisolone (Jap.), Encortolone (Pol.), Endoprenovis (Ital.), Hostacortin H (Germ.), Hydeltra, Hydeltrasol, Hydrocortancyl (Fr.),

Hydrocortidelt (Germ.), In-solone (G.B.), Keteocort H (Germ.), Marsolone (G.B.), Mecortolone (Pol.), Meticortelone, Nisolone (Span.), Panafcortelone (Austral.), Paracortol, Parisilon (G.B.), Precortalon (Swed.), Pre Cortisyl (G.B.), Prednelan (G.B.), Prednesol (G.B.), Predni-Coelin (Germ.), Predniretard (Fr.), Prednis, Prednisol (Ital.), Predonine (Jap.), Prelone (Austral.), Presolon (Jap.), Scherisolon (Austral., Germ.), Solu-Dacortin (Austral., Swed.), Solu-Decortin-H (Germ.), Sterane, Sterolone, Ulacort, Ultracorten-H (Germ.), Ultracortenol (G.B.); 15. Adasone (Austral.), Ancortone (Ital.), Anpisone (G.B.), Austrocort-P (Austral.), Betapar, Colisone (Canad.), Cortancyl (Fr.), Dacortin (Span.), Decortin (Germ.), DeCortisyl (G.B.), Delcortin (Denm.), Delta-Cortelan, Deltacortene (Ital.), Deltacortone (G.B.), Delta-Dome, Delta Prenovis (Ital.), Delta-Scheroson (Austral.), Deltasone, Deltastendiolo (Ital.), Deltatrione (Ital.), Di-Adreson (G.B.), Deltra, Encortone (Pol.), Hostacortin (Germ.), In-sone (G.B.), Keteocort (Germ.), Keysone, Lisacort, Marsone (G.B.), Meticorten, Nisone (Span.), Orasone, Panafcort (Austral.), Paracort, Parmenison (Aust.), Precortal (Swed.), Predniment Rectodelt (Germ.), Predni-tal (Ital.), Presone (Austral.), Scheroson-P (Austral.), Sterapred, Ultracorten (Germ.); 16. Adcortyl (G.B.), Aristocort, Aristospan, Delphicort (Germ.), Kenacort, Kenalog, Ledercort (G.B.), Polcortolone (Pol.), Tedarol (Fr.), Triamcort (Ital.), Volon (Germ.) *Ophthalmic:* 4. Cortistab (G.B.), Cortisyl (G.B.), Neosone; 6. Decadron, Maxidex; 8. FML Liquifilm, Oxylone; 10. Hydrocortistab (G.B.), HydroCortisyl (G.B.), Hydrocortone, Optef; 11. HMS Liquifilm, Medrocort; 12. Depo-Medrol; 14. Hydeltrasol, Inflamase, Optocort (Austral.), Predsol (G.B.), Sintisone (G.B.)

Primary Use: *Systemic:* These corticosteroids are effective in the replacement therapy of adrenocortical insufficiency and in the treatment of inflammatory and allergic disorders. *Ophthalmic:* These corticosteroids are effective in the treatment of ocular inflammatory and allergic disorders.

Ocular Side Effects

A. Systemic Administration
1. Decreased vision
2. Posterior subcapsular cataracts
3. Increased intraocular pressure
4. Decreased resistance to infection
5. Mydriasis — may precipitate narrow-angle glaucoma
6. Ptosis
7. Myopia
8. Exophthalmos
9. Papilledema secondary to pseudotumor cerebri
10. Diplopia
11. Paresis or paralysis of extraocular muscles
12. Problems with color vision — dyschromatopsia
13. Delayed healing of corneal wound
14. Visual fields
    a. Scotomas
    b. Enlarged blind spot

    15. Retinal edema
    16. Translucent blue sclera
    17. Eyelids or conjunctiva
        a. Hyperemia
        b. Edema
        c. Angioneurotic edema
        d. Lyell's syndrome
    18. Subconjunctival or retinal hemorrhages
    19. Blindness
    20. Macular degeneration (?)
    21. Central serous retinopathy (?)
    22. Congenital cataracts (?)

B. Local Ophthalmic Use or Exposure — Topical Application or Subconjunctival Injection
    1. Increased intraocular pressure
    2. Decreased resistance to infection
    3. Delayed healing of corneal or scleral wounds
    4. Mydriasis — may precipitate narrow-angle glaucoma
    5. Ptosis
    6. Posterior subcapsular cataracts
    7. Decreased vision
    8. Enhances lytic action of collagenase
    9. Paralysis of accommodation
    10. Visual fields
        a. Scotomas
        b. Constriction
        c. Enlarged blind spot
        d. Glaucoma field defect
    11. Problems with color vision
        a. Dyschromatopsia
        b. Colored haloes around lights
    12. Eyelids or conjunctiva
        a. Allergic reactions
        b. Petechiae
    13. Punctate keratitis
    14. Irritation
        a. Lacrimation
        b. Photophobia
        c. Ocular pain
        d. Burning sensation
        e. Anterior uveitis
    15. Corneal or scleral thickness
        a. Increased — initial
        b. Decreased
    16. Blindness
    17. Optic atrophy
    18. Granulomas

C. Inadvertent Ocular Exposure — Intraocular Injection
    1. Ocular pain
    2. Decreased vision
    3. Intraocular pressure
        a. Increased — initial
        b. Decreased
    4. Retinal hemorrhages
    5. Retinal degeneration
    6. Ascending optic atrophy
    7. Blindness
    8. Retinal detachment
    9. Global atrophy

Clinical Significance: Ocular side effects due to systemic or ocular administration of steroids are common and have significant clinical importance. The ocular side effects differ, depending on the route of administration. Systemic administration of steroids is more often implicated with posterior subcapsular cataracts, while ophthalmic administration of steroids is more common with drug-induced glaucoma. Adverse ocular effects are more likely to be dose-related than time-related. Age is also a factor since posterior subcapsular cataracts secondary to systemic administration of steroids are more frequent in children than in adults. In general, other than decreased resistance to infection, excluding herpes simplex virus, important adverse steroid drug reactions usually require a number of weeks of therapy to occur. The recent popularity of subconjunctival injections of steroids has brought additional drug reactions. Subconjunctival injections of steroids placed over a diseased cornea or sclera have been said to cause a thinning, and possibly rupture, at the site of the injection. Posterior subcapsular cataracts and subconjunctival granulomas have also been induced due to this mode of drug administration. Inadvertent intraocular steroid injections have caused blindness, probably as a result of direct drug toxicity to the retina or optic nerve.

Interactions with Other Drugs

A. Effect of Corticosteroids on Activity of Other Drugs
    1. Barbiturates ↑
    2. Sedatives and hypnotics ↑
    3. Tricyclic antidepressants ↑
    4. Anticholinesterases ↓
    5. Antiviral eye preparations ↓
    6. Salicylates ↓
B. Effect of Other Drugs on Activity of Corticosteroids
    1. Salicylates ↑
    2. Antihistamines ↓
    3. Barbiturates ↓
    4. Phenylbutazone ↓
    5. Sedatives and hypnotics ↓

References

Armaly, M. F.: Effect of corticosteroids on intraocular pressure and fluid dynamics. I. Effect of dexamethasone in the normal eye. Arch. Ophthalmol. 70:482, 1963.

Becker, B.: The side effects of corticosteroids. Invest. Ophthalmol. 3:492, 1964.

Crews, S. J.: Adverse reactions to corticosteroid therapy in the eye. Proc. R. Soc. Med. 58:533, 1965.

David, D. S., and Berkowitz, J. S.: Ocular effects of topical and systemic corticosteroids. Lancet 2:149, 1969.

Duke-Elder, S.: Systems of Ophthalmology. St. Louis, C. V. Mosby, Vol. XIV, Part 2, 1972, p. 1343.

Ey, R. C., et al.: Prevention of corneal vascularization. Am. J. Ophthalmol. 66:1118, 1968.

Fraunfelder, F. T., and Watson, P. G.: Evaluation of eyes enucleated for scleritis. To be published.

Grant, W. M.: Toxicology of the Eye. 2nd Ed., Springfield, Charles C Thomas, 1974, pp. 320–327.

Kraus, A. M.: Congenital cataract and maternal steroid ingestion. J. Pediatr. Ophthalmol. 12:107, 1975.

McKay, D. A. R., Watson, P. G., and Lyne, A. J.: Relapsing polychondritis and eye disease. Br. J. Ophthalmol. 58:600, 1974.

Schlagel, T. F., Jr., and Wilson, F. M.: Accidental intraocular injection of depot corticosteroids. Trans. Am. Acad. Ophthalmol. Otolaryngol. 78:847, 1974.

Walsh, F. B., and Hoyt, W. F.: Clinical Neuro-Ophthalmology. 3rd Ed., Baltimore, Williams & Wilkins, Vol. III, 1969, pp. 2501, 2701–2704.

* * * * * * * * * * * *

Class: Antithyroid Agents

Generic Name: 1. Carbimazole; 2. Methimazole; 3. Methylthiouracil; 4. Propylthiouracil

Proprietary Name: 1. Bimazol (G.B.), Neo-Mercazde (G.B.); 2. Tapazole; 3. Methiacil, Thimecil; 4. Propacil

Primary Use: These thioamides are effective in the treatment of hyperthyroidism and angina pectoris.

Ocular Side Effects

A. Systemic Administration
   1. Nystagmus (methylthiouracil)
   2. Keratitis
   3. Eyelids or conjunctiva
      a. Allergic reactions
      b. Conjunctivitis — nonspecific
      c. Depigmentation
      d. Urticaria
      e. Lupoid syndrome
      f. Exfoliative dermatitis

4. Decreased lacrimation (methylthiouracil)
5. Exophthalmos
6. Subconjunctival or retinal hemorrhages secondary to drug-induced anemia
7. Loss of eyelashes or eyebrows (?)

Clinical Significance: Ocular side effects secondary to these thioamides are rare. Nystagmus and decreased lacrimation have only been reported with methylthiouracil. Adverse ocular reactions are reversible and transitory after discontinued use of these drugs.

References

Frawley, T. F., and Koepf, G. F.: Neurotoxicity due to thiouracil and thiourea derivatives. J. Clin. Endocrinol. *10*:623, 1950.
Papadopoulos, S., and Harden, R. McG.: Hair loss in patients treated with carbimazole. Br. Med. J. 2:1502, 1966.
Prowse, C. B.: A toxic effect of thiouracil hitherto undescribed. Br. Med. J. 2:1312, 1960.
Schneeberg, N. G.: Loss of sense of taste due to methylthiouracil therapy. JAMA *149*:1091, 1952.
Stecher, P. G. (Ed.): The Merck Index: An Encyclopedia of Chemicals and Drugs. 8th Ed., Rahway, N. J., Merck and Co., Inc., 1968.
Willcox, P. H.: Antithyroid treatment. A personal series. Postgrad. Med. J. *43*:146, 1967.

* * * * * * * * * * * *

Generic Name: 1. Iodide and iodine solutions and compounds; 2. Radioactive iodides

Proprietary Name: *Systemic:* 1. Aqueous Iodine Solution, Compound Iodine Solution, Faringets (G.B.), Iodhema (G.B.), Lugol's Solution, Pima, Strong Iodine Solution; 2. Iodotope I-131, Oriodide-131, Theriodide-131 *Ophthalmic:* 1. Iodine Solution

Primary Use: *Systemic:* Iodide and iodine are effective in the diagnosis and management of thyroid disease, in the short-term management of respiratory tract disease, and in some instances, of fungal infections. *Ophthalmic:* Topical iodide and iodine solutions are used primarily as a chemical cautery in the treatment of herpes simplex.

Ocular Side Effects

A. Systemic Administration – Oral
 1. Decreased vision
 2. Exophthalmos
 3. Nonspecific ocular irritation
   a. Lacrimation
   b. Ocular pain
   c. Burning sensation
 4. Eyelids or conjunctiva
   a. Allergic reactions
   b. Hyperemia

  c. Conjunctivitis — nonspecific
  d. Edema
  e. Angioneurotic edema
 5. Punctate keratitis
 6. Hemorrhagic iritis
 7. Hypopyon
 8. Vitreous floaters
 9. Ocular teratogenic effects (radioactive iodides)
 10. Miosis (?)
 11. Paralysis of extraocular muscles (?)
 12. Retinal hemorrhages (?)
B. Systemic Administration — Intravenous
 1. Those mentioned for oral administration
 2. Visual fields
  a. Scotomas
  b. Constriction
  c. Hemianopsia
 3. Paralysis of accommodation
 4. Problems with color vision
  a. Dyschromatopsia
  b. Objects have green tinge
 5. Visual hallucinations
 6. Mydriasis
 7. Retinal degeneration
 8. Retinal or macular edema
 9. Retinal vasoconstriction
 10. Retrobulbar neuritis
 11. Blindness
 12. Optic atrophy
C. Local Ophthalmic Use or Exposure
 1. Decreased vision
 2. Keratitis bullosa
 3. Eyelids or conjunctiva
  a. Allergic reactions
  b. Blepharoconjunctivitis
  c. Edema
  d. Urticaria
 4. Irritation
  a. Lacrimation
  b. Hyperemia
  c. Ocular pain
  d. Edema
 5. Brown corneal discoloration
 6. Vascularization
 7. Stromal scarring
 8. Delayed healing of corneal wound

Clinical Significance: Few serious irreversible ocular side effects secondary to iodide or iodine administration have been reported except when these agents have been given intravenously. When they are given orally, retinal findings are exceedingly rare or nonexistent. Allergic reactions to these agents are of rapid onset and not uncommon. Most ocular side effects are dose-related.

References

Gerber, M.: Ocular reactions following iodide therapy. Am. J. Ophthalmol. *43*:879, 1957.

Goldberg, H. K.: Iodism with severe ocular involvement. Report of a case. Am. J. Ophthalmol. *22*:65, 1939.

Grant, W. M.: Toxicology of the Eye. 2nd Ed., Springfield, Charles C Thomas, 1974, pp. 586–588.

Havener, W. H.: Ocular Pharmacology. 2nd Ed., St. Louis, C. V. Mosby, 1970, pp. 343–344.

Walsh, F. B., and Hoyt, W. F.: Clinical Neuro-Ophthalmology. 3rd Ed., Baltimore, Williams & Wilkins, Vol. III, 1969, pp. 2558–2560.

* * * * * * * * * * * *

Class: Oral Contraceptives

Generic Name: Combination products of estrogens and progestogens.

Proprietary Name: Anovlar (G.B.), Conovid (G.B.), C-Quens, Demulen, Enavid (G.B.), Enovid, Gynformone (G.B.), Gynovlar (G.B.), Loestrin, Mentrinol (G.B.), Metrulen (G.B.), Minovlar (G.B.), Norinyl, Norlestrin, Norquen, Oracon, Orlest (G.B.), Ortho-Novum, Ovanon (G.B.), Ovral, Ovulen, Provest, Secrodyl (G.B.), Serial 28 (G.B.), Volidan, Zorane

Primary Use: These hormonal agents are used in the treatment of amenorrhea, dysfunctional uterine bleeding, premenstrual tension, dysmenorrhea, hypogonadism, and most commonly, as oral contraceptives.

Ocular Side Effects

A. Systemic Administration
1. Decreased vision
2. Retinal vascular disorders
    a. Thrombosis
    b. Occlusion
    c. Perivasculitis
3. Decreased tolerance to contact lenses
4. Papilledema secondary to pseudotumor cerebri
5. Flashing lights
6. Paralysis of extraocular muscles
7. Diplopia
8. Retrobulbar or optic neuritis
9. Retinal edema
10. Problems with color vision
    a. Dyschromatopsia

    b. Objects have blue tinge
    c. Colored haloes around lights — mainly blue
   11. Visual fields
    a. Scotomas — central
    b. Quadrantanopsia or hemianopsia
   12. Punctate keratitis
   13. Photophobia
   14. Decreased intraocular pressure
   15. Exophthalmos
   16. Proptosis secondary to pseudotumor of the orbit
   17. Myopia
   18. Central serous retinopathy
   19. Macular degeneration
   20. Eyelids or conjunctiva
    a. Allergic reactions
    b. Edema
    c. Urticaria
   21. Subconjunctival or retinal hemorrhages secondary to drug-induced anemia
   22. Orbital or periocular pain
   23. Pupils
    a. Mydriasis — may precipitate narrow-angle glaucoma
    b. Anisocoria
   24. Horner's syndrome
   25. Periorbital edema
   26. Optic atrophy
   27. Blindness

Clinical Significance: A significantly higher incidence of migraine, thrombophlebitis, and pseudotumor cerebri occurs in women taking oral contraceptives than in a comparable population. A higher incidence of ocular side effects associated with these three entities is therefore probable. There is no proved relationship between these drugs and other diseases of the eye even though a minimum of 80 reports in the literature concern themselves with this possiblity. There may be a relationship between women taking oral contraceptives and a decreased tolerance to wearing contact lenses. Most of the other ocular side effects listed are based on clinical reports of possible adverse reactions. Probably many of these are true ocular side effects, but at present most must be assumed to be only possibilities and await further documentation. In a few cases the courts have ruled that a cause and effect relationship between the use of oral contraceptives and retinal vascular abnormalities exists. Therefore, in most instances patients with retinal vascular abnormalities probably should not be given these medications. If retinal vascular abnormalities develop, the use of these drugs in that patient may need to be re-evaluated.

Interactions with Other Drugs

 A. Effect of Oral Contraceptives on Activity of Other Drugs
   1. Analgesics ↑

     2. Corticosteroids ↑
     3. Adrenergic blockers ↓
     4. Tricyclic antidepressants ↓
 B. Effect of Other Drugs on Activity of Oral Contraceptives
     1. Antihistamines ↓
     2. Barbiturates ↓
     3. Mineral oil ↓
     4. Phenylbutazone ↓
     5. Sedatives and hypnotics ↓

References

Chizek, D. J., and Franceschetti, A. T.: Oral contraceptives: Their side effects and ophthalmological manifestations. Surv. Ophthalmol. *14*:90, 1969.

Connell, E. B., and Kelman, C. D.: Eye examinations in patients taking oral contraceptives. Fertil. Steril. *20*:67, 1969.

Faust, J. M., and Tyler, E. T.: Ophthalmologic findings in patients using oral contraception. Fertil. Steril. *17*:1, 1966.

Fulmek, R.: Occlusion of a branch of the central retinal artery after prolonged use of ovulation inhibitors. Klin. Monatsbl. Augenheilkd. *164*:371, 1974.

Goren, S. B.: Retinal edema secondary to oral contraceptives. Am. J. Ophthalmol. *64*:447, 1967.

McGrand, J. C., and Cory, C. C.: Ophthalmic disease and the pill. Br. Med. J. *2*:187, 1969.

Salmon, M. L., Winkelman, J. Z., and Gay, A. J.: Neuro-ophthalmic sequelae in users of oral contraceptives. JAMA *206*:85, 1968.

Walsh, F. B., et al.: Oral contraceptives and neuro-ophthalmologic interest. Arch. Ophthalmol. *74*:628, 1965.

* * * * * * * * * * * *

Class: Ovulatory Agents

Generic Name: Clomiphene

Proprietary Name: Clomid

Primary Use: This synthetic nonsteroidal agent is effective in the treatment of anovulation.

Ocular Side Effects

 A. Systemic Administration
     1. Decreased vision
     2. Mydriasis
     3. Visual sensations
        a. Flashing lights
        b. Scintillating scotomas
        c. Distortion of images secondary to sensations of waves or glare
        d. Various colored lights — mainly silver
        e. Phosphene stimulation

       f. Prolongation of after image
4. Visual fields
       a. Scotomas — central
       b. Constriction
5. Photophobia
6. Diplopia
7. Eyelids or conjunctiva
       a. Allergic reactions
       b. Urticaria
8. Retinal vasospasms (?)
9. Detachment posterior vitreous (?)
10. Posterior subcapsular cataracts (?)

Clinical Significance: Ocular side effects are seen in 5 to 10 percent of patients taking clomiphene. Ocular symptoms are severe enough to require some to discontinue the use of this drug. Except for detachment of the posterior vitreous and posterior subcapsular cataracts, which are both questionable side effects, all others are reversible with discontinuation of the drug.

References

Beck, P., et al.: Induction of ovulation with clomiphene. Report of a study including comparison with intravenous estrogen and human chorionic gonadotropin. Obstet. Gynecol. 27:54, 1966.

Grant, W. M.: Toxicology of the Eye. 2nd Ed., Springfield, Charles C Thomas, 1974, p. 301.

Roch, L. M., II, et al.: Visual changes associated with clomiphene citrate therapy. Arch. Ophthalmol. 77:14, 1967.

Today's Drugs. Clomiphene citrate. Br. Med. J. 1:363, 1968.

Walsh, F. B., and Hoyt, W. F.: Clinical Neuro-Ophthalmology. 3rd Ed., Baltimore, Williams & Wilkins, Vol. III, 1969, pp. 2686–2687.

* * * * * * * * * * * *

Class: Thyroid Hormones

Generic Names: 1. Dextrothyroxine; 2. Thyroid

Proprietary Name: 1. Choloxin, Choloxon (G.B.), Dethyron (Denm.), Dethyrona (Norw.); 2. S-P-T, Thyranon (Swed.), Thyrar, Thyreototal (Swed.)

Primary Use: These thyroid hormones are effective in the replacement therapy of thyroid deficiencies such as hypothyroidism and simple goiter. Dextrothyroxine is also effective in the management of hypercholesterolemia.

Ocular Side Effects

A. Systemic Administration
1. Decreased vision (thyroid)
2. Conjunctival hyperemia (thyroid)
3. Ptosis (dextrothyroxine)
4. Loss of eyelashes or eyebrows (?) (dextrothyroxine)
5. Exophthalmos (?) (thyroid)
6. Scotomas — central (?) (thyroid)
7. Optic neuritis (?) (thyroid)
8. Optic atrophy (?) (thyroid)

Clinical Significance: There have been no reports in the past three decades of ocular side effects of any consequence related to these drugs. Ptosis and loss of eyelashes or eyebrows have only been reported with dextrothyroxine, while the other listed ocular side effects have only been reported with thyroid.

Interactions with Other Drugs

A. Effect of Thyroid Hormones on Activity of Other Drugs
1. Analgesics ↑
2. Sympathomimetics ↑
3. Tricyclic antidepressants ↑
4. Adrenergic blockers ↓
5. Barbiturates ↓
B. Effect of Other Drugs on Activity of Thyroid Hormones
1. Barbiturates ↑
2. Tricyclic antidepressants ↑

References

Brain, W. R.: Exophthalmos following administration of thyroid extract. Lancet *1*:182, 1936.

Grant, W. M.: Toxicology of the Eye. 2nd Ed., Springfield, Charles C Thomas, 1974, pp. 1014–1015.

Uenoyama, E.: Atrophia nervi optici after taking an anti-fat remedy. (Thyreoidine ?) Jahresbericht Ophthalmol. *63*:147, 1936.

Walsh, F. B., and Hoyt, W. F.: Clinical Neuro-Ophthalmology. 3rd Ed., Baltimore, Williams & Wilkins, Vol. III, 1969, p. 2592.

* * * * * * * * * * * *

VIII. Agents Affecting Blood Formation and Coagulability

Class: Agents Used to Treat Deficiency Anemias

Generic Name: Cobalt

Proprietary Name: Cobalt

Primary Use: This agent is used in the treatment of iron-deficiency anemia.

Ocular Side Effects

A. Systemic Administration
1. Decreased vision
2. Cataracts
3. Visual fields (?)
   a. Scotomas — central or paramacular
   b. Constriction
4. Retinal hemorrhages (?)
5. Optic atrophy (?)
6. Retinal edema (?)
7. Choroidal pigmentary changes (?)
8. Decreased choroidal profusion (?)

Clinical Significance: Cobalt is now only occasionally used since significant systemic side effects occur and safer drugs are currently available. Only rarely are ocular side effects due to cobalt therapy seen, and decreased vision is most common. Recently a case suggestive of cobalt-induced optic atrophy with retinal and choroidal changes was reported.

References

Goodman, L. S., and Gilman, A. (Eds.): The Pharmacological Basis of Therapeutics. 4th Ed., New York, Macmillan, 1970, p. 1409.
Light, A., Oliver, M., and Rachmilewitz, E. A.: Optic atrophy following treatment with cobalt chloride in a patient with pancytopenia and hypercellular marrow. Isr. J. Med. Sci. 8:61, 1972.
Walsh, F. B., and Hoyt, W. F.: Clinical Neuro-Ophthalmology. 3rd Ed., Baltimore, Williams & Wilkins, Vol. III, 1969, pp. 2686–2687.

* * * * * * * * * * * *

Generic Name: 1. Ferrocholinate; 2. Ferrous Fumarate; 3. Ferrous Gluconate; 4. Ferrous Succinate; 5. Ferrous Sulfate; 6. Iron Dextran; 7. Iron Sorbitex; 8. Polysaccharide-Iron Complex

Proprietary Name: 1. Ferrolip; 2. Feostat, Feramal (Austral.), Feroton (Canad.), Ferrofume (Canad.), Fersaday (G.B.), Fersamal (G.B.), Fumiron (Austral.), Ircon, Laud-Iron, Palafer (Canad.), Span-FF, Toleron, Tolifer (Canad.); 3. Ferate (Austral.), Fergon, Ferrin-55 (Austral.), Ferro-G (Austral.), Ferronicum (Austral.), Ferrose (Austral.), Glistron (G.B.), Gluciron (Austral.), Glucohaem (Austral.), Ironate (Austral.); 4. Ferromyn (G.B.); 5. Feosol, Feospan (G.B.), Fer-In-Sol, Ferri-Vita (Austral.), Fero-Grad-500, Fero-Gradumet, Haemofort (Austral.), Polyhaemen (Austral.), Slow-Fe (G.B.), Toniron (G.B.); 6. Direx (G.B.), Imferon, Ironorm (G.B.); 7. Jectofer; 8. Hytinic, Niferex, Nu-Iron

Primary Use: These iron preparations are effective in the prophylaxis and treatment of iron-deficiency anemias.

Ocular Side Effects

A. Systemic Administration
1. Decreased vision (iron dextran)
2. Yellow-brown discoloration
   a. Sclera
   b. Choroid
3. Eyelids or conjunctiva (iron dextran)
   a. Erythema
   b. Edema
   c. Angioneurotic edema
4. Retinal degeneration
5. Optic neuritis (?)
6. Optic atrophy (?)
7. Problems with color vision — dyschromatopsia (?)
B. Inadvertent Ocular Exposure
1. Irritation
   a. Hyperemia
   b. Photophobia
2. Yellow-brown discoloration or deposits
   a. Eyelids
   b. Conjunctiva
   c. Cornea
   d. Sclera
3. Hypopyon
4. Ulceration
   a. Eyelids
   b. Conjunctiva
   c. Cornea

Clinical Significance: Systemically administered iron preparations seldom cause ocular side effects. Adverse ocular reactions have been reported after multiple blood transfusions (over 100), unusually large amounts of iron in the diet, or markedly prolonged iron therapy. A few cases of retinitis pigmentosa-like fundal degeneration have been reported. Direct ocular exposure to acidic ferrous salts can cause ocular irritation, but significant ocular side effects rarely occur.

Interactions with Other Drugs

- A.   Effect of Iron on Activity of Other Drugs
    1. Tetracyclines ↓
- B.   Effect of Other Drugs on Activity of Iron
    1. Antacids ↓
    2. Chloramphenicol ↓

References

Chisholm, J. F.: Iron pigmentation of the palpebral conjunctiva. Am. J. Ophthalmol. *33*:1108, 1950.

Duke-Elder, S.: Systems of Ophthalmology. St. Louis, C. V. Mosby, Vol. XIV, Part 2, 1972, p. 1099.

Grant, W. M.: Toxicology of the Eye. 2nd Ed., Springfield, Charles C Thomas, 1974, pp. 594–605.

Lane, R. S.: Intravenous infusion of iron-dextran complex for iron-deficiency anaemia. Lancet *1*:852, 1964.

Meyler, L., and Herxheimer, A. (Eds.): Side Effects of Drugs. Amsterdam, Excerpta Medica, Vol. VII, 1972, pp. 320–322.

Zuckerman, B. D., and Lieberman, T. W.: Corneal rust ring. Arch. Ophthalmol. *63*:254, 1960.

* * * * * * * * * * * *

Generic Name: Methylene Blue (Methylthionine)

Proprietary Name: M-B Tabs, Urolene Blue

Primary Use: *Systemic:* Methylene blue is a weak germicidal agent used in the treatment of methemoglobinemia and "cyanosis anemia" and as a urinary or gastrointestinal antiseptic. It is also used as a dye to demonstrate cerebrospinal fluid fistulae or blocks. *Ophthalmic:* Methylene blue is used as a tissue marker during ocular or lacrimal surgery and has been applied to the conjunctiva to decrease glare during microsurgery.

Ocular Side Effects

- A.   Systemic Administration
    1. Decreased vision
    2. Decreased accommodation
    3. Mydriasis
    4. Papilledema
    5. Diplopia
    6. Paresis of extraocular muscles
    7. Accommodative spasm

8. Optic atrophy
9. Blindness
10. Blue-gray discoloration of ocular tissue — especially vitreous and retina
11. Problems with color vision — objects have blue tinge
12. Subconjunctival or retinal hemorrhages secondary to drug-induced anemia
B. Local Ophthalmic Use or Exposure
1. Burning sensation
2. Stains corneal nerves

Clinical Significance: Severe ocular side effects due to methylene blue have only been reported with intrathecal or intraventricular injections. The most common ocular side effects after intravenous administration other than cyanopsia or blue-gray discoloration of ocular tissue are decreased vision, mydriasis, and decreased accommodation. Topical ocular application in low concentrations (1%) is almost free of ocular side effects; however, irritation is so severe that a local anesthetic is required for the patient's comfort.

References

Evans, J. P., and Keegan, H. R.: Danger in the use of intrathecal methylene blue. JAMA *174*:856, 1960.
Gerber, A., and Lambert, R. K.: Blue appearance of fundus caused by prolonged ingestion of methylthionine chloride. Arch. Ophthalmol. *16*:443, 1936.
Lubeck, M. J.: Effects of drugs on ocular muscles. Int. Ophthalmol. Clin. *11*(2):35, 1971.
Norn, M. S.: Methylene blue (Methylthionine) vital staining of the cornea and conjunctiva. Acta Ophthalmol. *45*:347, 1967.
Walsh, F. B., and Hoyt, W. F.: Clinical Neuro-Ophthalmology. 3rd Ed., Baltimore, Williams & Wilkins, Vol. III, 1969, pp. 2706–2707.

* * * * * * * * * * * *

Class: Anticoagulants

Generic Name: 1. Acenocoumarin; 2. Bishydroxycoumarin (Dicoumarol); 3. Phenprocoumon; 4. Warfarin

Proprietary Name: 1. Nicoumalone (G.B.), Sinthrome (G.B.), Sintrom; 2. Dicumarol; 3. Liquamar, Marcoumar (G.B.); 4. Athrombin-K, Coumadin, Mareran (G.B.), Panwarfin, Prothromadin

Primary Use: These coumarin derivatives are used as anticoagulants in the prophylaxis and treatment of venous thrombosis.

Ocular Side Effects

A.   Systemic Administration
1.   Subconjunctival or retinal hemorrhages
a.   Secondary to drug-induced anticoagulation
b.   Secondary to drug-induced anemia
2.   Eyelids or conjunctiva
a.   Allergic reactions
b.   Conjunctivitis — nonspecific
c.   Urticaria
3.   Lacrimation (bishydroxycoumarin)
4.   Blindness (bishydroxycoumarin)
5.   Loss of eyelashes or eyebrows (?)
6.   Congenital optic atrophy (?)

Clinical Significance: Ocular side effects due to coumarin anticoagulants are rare. Massive retinal hemorrhages, especially in diseased tissue with possible capillary fragility (disciform degeneration of the macula), have been reported. Even so, as extensively as this group of agents has been used, only a few adverse ocular side effects have been reported. These drugs should be discontinued prior to ocular surgery to prevent increased hemorrhaging, especially in patients with diabetes or hypertension.

Interactions with Other Drugs

A.   Effect of Other Drugs on Activity of Coumarins
1.   Adrenergic blockers ↑
2.   Analgesics ↑
3.   Antibiotics ↑
(Chloramphenicol, Kanamycin, Neomycin, Penicillins, Streptomycin, Sulfonamides, Tetracyclines)
4.   Chymotrypsin-trypsin ↑
5.   General anesthetics ↑
6.   Monoamine oxidase inhibitors ↑
7.   Oxyphenbutazone ↑
8.   Phenylbutazone ↑
9.   Salicylates ↑
10.   Urea ↑
11.   Alcohol ↑↓
12.   Corticosteroids ↑↓
13.   Antacids ↓
14.   Antihistamines ↓
15.   Barbiturates ↓
16.   Diuretics ↓
17.   Phenothiazines ↓
18.   Sedatives and hypnotics ↓

References

Feman, S. S., et al.: Intraocular hemorrhage and blindness associated with systemic anticoagulation. JAMA *220*:1354, 1972.

Gordon, D. M., and Mead, J.: Retinal hemorrhage with visual loss during anticoagulant therapy: Case report. J. Am. Geriatr. Soc. *16*:99, 1968.
Klingensmith, W., and Oles, P.: Surgical complications of Dicumarol therapy. Am. J. Surg. *108*:640, 1964.
Physicians' Desk Reference. 28th Ed., Oradell, N. J., Medical Economics Co., 1974, pp. 504, 532, 775.
Walsh, F. B., and Hoyt, W. F.: Clinical Neuro-Ophthalmology. 3rd Ed., Baltimore, Williams & Wilkins, Vol. III, 1969, pp. 2683–2684.

* * * * * * * * * * * * *

Generic Name: 1. Anisindione; 2. Diphenadione; 3. Phenindione

Proprietary Name: 1. Miradon; 2. Dipaxin; 3. Acluton (Austral.), Danilone, Dindevan (G.B.), Eridione, Haemopan (Austral.), Hedulin, Theradione (G.B.)

Primary Use: These indandione derivatives are used as anticoagulants in the prophylaxis and treatment of venous thrombosis.

Ocular Side Effects

A. Systemic Administration
1. Subconjunctival or retinal hemorrhages
   a. Secondary to drug-induced anticoagulation
   b. Secondary to drug-induced anemia
2. Decreased vision
3. Paralysis of accommodation
4. Eyelids or conjunctiva
   a. Allergic reactions
   b. Conjunctivitis — nonspecific
   c. Urticaria
   d. Exfoliative dermatitis
5. Loss of eyelashes or eyebrows (?)

Clinical Significance: The most common adverse ocular reaction due to these indandione anticoagulants is ocular hemorrhage, which is just an extension of the intended pharmacologic activity of these drugs. This is probably more common in ocular conditions with associated capillary fragility such as disciform macular degeneration. Most other ocular side effects are uncommon, insignificant, and reversible.

Interactions with Other Drugs

A. Effect of Other Drugs on Activity of Indandiones
1. Adrenergic blockers ↑
2. Analgesics ↑
3. Antibiotics ↑
   (Chloramphenicol, Kanamycin, Neomycin, Penicillins, Streptomycin, Sulfonamides, Tetracyclines)
4. Chymotrypsin — trypsin ↑
5. General anesthetics ↑
6. Monoamine oxidase inhibitors ↑

    7.   Oxyphenbutazone ↑
    8.   Phenylbutazone ↑
    9.   Salicylates ↑
  10.   Urea ↑
  11.   Alcohol ↑↓
  12.   Corticosteroids ↑↓
  13.   Antacids ↓
  14.   Antihistamines ↓
  15.   Barbiturates ↓
  16.   Diuretics ↓
  17.   Phenothiazines ↓
  18.   Sedatives and hypnotics ↓

References

American Hospital Formulary Service. Washington, D.C., American Society of Hospital Pharmacists, Vol. 1, 20:12.04, 1973.

Blacow, N. W. (Ed.): Martindale: The Extra Pharmacopoeia. 26th Ed., London, Pharmaceutical Press, 1972, pp. 867, 869–874.

Goodman, L. S., and Gilman, A. (Eds.): The Pharmacological Basis of Therapeutics. 4th Ed., New York, Macmillan, 1970, pp. 1451–1459.

Physicians' Desk Reference. 28th Ed., Oradell, N. J., Medical Economics Co., 1974, p. 1311.

* * * * * * * * * * * *

Generic Name: Heparin

Proprietary Name: Depo-Heparin, Hepathrom, Lipo-Hepin, Liquaemin, Panheprin, Pularin (G.B.)

Primary Use: This complex organic acid inhibits the blood clotting mechanism and is used in the prophylaxis and treatment of venous thrombosis.

Ocular Side Effects

  A.   Systemic Administration
    1.   Subconjunctival or retinal hemorrhages
      a.   Secondary to drug-induced anticoagulation
      b.   Secondary to drug-induced anemia
    2.   Eyelids or conjunctiva
      a.   Allergic reactions
      b.   Conjunctivitis — nonspecific
      c.   Angioneurotic edema
      d.   Urticaria
    3.   Lacrimation
    4.   Loss of eyelashes or eyebrows (?)
  B.   Local Ophthalmic Use or Exposure — Subconjunctival Injection
    1.   Subconjunctival or periocular hemorrhages
    2.   Subconjunctival scarring
    3.   Exacerbation of primary disease
    4.   Decreased intraocular pressure — minimal

Clinical Significance: Ocular side effects due to systemic heparin are few and usually of little consequence. Ocular hemorrhage is the most serious adverse reaction and is probably more common in ocular conditions with increased capillary fragility. Subconjunctival or periocular hemorrhage is the most common adverse reaction due to subconjunctival heparin injections. It is more common after the third or fourth injection and seldom prevents continuation of this mode of heparin therapy.

Interactions with Other Drugs

   A. Effect of Other Drugs on Activity of Heparin
        1. EDTA ↑
        2. Salicylates ↑
        3. Antihistamines ↓
        4. Penicillins ↓
        5. Phenothiazines ↓
        6. Tetracyclines ↓

References

Aronson, S. B., and Elliott, J. H.: Ocular Inflammation. St. Louis, C. V. Mosby, 1972, pp. 91–92.
Goodman, L. S., and Gilman, A., (Eds.): The Pharmacological Basis of Therapeutics. 4th Ed., New York, Macmillan, 1970, pp. 1446–1451.
Lipson, M. L.: Toxicity of systemic agents. Int. Ophthalmol. Clin. 11(2):159, 1971.
Physicians' Desk Reference. 28th Ed., Oradell, N. J., Medical Economics Co., 1974, pp. 531, 1192.
Turcotte, J. G., Kraft, R. O., and Fry, W. J.: Heparin reactions in patients with vascular disease. Arch. Surg. 90:375, 1965.

* * * * * * * * * * * * *

Class: Oxytocic Agents

Generic Name: Ergot

Proprietary Name: Ergoapiol (G.B.)

Primary Use: This drug is used to control postpartum and illegal abortion hemorrhages.

Ocular Side Effects

   A. Systemic Administration
        1. Decreased vision
        2. Paralysis of accommodation
        3. Hypermetropia

4. Pupils
   a.   Mydriasis — acute
   b.   Miosis
   c.   Decreased reaction to light
5. Blindness
6. Visual fields
   a.   Scotomas
   b.   Constriction
   c.   Enlarged blind spot
7. Retinal edema
8. Retinal vasoconstriction
9. Scintillating scotomas (?)
10. Diplopia (?)
11. Nystagmus (?)
12. Optic atrophy (?)
13. Cataracts (?)

Clinical Significance: Ergot preparations have caused numerous ocular side effects, primarily in overdose situations for attempted abortions. In general, these adverse ocular reactions are usually transitory and rarely permanent. While blindness may occur, it is in most instances reversible. Cataracts have not been reported with medically administered ergot. In an unusual form of epidemic ergot intoxication due to contaminated grain, cataracts, diplopia, nystagmus, and scintillating scotomas were commonly seen.

Interactions with Other Drugs

A.   Synergistic Activity
   1.   Sympathomimetics

References

Blacow, N. W. (Ed.): Martindale: The Extra Pharmacopoeia. 26th Ed., London, Pharmaceutical Press, 1972, pp. 697–698.

Grant, W. M.: Toxicology of the Eye. 2nd Ed., Springfield, Charles C Thomas, 1974, pp. 454–456.

Kravitz, D.: Neuroretinitis associated with symptoms of ergot poisoning: Report of a case. Arch. Ophthalmol. *73*:201, 1935.

Schneider, P.: Beiderseitige Ophthalmoplegia interna, hervorgerufen durch Extractum Secalis cornuti. Munch. Med. Wochenschr. *49*:1620, 1902.

Scott, J. G.: Does ergot cause cataract? Med. Proc. *8*:4, 1962.

* * * * * * * * * * * * *

IX. Homeostatic and Nutrient Agents

Class: Agents Used to Treat Hyperglycemia

Generic Name: 1. Acetohexamide; 2. Chlorpropamide; 3. Tolazamide; 4. Tolbutamide

Proprietary Name: 1. Dimelor (G.B.), Dymelor; 2. Diabinese, Dialane (Ind.) 3. Tolanase (G.B.), Tolinase; 4. Arcosal (Denm.), Dolipol (Fr.), Ipoglicone (Ital.), Mobenol (Canad.), Orinase, Rastinon (G.B.), Tol 500 (Canad.), Tolbugen (Canad.), Tolbutol (Canad.), Tolbutone (Canad.)

Primary Use: These oral hypoglycemic sulfonylureas are effective in the management of selected cases of diabetes mellitus.

Ocular Side Effects

A. Systemic Administration
1. Decreased vision
2. Paresis of extraocular muscles
3. Diplopia
4. Eyelids or conjunctiva
   a. Allergic reactions
   b. Hyperemia
   c. Conjunctivitis — nonspecific
   d. Edema
   e. Photosensitivity
   f. Purpura
   g. Erythema multiforme
   h. Stevens-Johnson syndrome
   i. Exfoliative dermatitis
5. Photophobia
6. Subconjunctival or retinal hemorrhages secondary to drug-induced anemia
7. Scotomas — central or centrocecal (?) (chlorpropamide)
8. Retrobulbar or optic neuritis (?)
9. Hypermetropia (?) (tolbutamide)
10. Loss of eyelashes or eyebrows (?)

Clinical Significance: As with other hypoglycemics, the sulfonylureas have few documented toxic effects on the eyes. Adverse ocular reactions are mainly due to drug-induced hypoglycemic attacks. Chlorpropamide has a 6 percent incidence of untoward reactions, while the incidence of acetohexamide, tolazamide, and tolbutamide is around 3 percent. Cutaneous reactions due to these drugs are not unusual. While optic nerve disease has been reported, differentiation of which changes are due to diabetes and which are due to a toxic drug effect is difficult. There are two case reports implicating chlorpropamide with scotomas and decreased vision.

Interactions with Other Drugs

   A. Effect of Sulfonylureas on Activity of Other Drugs
        1. Barbiturates ↑
        2. Phenylbutazone ↑
        3. Salicylates ↑
        4. Sedatives and hypnotics ↑
        5. Sulfonamides ↑
   B. Effect of Other Drugs on Activity of Sulfonylureas
        1. Adrenergic blockers ↑
        2. Analgesics ↑
        3. Chloramphenicol ↑
        4. Monoamine oxidase inhibitors ↑
        5. Oxyphenbutazone ↑
        6. Phenylbutazone ↑
        7. Salicylates ↑
        8. Sulfonamides ↑
        9. Alcohol ↑↓
      10. Phenothiazines ↑↓
      11. Corticosteroids ↓
      12. Diuretics ↓
      13. Sympathomimetics ↓

References

Catros, A., et al.: Nevrite optique axiale bilaterale au cours d'un traitement par le D860. Rev. Otoneuroophtalmol. *30*:253, 1958.

Davidson, S. I.: Report of ocular adverse reactions. Trans. Ophthalmol. Soc. U. K. *93*:495, 1973.

George, C. W.: Central scotomata due to chlorpropamide (Diabenese). Arch. Ophthalmol. *69*:773, 1963.

Givner, I.: Centrocecal scotomas due to chlorpropamide. Arch. Ophthalmol. *66*:64, 1961.

Kapetansky, F. M.: Refractive changes with tolbutamide. Ohio State Med. J. *59*:275, 1963.

Meyler, L., and Herxheimer, A. (Eds.): Side Effects of Drugs. Amsterdam, Excerpta Medica, Vol. VII, 1972, pp. 583–587.

* * * * * * * * * * * *

Generic Name: Insulin

Proprietary Name: Lente, NPH, Regular, Semilente, Ultralente (Iletin or Insulin)

Primary Use: This hypoglycemic agent is effective in the management of diabetes mellitus.

Ocular Side Effects

A. Systemic Administration
1. Decreased vision
2. Nystagmus
3. Paresis of extraocular muscles
4. Diplopia
5. Pupils
  a. Mydriasis
  b. Absence of reaction to light
6. Eyelids or conjunctiva
  a. Allergic reactions
  b. Blepharoconjunctivitis
  c. Angioneurotic edema
7. Strabismus
8. Decreased intraocular pressure
9. Anosognosia (?)

Clinical Significance: Insulin has no direct toxic effect on the eyes. The ocular side effects due to insulin are probably secondary to hypoglycemic attacks. Nearly all ocular side effects are reversible; however, some may take weeks to resolve.

Interactions with Other Drugs

A. Effect of Insulin on Activity of Other Drugs
1. Sympathomimetics ↓
B. Effect of Other Drugs on Activity of Insulin
1. Alcohol ↑
2. Analgesics ↑
3. Chloramphenicol ↑
4. Monoamine oxidase inhibitors ↑
5. Oxyphenbutazone ↑
6. Phenylbutazone ↑
7. Salicylates ↑
8. Sulfonamides ↑
9. Corticosteroids ↓
10. Diuretics ↓
11. Sympathomimetics ↓

References

AMA Drug Evaluations. 2nd Ed., Acton, Mass., Publishing Sciences Group, 1973, pp. 126–129.

Gralnick, A.: The retina and intraocular tension during prolonged insulin coma with autopsy eye findings. Am. J. Ophthalmol. 24:1174, 1941.

Grant, W. M.: Toxicology of the Eye. 2nd Ed., Springfield, Charles C Thomas, 1974, pp. 579–580.

Walsh, F. B., and Hoyt, W. F.: Clinical Neuro-Ophthalmology. 3rd Ed., Baltimore, Williams & Wilkins, Vol. III, 1969, pp. 2684–2685.

* * * * * * * * * * * *

Generic Name: Phenformin

Proprietary Name: DBI, Dibotin (G.B.), Insoral (Austral.), Meltrol

Primary Use: This biguanide derivative is effective in the management of selected cases of diabetes mellitus.

Ocular Side Effects

  A. Systemic Administration
  1. Decreased vision
  2. Myopia
  3. Diplopia
  4. Subconjunctival or retinal hemorrhages secondary to drug-induced anemia

Clinical Significance: Adverse ocular reactions due to phenformin are quite rare, transient, and usually insignificant. Like many other hypoglycemics, phenformin has no documented toxic effect on the eyes, and adverse ocular reactions are primarily due to drug-induced hypoglycemic attacks.

Interactions with Other Drugs

  A. Effect of Phenformin on Activity of Other Drugs
  1. Sympathomimetics ↑
  B. Effect of Other Drugs on Activity of Phenformin
  1. Corticosteroids ↓
  2. Diuretics ↓

References

Blacow, N. W. (Ed.): Martindale: The Extra Pharmacopoeia. 26th Ed., London, Pharmaceutical Press, 1972, pp. 969–972.
Grant, W. M.: Toxicology of the Eye. 2nd Ed., Springfield, Charles C Thomas, 1974, p. 806.
Physicians' Desk Reference. 28th Ed., Oradell, N. J., Medical Economics Co., 1974, p. 774.
Scialdone, D., and Artifoni, E.: Miopia transitoria in corso di terapia con Debinyl. G. Ital. Oftal. 16:92, 1963.

* * * * * * * * * * * *

Class: Vitamins

Generic Name: Vitamin A

Proprietary Name: Acon, Alphalin, Aquasol A, Atamin Forte (Austral.), Carotin (Austral.), DispAtabs, Resistovites, Ro-A-Vit (G.B.), Super A Vitamin, Testavol-S, Vi-Dom-A, Vio-A

Primary Use: Vitamin A is used as a dietary supplement and in the management of vitamin A-deficient states.

Ocular Side Effects

A. Systemic Administration
1. Nystagmus
2. Loss of eyelashes or eyebrows
3. Paresis or paralysis of extraocular muscles
4. Diplopia
5. Yellow discoloration of eyelids
6. Papilledema secondary to pseudotumor cerebri
7. Miosis
8. Exophthalmos
9. Strabismus
10. Decreased intraocular pressure
11. Enlarged blind spot
12. Problems with color vision
    a. Objects have yellow tinge
    b. Improves red achromatopsia
13. Subconjunctival or retinal hemorrhages secondary to drug-induced anemia
14. Cataracts (?)

Clinical Significance: Ocular side effects due to hypervitaminosis A are much more frequent and extensive in infants and children than in adults. Nearly all ocular side effects are rapidly reversible after the vitamin therapy is discontinued; however, in some instances it may be several months before these effects are completely resolved, probably because of the extensive storage of vitamin A in the liver. If exophthalmos occurs, it may be secondary to thyroid changes since vitamin A has antithyroid activity.

Interactions with Other Drugs

A. Effect of Vitamin A on Activity of Other Drugs
1. Corticosteroids ↓

References

DiBenedetto, R. J.: Chronic hypervitaminosis A in an adult. JAMA 201:700, 1967.
Lascari, A. D., and Bell, W. E.: Pseudotumor cerebri due to hypervitaminosis A. Clin. Pediatr. 9:627, 1970.
Muenter, M. D., Perry, H. O., and Ludwig, J.: Chronic vitamin A intoxication in adults. Hepatic, neurologic and dermatologic complications. Am. J. Med. 50:129, 1971.
Oliver, T. K., and Havener, W. H.: Eye manifestations of chronic vitamin A intoxication. Arch. Ophthalmol. 60:19, 1958.
Turtz, C. A., and Turtz, A. I.: Vitamin-A intoxication. Am. J. Ophthalmol. 50:165, 1960.

* * * * * * * * * * * *

Generic Name: 1. Vitamin D; 2. Vitamin D_2 (Ergocalciferol); 3. Vitamin D_3

Proprietary Name: 1. Vitamin D; 2. Calciferol (G.B.), Deltalin, Deltavit (Ital.), Drisdol, Sterogyl-15 (G.B.); 3. Cholecalciferol (G.B.), D_3-Vicotrat (Germ.), Vi-De-3 Hydrosol (Germ.), Vigantol (Germ.), Vigantoletten (Germ.)

Primary Use: Vitamin D is used as a dietary supplement and in the management of vitamin D-deficient states and hypoparathyroidism.

Ocular Side Effects

A.   Systemic Administration
1. Esotropia
2. Epicanthus
3. Calcium deposits or band keratopathy
   a. Conjunctiva
   b. Cornea
   c. Sclera
4. Nystagmus
5. Decreased pupillary reaction to light
6. Narrowed optic foramina
7. Papilledema
8. Optic atrophy
9. Small optic discs
10. Visual hallucinations
11. Subconjunctival or retinal hemorrhages secondary to drug-induced anemia
12. Paresis of extraocular muscles (?)
13. Optic neuritis (?)
14. Cataracts (?)
15. Hemianopsia (?)

Clinical Significance: Severe adverse ocular reactions due to vitamin D are either caused by a direct toxicity or an unusual sensitivity and are primarily seen in infants. Calcium deposits in or around the optic canal cause narrowing of the optic foramina, which may in turn cause papilledema. If the vitamin intake is not discontinued, optic atrophy may result. Children with these toxic effects often have elfin-like faces and prominent epicanthal folds. In adults, the toxic effects are few and the calcium deposits in ocular tissue appear to be the main adverse reaction. One case of a presumed basilar artery insufficiency with hemianopsia due to vitamin D intake has been reported.

References

Cogan, D. G., Albright, F., and Bartter, F. C.: Hypercalcemia and band keratopathy. Arch. Ophthalmol. *40*:624, 1948.

Gartner, S., and Rubner, K.: Calcified scleral nodules in hypervitaminosis D. Am. J. Ophthalmol. *39*:658, 1955.

Harley, R. D., et al.: Idiopathic hypercalcemia of infancy: Optic atrophy and other ocular changes. Trans. Am. Acad. Ophthalmol. Otolaryngol. *69*:977, 1965.

Meyler, L., and Herxheimer, A. (Eds.): Side Effects of Drugs. Amsterdam, Excerpta Medica, Vol. VII, 1972, pp. 510–512.

Wagener, H. P.: The ocular manifestations of hypercalcemia. Am. J. Med. Sci. *231*:218, 1956.

* * * * * * * * * * * *

X. Agents Used to Treat Allergic and Neuromuscular Disorders

Class: Agents Used to Treat Myasthenia Gravis

Generic Name: 1. Ambenonium; 2. Edrophonium; 3. Pyridostigmine

Proprietary Name: 1. Mytelase; 2. Tensilon; 3. Mestinon

Primary Use: These anticholinesterase agents are effective in the treatment of myasthenia gravis. Edrophonium is primarily used as an antidote for curariform agents and as a diagnostic test for myasthenia gravis.

Ocular Side Effects
A. Systemic Administration
   1. Miosis
   2. Decreased vision
   3. Diplopia
   4. Lacrimation
   5. Blepharoclonus
B. Local Ophthalmic Use or Exposure — Edrophonium
   1. Photophobia
   2. Eyelids or conjunctiva
      a. Allergic reactions
      b. Conjunctivitis — nonspecific
   3. Iritis
   4. Iris cysts
   5. Decreased anterior chamber depth
   6. Vitreous hemorrhages
   7. Cataracts

Clinical Significance: Ocular side effects due to these anticholinesterase agents are rare and seldom of clinical significance. All adverse ocular reactions are reversible with discontinued drug use. Blepharoclonus is only seen in overdose situations.

Interactions with Other Drugs
A. Effect of Anticholinesterases on Activity of Other Drugs
   1. Antibiotics ↓ (edrophonium)
      (Kanamycin, Neomycin, Streptomycin)

B.   Effect of Other Drugs on Activity of Anticholinesterases
    1.   Antihistamines ↑
    2.   Monoamine oxidase inhibitors ↑
    3.   Phenothiazines ↑
    4.   Tricyclic antidepressants ↑

References

AMA Drug Evaluations. 2nd Ed., Acton, Mass., Publishing Sciences Group, 1973, pp. 751–752.

American Hospital Formulary Service. Washington, D. C., American Society of Hospital Pharmacists, Vol. 1, 12:04, 1959–1961.

Goodman, L. S., and Gilman, A. (Eds.): The Pharmacological Basis of Therapeutics. 4th Ed., New York, Macmillan, 1970, pp. 442–465.

Leopold, I. H. (Ed.): Glaucoma Drug Therapy: Monograph 1, Parasympathetic Agents. Irvine, Calif., Allergan Pharmaceuticals, 1975, pp. 19–21.

Meyler, L., and Herxheimer, A.: Side Effects of Drugs. Amsterdam, Excerpta Medica, Vol. VII, 1972, pp. 239, 241.

Physicians' Desk Reference. 28th Ed., Oradell, N. J., Medical Economics Co., 1974, p. 1230.

* * * * * * * * * * * *

Class: Antihistamines

Generic Name: 1. Brompheniramine; 2. Chlorpheniramine; 3. Dexbrompheniramine; 4. Dexchlorpheniramine; 5. Dimethindene

Proprietary Name: 1. Dimegan (Fr.), Dimetane, Dimotane (G.B.); 2. Allerbid, Allergex (Austral.), Antagonate, Chlo-Amine, Chloramate, Chlor-Trimeton, Drize, Enamine (Austral.), Haynon (G.B.), Histadur, Histafen (G.B.), Histaids (Austral.), Histaspan, Histrey, Piranex (Austral.), Piriton (G.B.), Teldrin; 3. Disomer; 4. Polaramine; 5. Fenostil (G.B.), Forhistal, Triten

Primary Use: These alkylamine antihistamines are used in the symptomatic relief of allergic or vasomotor rhinitis, allergic conjunctivitis, and allergic skin manifestations.

Ocular Side Effects

A.   Systemic Administration
    1.   Decreased vision
    2.   Pupils
       a.   Mydriasis — may precipitate narrow angle glaucoma
       b.   Decreased or absent reaction to light
    3.   Decreased tolerance to contact lenses
    4.   Diplopia
    5.   Photosensitivity (brompheniramine)
    6.   Visual hallucinations (chlorpheniramine)

7. Subconjunctival or retinal hemorrhages secondary to drug-induced anemia

Clinical Significance: Ocular side effects due to these antihistamines are rare and frequently disappear even if use of the drug is continued. These antihistamines have a weak atropine action which accounts for the pupillary changes. They probably also cause a decrease in mucoid and lacrimal secretions, which may account for decreased contact lens tolerance. Lack of pupillary responses or visual hallucinations occur only in severely toxic states due to drug overdose. The alkylamines seem to have a lower incidence of ocular side effects than do other antihistamines, with dexchlorpheniramine having the fewest reported side effects.

Interactions with Other Drugs

A. Effect of Antihistamines on Activity of Other Drugs
   1. Alcohol ↑
   2. Anticholinergics ↑
   3. Sedatives and hypnotics ↑
   4. Sympathomimetics ↑
   5. Adrenergic blockers ↓
   6. Barbiturates ↓
   7. Corticosteroids ↓
   8. Phenylbutazone ↓
B. Effect of Other Drugs on Activity of Antihistamines
   1. Monoamine oxidase inhibitors ↑
   2. Phenothiazines ↑
   3. Adrenergic blockers ↓
   4. Barbiturates ↓
   5. Phenylbutazone ↓

References

General Practitioner Research Group: A new antihistaminic and mucoinhibitory drug. Practitioner *192*:682, 1964.

Goodman, L. S., and Gilman, A. (Eds.): The Pharmacological Basis of Therapeutics. 4th Ed., New York, Macmillan, 1970, pp. 635–645.

Grant, W. M.: Toxicology of the Eye. 2nd Ed., Springfield, Charles C Thomas, 1974, pp. 281, 355.

Miller, D.: Role of the tear film in contact lens wear. Int. Ophthalmol. Clin. *13*(1):247, 1973. ·

Soleymanikashi, Y., and Weiss, N. S.: Antihistaminic reaction: A review and presentation of two unusual examples. Ann. Allergy *28*:486, 1970.

* * * * * * * * * * * *

Generic Name: 1. Carbinoxamine; 2. Diphenhydramine; 3. Diphenylpyraline; 4. Tripelennamine

Proprietary Name: 1. Clistin; 2. Alergicap (Austral.), Benadryl, Bidramine (Austral.), Histergan (G.B.), Histex (G.B.); 3. Anti-Hist (Austral.), Diafen, Hispril, Histalert (Austral.), Histryl (G.B.), Lergoban (G.B.); 4. Pyribenzamine

Primary Use: These ethanolamine antihistamines are used in the symptomatic relief of allergic or vasomotor rhinitis, allergic conjunctivitis, and allergic skin manifestations.

Ocular Side Effects

   A. Systemic Administration
      1. Decreased vision
      2. Pupils
         a. Mydriasis — may precipitate narrow-angle glaucoma
         b. Decreased or absent reaction to light
      3. Decreased tolerance to contact lenses
      4. Photosensitivity
      5. Diplopia
      6. Visual hallucinations
      7. Decrease or paralysis of accommodation
      8. Nystagmus
      9. Strabismus (diphenhydramine)
    10. Blindness
    11. Subconjunctival or retinal hemorrhages secondary to drug-induced anemia

Clinical Significance: Ocular side effects due to these antihistamines are rare and frequently disappear even if use of the drug is continued. These ethanolamines have a weak atropine action which accounts for the pupillary and ciliary body changes. These drugs also possibly cause a decrease in mucoid and lacrimal secretions, which may account for the decreased contact lens tolerance. Lack of pupillary responses, visual hallucinations, and transitory blindness only occur in severe toxic states due to drug overdose. Most of the ocular side effects in this group have been attributed to diphenhydramine and tripelennamine; however, these two drugs are the ones most commonly used.

Interactions with Other Drugs

   A. Effect of Antihistamines on Activity of Other Drugs
      1. Alcohol ↑
      2. Anticholinergics ↑
      3. Sedatives and hypnotics ↑
      4. Sympathomimetics ↑
      5. Adrenergic blockers ↓
      6. Barbiturates ↓
      7. Corticosteroids ↓
      8. Phenylbutazone ↓
   B. Effect of Other Drugs on Activity of Antihistamines
      1. Monoamine oxidase inhibitors ↑
      2. Phenothiazines ↑
      3. Adrenergic blockers ↓
      4. Barbiturates ↓
      5. Phenylbutazone ↓

References

Goodman, L. S., and Gilman, A. (Eds.): The Pharmacological Basis of Therapeutics. 4th Ed., New York, Macmillan, 1970, pp. 635–645.

Grant, W. M.: Toxicology of the Eye. 2nd Ed., Springfield, Charles C Thomas, 1974, pp. 149, 417, 1065.

Miller, D.: Role of the tear film in contact lens wear. Int. Ophthalmol. Clin. 13(1):247, 1973.

Nigro, S. A.: Toxic psychosis due to diphenhydramine hydrochloride. JAMA 203:301, 1968.

Physicians' Desk Reference. 28th Ed., Oradell, N. J., Medical Economics Co., 1974, pp. 688, 1084, 1187, 1365.

Rinker, J. R., and Sullivan, J. H.: Drug reactions following urethral instillation of tripelennamine (Pyribenzamine). J. Urol. 91:433, 1964.

Schipior, P. G.: An unusual case of antihistamine intoxication. J. Pediatr. 71:589, 1967.

Wyngaarden, V. B., and Seevers, M. H.: Toxic effects of antihistaminic drugs. JAMA 145:277, 1951.

* * * * * * * * * * * *

Generic Name: Cyproheptadine

Proprietary Name: Antegan (Austral.), Periactin

Primary Use: This potent histamine and 5-hydroxytryptamine antagonist is used in the symptomatic relief of allergic or vasomotor rhinitis, allergic conjunctivitis, and allergic skin manifestations.

Ocular Side Effects

A. Systemic Administration
 1. Decreased vision
 2. Mydriasis — may precipitate narrow-angle glaucoma
 3. Decreased tolerance to contact lenses
 4. Diplopia
 5. Photosensitivity
 6. Visual hallucinations
 7. Subconjunctival or retinal hemorrhages secondary to drug-induced anemia

Clinical Significance: Ocular side effects due to cyproheptadine are rare and frequently disappear even if use of the drug is continued. Cyproheptadine has atropine-like effects such as mydriasis and decreased secretions. Possible decreased lacrimal or mucoid secretion has been suggested as the cause of decreased tolerance to contact lenses.

Interactions with Other Drugs

A. Effect of Cyproheptadine on Activity of Other Drugs
 1. Alcohol ↑
 2. Anticholinergics ↑
 3. Sedatives and hypnotics ↑
 4. Sympathomimetics ↑

    5. Adrenergic blockers ↓
    6. Analgesics ↓
    7. Barbiturates ↓
    8. Corticosteroids ↓
    9. Phenylbutazone ↓
  B. Effect of Other Drugs on Activity of Cyproheptadine
    1. Monoamine oxidase inhibitors ↑
    2. Phenothiazines ↑
    3. Adrenergic blockers ↓
    4. Barbiturates ↓
    5. Phenylbutazone ↓

References

American Hospital Formulary Service. Washington, D. C., American Society of Hospital Pharmacists, Vol. II, 92:00, 1971.

Goodman, L. S., and Gilman, A. (Eds.): The Pharmacological Basis of Therapeutics. 4th Ed., New York, Macmillan, 1970, p. 657.

Grant, W. M.: Toxicology of the Eye. 2nd Ed., Springfield, Charles C Thomas, 1974, p. 346.

Miller, D.: Role of the tear film in contact lens wear. Int. Ophthalmol. Clin. 13(1):247, 1973.

Physicians' Desk Reference. Supplement A. Oradell, N. J., Medical Economics Co., 1974, p. A18.

* * * * * * * * * * * *

Class: Antiparkinsonism Agents

Generic Name: Amantadine

Proprietary Name: Symmetrel

Primary Use: This synthetic antiviral agent is used in the treatment of Parkinson's disease and in the prophylaxis of influenza A_2 (Asian) virus infections.

Ocular Side Effects

  A. Systemic Administration
    1. Decreased vision
    2. Visual hallucinations
    3. Oculogyric crises
    4. Eyelids or conjunctiva — eczema

Clinical Significance: Ocular side effects due to amantadine are rare except for decreased vision, which is transitory and seldom significant. All ocular effects appear to be dose-related and are reversible with discontinued amantadine usage.

Interactions with Other Drugs

    A. Effect of Amantadine on Activity of Other Drugs
        1. Anticholinergics ↑

References

AMA Drug Evaluations. 2nd Ed., Acton, Mass., Publishing Sciences Group, 1973, pp. 747–748.
American Hospital Formulary Service. Washington, D. C., American Society of Hospital Pharmacists, Vol. 1, *8*:40, 1967.
Blacow, N. W. (Ed.): Martindale: The Extra Pharmacopoeia. 26th Ed., London, Pharmaceutical Press, 1972, pp. 1065–1067.
Goodman, L. S., and Gilman, A. (Eds.): The Pharmacological Basis of Therapeutics. 4th Ed., New York, Macmillan, 1970, pp. 1305–1306.
Grant, W. M.: Toxicology of the Eye. 2nd Ed., Springfield, Charles C Thomas, 1974, p. 112.
Physicians' Desk Reference. 28th Ed., Oradell, N. J., Medical Economics Co., 1974, p. 755.

* * * * * * * * * * * *

Generic Name: 1. Benztropine; 2. Biperiden; 3. Chlorphenoxamine; 4. Cycrimine; 5. Procyclidine; 6. Trihexyphenidyl

Proprietary Name: 1. Cogentin; 2. Akineton; 3. Clorevan (G.B.), Phenoxene, Systral (Swed.); 4. Pagitane; 5. Kemadrin; 6. Anti-Spas (Austral.), Artane, Benzhexol (G.B.), Pargitan (Swed.), Peragit (Denm., Norw.), Pipanol, Tremin, Trinol (G.B.)

Primary Use: These anticholinergic agents are used in the management of Parkinson's disease and in the control of extrapyramidal disorders due to central nervous system drugs such as reserpine or the phenothiazines.

Ocular Side Effects

    A. Systemic Administration
        1. Mydriasis — may precipitate narrow-angle glaucoma
        2. Decreased vision
        3. Decrease or paralysis of accommodation
        4. Visual hallucinations

Clinical Significance: The degree of anticholinergic activity of these drugs which induce ocular side effects varies with each agent. With benztropine adverse ocular reactions are common while with biperiden they are rare. In the younger age groups, decreased accommodation may cause considerable inconveniences which may be partially reversed by topical ocular application of a weak, long-acting anticholinesterase. Significant mydriasis and visual hallucinations are primarily seen in overdose situations.

Interactions with Other Drugs

    A. Effect of Anticholinergics on Activity of Other Drugs
        1. Barbiturates ↑ (chlorphenoxamine)
    B. Effect of Other Drugs on Activity of Anticholinergics
        1. Antihistamines ↑

2. Monoamine oxidase inhibitors ↑
3. Phenothiazines ↑
4. Tricyclic antidepressants ↑

References

AMA Drug Evaluations. 2nd Ed., Acton, Mass., Publishing Sciences Group, 1973, pp. 744–746.
Grant, W. M.: Toxicology of the Eye. 2nd Ed., Springfield, Charles C Thomas, 1974, pp. 180, 190, 346, 1058.
Medina, C., Kramer, M. D., and Kurland, A. A.: Biperiden in the treatment of phenothiazine-induced extrapyramidal reactions. JAMA 182:1127, 1962.
Physicians' Desk Reference. 28th Ed., Oradell, N. J., Medical Economics Co., 1974, pp. 652, 812, 839, 1007, 1326, 1591.
Walsh, F. B., and Hoyt, W. F.: Clinical Neuro-Ophthalmology. 3rd Ed., Baltimore, Williams & Wilkins, Vol. III, 1969, pp. 2618, 2661, 2664.

* * * * * * * * * * * *

Generic Name: Caramiphen

Proprietary Name: Panparnit

Primary Use: This anticholinergic agent is used in the treatment of Parkinson's disease.

Ocular Side Effects

A. Systemic Administration
    1. Mydriasis — may precipitate narrow-angle glaucoma
    2. Paralysis of accommodation
    3. Retrobulbar neuritis (?)
    4. Scotomas (?)

Clinical Significance: Significant ocular side effects due to caramiphen are very rare. Only one case of retrobulbar neuritis has been reported; however, it was well documented. The retrobulbar neuritis occurred each time caramiphen therapy was restarted.

Interactions with Other Drugs

A. Effect of Other Drugs on Activity of Caramiphen
    1. Antihistamines ↑
    2. Monoamine oxidase inhibitors ↑
    3. Phenothiazines ↑
    4. Tricyclic antidepressants ↑

References

Bruckner, R.: Über pharmakologische Beeinflussung des Augendruckes bei verschiedenen Körperlagen. Ophthalmologica 116:200, 1948.
Grant, W. M.: Toxicology of the Eye. 2nd Ed., Springfield, Charles C Thomas, 1974, p. 228.
Hermans, G.: Le systeme moteur. Bull. Soc. Belge Ophtalmol. 160:97–106, 1972.

Leibold, J. E.: Drugs having a toxic effect on the optic nerve. Int. Ophthalmol. Clin. *11*(2):137–157, 1971.
Lubeck, M. J.: Effects of drugs on ocular muscles. Int. Ophthalmol. Clin. *11*(2):35–62, 1971.
Walsh, F. B., and Hoyt, W. F.: Clinical Neuro-Ophthalmology. 3rd Ed., Baltimore, Williams & Wilkins, Vol. III, 1969, p. 2664.

* * * * * * * * * * * * *

Generic Name: Levodopa

Proprietary Name: Bendopa, Brocadopa (G.B.), Dopar, Larodopa, Veldopa (G.B.)

Primary Use: This beta-adrenergic blocking agent is used in the management of Parkinson's disease.

Ocular Side Effects

A. Systemic Administration
    1. Pupils
        a. Mydriasis – may precipitate narrow angle glaucoma
        b. Miosis
    2. Widening of palpebral fissure
    3. Decreased vision
    4. Diplopia
    5. Blepharospasm
    6. Horner's syndrome
    7. Paresis of extraocular muscles – especially V cranial nerve
    8. Blepharoclonus
    9. Visual hallucinations
    10. Oculogyric crises
    11. Eyelids or conjunctiva
        a. Allergic reactions
        b. Edema
    12. Subconjunctival or retinal hemorrhages secondary to drug-induced anemia
    13. Loss of eyelashes or eyebrows (?)

Clinical Significance: While numerous ocular side effects due to levodopa are known, they appear to be dose-dependent, reversible, and of little clinical significance. Pupillary side effects are variable. Initially, slight mydriasis may occur which possibly has the potential to precipitate narrow-angle glaucoma. After a few weeks of levodopa therapy, miosis is not uncommon. Oculogyric crises have been precipitated by levodopa, primarily in patients with a prior history of encephalitis.

Interactions with Other Drugs

A. Effect of Levodopa on Activity of Other Drugs
    1. Sympathomimetics ↓

B.   Effect of Other Drugs on Activity of Levodopa
1.   Anticholinergics ↑
2.   Tricyclic antidepressants ↑
3.   Adrenergic blockers ↓
4.   Phenothiazines ↓

References

Meyler, L., and Herxheimer, A.: Side Effects of Drugs. Amsterdam, Excerpta Medica, Vol. VII, 1972, pp. 231–235.
Physicians' Desk Reference. 28th Ed., Oradell, N. J., Medical Economics Co., 1974, pp. 738, 799, 1223.
Spiers, A. S. D.: Mydriatic responses to sympathomimetic amines in patients treated with L-Dopa. Lancet, 2:1301, 1969.
Spiers, A. S. D., Calne, D. B., and Fayers, P. M.: Miosis during L-Dopa therapy. Br. Med. J. 2:639, 1970.
Yahr, M. D., et al.: Treatment of parkinsonism with levodopa. Arch. Neurol. 21:343, 1969.

* * * * * * * * * * * * *

Class: Cholinesterase Reactivators

Generic Name: Pralidoxime

Proprietary Name: Contrathion (Fr.), Protopam

Primary Use: This cholinesterase reactivator is used as an antidote for poisoning due to organophosphate pesticides or other chemicals which have anticholinesterase activity. It is also of value in the control of overdosage by anticholinesterase agents used in the treatment of myasthenia gravis.

Ocular Side Effects

A.   Systemic Administration
1.   Decreased vision
2.   Diplopia
3.   Decreased accommodation
B.   Local Ophthalmic Use or Exposure — Subconjunctival Injection
1.   Irritation
a.   Hyperemia
b.   Burning sensation
2.   Subconjunctival hemorrhages
3.   Iritis
4.   Reverses miosis
5.   Reverses accommodative spasms

Clinical Significance: Pralidoxime commonly causes adverse ocular reactions after systemic administration. These effects are of rapid onset, seldom last over half an hour, and are completely reversible. Ocular side effects from subconjunctival injection are also transitory and reversible.

Interactions with Other Drugs

    A. Effect of Pralidoxime on Activity of Other Drugs
        1. Anticholinesterases ↓
    B. Contraindications
        1. Analgesics
        2. Phenothiazines
        3. Succinylcholine

References

AMA Drug Evaluations. 2nd Ed., Acton, Mass., Publishing Sciences Group, 1973, pp. 728, 904–905.

Byron, H. M., and Posner, H.: Clinical evaluation of Protopam. Am. J. Ophthalmol. *57*:409, 1964.

Dekking, H. M.: Stopping the action of strong miotics. Ophthalmologica *148*:428, 1964.

Jager, B. V., and Stagg, G. N.: Toxicity of diacetyl monoxime and of pyridine-2-aldoxime methiodide in man. Bull. Johns Hopkins Hosp. *102*:203, 1958.

Taylor, W. J. R., et al.: Effects of a combination of atropine, metaraminol and pyridine aldoxime methanesulfonate (AMP therapy) on normal human subjects. Can. Med. Assoc. J. *93*:957, 1965.

* * * * * * * * * * * *

Class: Muscle Relaxants

Generic Name: 1. Mephenesin; 2. Methocarbamol

Proprietary Name: 1. Decontractyl (Fr.), Myanesin, Rhex (Germ.), Tolserol, Tolseram; 2. Lumirelax (Fr.), Robaxin, Tresortil (Denm.)

Primary Use: These centrally acting muscle relaxants are used in the treatment of acute musculoskeletal disorders. Mephenesin has also been used as an adjunct to anesthesia and in the treatment of Parkinson's disease and tetanus.

Ocular Side Effects

    A. Systemic Administration
        1. Decreased vision
        2. Nystagmus — horizontal, vertical, or rotatory
        3. Diplopia
        4. Ptosis (mephenesin)

5. Ciliary hyperemia (mephenesin)
6. Decreased intraocular pressure (mephenesin)
7. Paresis of extraocular muscles (mephenesin)
8. Conjunctivitis — nonspecific (methocarbamol)

Clinical Significance: Ocular side effects due to these muscle relaxants are much more common after intravenous administration than when given orally. Adverse ocular reactions are transitory and usually of little consequence. Ptosis, ciliary hyperemia, decreased intraocular pressure, and paresis of extraocular muscles are only seen with mephenesin, while nonspecific conjunctivitis has only been reported with methocarbamol.

Interactions with Other Drugs

A. Effect of Muscle Relaxants on Activity of Other Drugs
    1. Barbiturates ↑
    2. Phenothiazines ↑
    3. Sedatives and hypnotics ↑

References

Goodman, L. S., and Gilman, A. (Eds.): The Pharmacological Basis of Therapeutics. 4th Ed., New York, Macmillan, 1970, pp. 227–228.
Grant, W. M.: Toxicology of the Eye. 2nd Ed., Springfield, Charles C Thomas, 1974, pp. 646, 677.
Schlesinger, E. B., Drew, A. L., and Wood, B.: Clinical studies in the use of Myanesin. Am. J. Med. 4:365, 1948.
Stephen, C. R., and Chandy, J.: Clinical and experimental studies with Myanesin. Can. Med. Assoc. J. 57:463, 1947.
Walsh, F. B., and Hoyt, W. F.: Clinical Neuro-Ophthalmology. 3rd Ed., Baltimore, Williams & Wilkins, Vol. III, 1969, p. 2648.

* * * * * * * * * * * *

Generic Name: Orphenadrine

Proprietary Name: Disipal, Mephenamin (Germ.), Norflex

Primary Use: This antihistaminic agent is used in the treatment of skeletal muscle spasm and the associated pain of parkinsonism.

Ocular Side Effects

A. Systemic Administration
    1. Pupils
        a. Mydriasis — may precipitate narrow-angle glaucoma
        b. Absence of reaction to light
    2. Decreased vision
    3. Paralysis of accommodation
    4. Diplopia
    5. Subconjunctival or retinal hemorrhages secondary to drug-induced anemia
    6. Decreased tolerance to contact lenses (?)

Clinical Significance: Ocular side effects due to orphenadrine are transient and probably the result of its weak anticholinergic effect. These are seldom a significant clinical problem, although narrow-angle glaucoma has been precipitated secondary to drug-induced mydriasis. Nonreactive dilated pupils are only seen in overdose situations.

Interactions with Other Drugs

A. Effect of Orphenadrine on Activity of Other Drugs
   1. Anticholinergics ↑
   2. Phenothiazines ↑
   3. Phenylbutazone ↓
B. Effect of Other Drugs on Activity of Orphenadrine
   1. Antihistamines ↑
   2. Monoamine oxidase inhibitors ↑
   3. Phenothiazines ↑
   4. Tricyclic antidepressants ↑

References

AMA Drug Evaluations. 2nd Ed., Acton, Mass., Publishing Sciences Group, 1973, pp. 342–343, 746–747.

Curry, A. S.: Twenty-one uncommon cases of poisoning. Br. Med. J. 1:687, 1962.

Davidson, S. I.: Reports of ocular adverse reactions. Trans. Ophthalmol. Soc. U. K. 93:495–510, 1973.

Goodman, L. S., and Gilman, A. (Eds.): The Pharmacological Basis of Therapeutics. 4th Ed., New York, Macmillan, 1970, p. 232.

Heinonen, J., et al.: Orphenadrine poisoning. A case report supplemented with animal experiments. Arch. Toxikol. 23:264, 1968.

Physicians' Desk Reference. 28th Ed., Oradell, N. J., Medical Economics Co., 1974, pp. 1188, 1190.

Stoddart, J. C., Parkin, J. M., and Wynne, N. A.: Orphenadrine poisoning. A case report. Br. J. Anaesth. 40:789, 1968.

* * * * * * * * * * * *

XI. Oncolytic Agents

Class: Antineoplastic Agents

Generic Name: 1. Actinomycin C; 2. Aminopterin; 3. Bleomycin; 4. Dactinomycin; 5. Dromostanolone; 6. Fluoxymesterone; 7. Pipobroman; 8. Testolactone; 9. Testosterone

Proprietary Name: 1. Sanamycin (G.B.); 2. Aminopterin; 3. Blenoxane; 4. Cosmegen; 5. Drolban, Masteril (G.B.), Masterone; 6. Halotestin, Ora-Testryl, Oratestin (Canad.), Ultandren; 7. Vercyte; 8. Teslac; 9. Andronate, Andrusol-P, Andronaq, Delatestryl, Masenate, Neo-Hombreol, Oreton, Perandren, Testrol (G.B.), Testoviron (Germ.)

Primary Use: These various anticancer agents are used in a variety of malignant conditions. Dromostanolone, fluoxymesterone, testolactone, and testosterone are androgen derivatives used in the management of carcinoma of the breast. Pipobroman is a neutral amide used in the management of polycythemia vera and chronic granulocytic leukemia. Bleomycin is a polypeptide antibiotic used in the management of squamous cell carcinomas, lymphomas, and testicular carcinomas. Actinomycin C and dactinomycin are antibiotics used in the management of choriocarcinoma, rhabdomyosarcoma, Wilms' tumor, testicular neoplasma, and carcinoid syndrome. Aminopterin is a folic acid antagonist used in the treatment of acute leukemia.

Ocular Side Effects

A. Systemic Administration
1. Eyelids or conjunctiva
   a. Allergic reactions
   b. Erythema
   c. Edema
   d. Hyperpigmentation
2. Subconjunctival or retinal hemorrhages secondary to drug-induced anemia
3. Loss of eyelashes or eyebrows (?)
4. Increased intraocular pressure (?) (testosterone)
5. Ocular teratogenic effects (?)

Clinical Significance: Ocular side effects due to these drugs are in general reversible and transitory, except for their teratogenic effects. Small protuberant eyes, underdeveloped orbital ridges, and congenital myopia have been seen in offspring of mothers exposed to aminopterin. Loss of eyelashes or eyebrows has been seen due to actinomycin C and dactinomycin usage and it has been suspected with the other antineoplastic agents.

References

Apt, L., and Gaffney, W. L.: Congenital eye abnormalities from drugs during pregnancy. In Leopold, I. H. (Ed.): Symposium on Ocular Therapy. St. Louis, C. V. Mosby, Vol. VII, 1974, pp. 1–22.

Blacow, N. W. (Ed.): Martindale: The Extra Pharmacopoeia. 26th Ed., London, Pharmaceutical Press, 1972, pp. 1181–1183, 1187, 1221, 1649, 1655, 1688–1690.

Meyler, L., and Herxheimer, A.: Side Effects of Drugs. Amsterdam, Excerpta Medica, Vol. VII, 1972, pp. 540–544, 601–602, 612, 622–623.

Shaw, E. B., and Steinbach, H. L.: Aminopterin-induced fetal malformation. Am. J. Dis. Child. 115:477, 1968.

* * * * * * * * * * * *

Generic Name: 1. Busulfan; 2. Chlorambucil; 3. Cyclophosphamide; 4. Mechlorethamine; 5. Melphalan; 6. Triethylenemelamine; 7. Uracil Mustard

Proprietary Name: 1. Myleran; 2. Chloraminophene (Fr.), Leukeran; 3. Cytoxan, Endoxan, Endoxana (G.B.), Enduxan (Braz.), Genoxal (Span.), Procytox (Canad.), Sendoxan (Norw., Swed.); 4. Mustargen, Mustine (G.B.); 5. Alkeran, Sarcolysin (U.S.S.R.); 6. TEM; 7. Uracil Mustard

Primary Use: These alkylating agents are used in the treatment of Hodgkin's disease, lymphomas, multiple myeloma, leukemia, neuroblastoma, and retinoblastoma. All are nitrogen mustard derivatives except for triethylenemelamine, which is an ethylenimine derivative, and busulfan, which is an alkyl sulfonate derivative.

Ocular Side Effects

A. Systemic Administration
    1. Eyelids or conjunctiva
        a. Allergic reactions
        b. Erythema
        c. Conjunctivitis — nonspecific
        d. Hyperpigmentation (busulfan, cyclophosphamide, and uracil mustard)
        e. Exfoliative dermatitis
        f. Lyell's syndrome
    2. Decreased vision
    3. Subconjunctival or retinal hemorrhages secondary to drug-induced anemia
    4. Nonspecific ocular irritation (cyclophosphamide)
        a. Hyperemia
        b. Ocular pain
        c. Edema
    5. Cataracts (busulfan)
    6. Keratitis (chlorambucil)
    7. Loss of eyelashes or eyebrows (?)

8. Corneal opacities (?)
9. Ocular teratogenic effects (?)

Clinical Significance: Ocular side effects due to these alkylating agents are uncommon, transitory, and seldom of major significance; however, in high dosages busulfan has caused cataracts. Hyperpigmentation of the skin and mucous membranes seen with some of these agents is an indication for discontinued drug use and is reversible. Loss of eyelashes or eyebrows is almost always seen only with severe drug-induced alopecia. Inadvertent ocular exposure with these agents has caused severe conjunctival irritation and has been suspected of causing corneal opacities.

References

Apt, L., and Gaffney, W. L.: Congenital eye abnormalities from drugs during pregnancy. In Leopold, I. H. (Ed.): Symposium on Ocular Therapy. St. Louis, C. V. Mosby Co., 1974, Vol. VII, pp. 1–22.

Blacow, N. W. (Ed.): Martindale: The Extra Pharmacopoeia. 26th Ed. London, Pharmaceutical Press, 1972, pp. 1187–1191, 1193–1197, 1206–1208, 1219–1221, 1225–1227.

Ellis, P. P., and Smith, D. L.: Handbook of Ocular Therapeutics and Pharmacology. 4th Ed. St. Louis, C. V. Mosby, 1973, pp. 182–183, 202–203, 221.

Goodman, L. S., and Gilman, A. (Eds.): The Pharmacological Basis of Therapeutics. 4th Ed. New York, Macmillan, 1970, pp. 1346–1360.

Green, A. A., and Naiman, J. L.: Chlorambucil poisoning. Am. J. Dis. Child. *116*:190, 1968.

Havener, W. H.: Ocular Pharmacology. 2nd Ed. St. Louis, C. V. Mosby, 1970, pp. 155–156.

Johnson, D. R., and Burns, R. P.: Blepharoconjunctivitis associated with cancer chemotherapy. Trans. Pac. Coast Oto-Ophthalmol. Soc. *46*:43, 1965.

Rugh, R., and Skaredoff, L.: Radiation and radiomimetic chlorambucil and the fetal retina. Arch. Ophthalmol. *74*:382, 1965.

* * * * * * * * * * * * *

Generic Name: Cytarabine. See under *Class: Antiviral Agents.*

* * * * * * * * * * * * *

Generic Name: 1. Floxuridine; 2. Fluorouracil

Proprietary Name: *Systemic:* 1. FUDR; 2. Fluorouracil *Topical:* 2. Efudex, Fluoroplex

Primary Use: These fluorinated pyrimidine antimetabolites are used in the management of carcinoma of the colon, rectum, breast, stomach, and pancreas. Fluorouracil is also used topically for actinic keratoses or skin cancer.

Ocular Side Effects

A. Systemic Administration
    1. Nonspecific ocular irritation
        a. Lacrimation
        b. Hyperemia
        c. Photophobia
        d. Ocular pain

   e. Edema
   f. Burning sensation
  2. Decreased vision
  3. Eyelids or conjunctiva
   a. Erythema
   b. Edema
   c. Hyperpigmentation
   d. Photosensitivity
   e. Ulceration
  4. Nystagmus
  5. Subconjunctival or retinal hemorrhages secondary to drug-induced anemia
  6. Decreased accommodation
  7. Loss of eyelashes or eyebrows (?)
  8. Ocular teratogenic effects (?)
 B. Topical Administration
  1. Irritation
   a. Lacrimation
   b. Ocular pain
   c. Edema
   d. Burning sensation
  2. Eyelids or conjunctiva
   a. Allergic reactions
   b. Hyperpigmentation
   c. Photosensitivity
  3. Periorbital edema
  4. Subconjunctival or retinal hemorrhages
 C. Inadvertent Ocular Exposure -- Fluorouracil
  1. Irritation
   a. Hyperemia
   b. Burning sensation

Clinical Significance: Systemic floxuridine or fluorouracil causes frequent adverse ocular reactions since its therapeutic dose often is close to its toxic level. Ocular irritation is the most common side effect for both systemic and topical therapy. All adverse ocular reactions due to systemic therapy are reversible and seldom interfere with continued therapy. Ointments containing fluorouracil used in the treatment of skin lesions near the eye have caused significant ocular irritation requiring discontinuation of this form of therapy. Ocular side effects due to local therapy are usually reversible if the eye had only limited exposure.

References
Blacow, N. W. (Ed.): Martindale: The Extra Pharmacopoeia. 26th Ed., London, Pharmaceutical Press, 1972, pp. 1202–1205.
Goodman, L. S., and Gilman, A. (Eds.): The Pharmacological Basis of Therapeutics. 4th Ed., New York, Macmillan, 1970, pp. 1364–1369.
Hamersley, J., et al.: Excessive lacrimation from fluorouracil treatment. JAMA 225:747, 1973.
Meyler, L., and Herxheimer, A.: Side Effects of Drugs. Amsterdam, Excerpta Medica, Vol. VII, 1972, pp. 617–618.

Physicians' Desk Reference. 28th Edition. Oradell, N. J., Medical Economics Co., 1974, pp. 791, 1217–1219.

* * * * * * * * * * * *

Generic Name: Hydroxyurea

Proprietary Name: Hydrea

Primary Use: This substituted urea preparation is used in the management of chronic granulocytic leukemia, carcinoma of the ovary, and malignant melanoma.

Ocular Side Effects

A. Systemic Administration
1. Subconjunctival or retinal hemorrhages secondary to drug-induced anemia
2. Eyelids – erythema
3. Visual hallucinations
4. Loss of eyelashes or eyebrows (?)
5. Ocular teratogenic effects (?)

Clinical Significance: Adverse ocular reactions due to hydroxyurea are quite rare. Ocular side effects other than teratogenic effects are reversible and transitory after the drug is discontinued.

References

Apt, L., and Gaffney, W. L.: Congenital eye abnormalities from drugs during pregnancy. In Leopold, I. H. (Ed.): Symposium on Ocular Therapy. St. Louis, C. V. Mosby, Vol. VII, 1974, pp. 1–22.
Goodman, L. S., and Gilman, A. (Eds.): The Pharmacological Basis of Therapeutics. 4th Ed., New York, Macmillan, 1970, pp. 1381–1382.
Meyler, L., and Herxheimer, A.: Side Effects of Drugs. Amsterdam, Excerpta Medica, Vol. VII, 1972, pp. 599, 627.
Physicians Desk Reference. 28th Ed., Oradell, N. J., Medical Economics Co., 1974, p. 1402.

* * * * * * * * * * * *

Generic Name: 1. Mercaptopurine; 2. Thioguanine

Proprietary Name: 1. Purinethol; 2. Thioguanine

Primary Use: These purine analogs are used in the treatment of acute and some forms of chronic leukemias.

Ocular Side Effects

A. Systemic Administration
1. Eyelids or conjunctiva – hyperpigmentation
2. Subconjunctival or retinal hemorrhages secondary to drug-induced anemia

3. Ocular teratogenic effects (?)

Clinical Significance: Ocular side effects due to these antimetabolites are rare and seldom of clinical importance.

Interactions with Other Drugs
A. Effect of Other Drugs on Activity of Purine Analogs
   1. Salicylates ↑
   2. Sulfonamides ↑

References
AMA Drug Evaluations. 2nd Ed., Acton, Mass., Publishing Sciences Group, 1973, pp. 847–849.

Apt, L., and Gaffney, W. L.: Congenital eye abnormalities from drugs during pregnancy. In Leopold, I. H. (Ed.): Symposium on Ocular Therapy. St. Louis, C. V. Mosby, Vol. VII, 1974, pp. 1–22.

Goodman, L. S., and Gilman, A. (Eds.): The Pharmacological Basis of Therapeutics. 4th Ed., New York, Macmillan, 1970, pp. 1346, 1371–1375.

Meyler, L., and Herxheimer, A.: Side Effects of Drugs. Amsterdam, Excerpta Medica, Vol. VII, 1972, pp. 618, 622, 644.

* * * * * * * * * * * * *

Generic Name: Methotrexate

Proprietary Name: Methotrexate

Primary Use: This folic acid antagonist is effective in the treatment of certain neoplastic diseases and in the management of psoriasis.

Ocular Side Effects
A. Systemic Administration
   1. Eyelids or conjunctiva
      a. Allergic reactions
      b. Erythema
      c. Blepharoconjunctivitis
      d. Depigmentation
      e. Hyperpigmentation
      f. Photosensitivity
      g. Urticaria
      h. Lyell's syndrome
   2. Decreased vision
   3. Nonspecific ocular irritation
      a. Lacrimation
      b. Hyperemia
      c. Photophobia
      d. Ocular pain
      e. Burning sensation
   4. Subconjunctival or retinal hemorrhages secondary to drug-induced anemia

5. Keratitis
6. Loss of eyelashes or eyebrows (?)
7. Ocular teratogenic effects (?)

Clinical Significance: Systemic side effects due to methotrexate are common; however, ocular side effects are rare and seldom of clinical significance. In spite of minimal blepharoconjunctivitis, occasional patients have marked subjective complaints. A cause and effect relationship due to drug usage has not been firmly established, however.

Interactions with Other Drugs

A. Effect of Other Drugs on Activity of Methotrexate
1. Analgesics ↑
2. Salicylates ↑
3. Sulfonamides ↑

References

American Hospital Formulary Service. Washington, D. C., American Society of Hospital Pharmacists, Vol. 1, 1973.
Grant, W. M.: Toxicology of the Eye. 2nd Ed. Springfield, Ill., Charles C Thomas, 1974, p. 677.
Havener, W. H.: Ocular Pharmacology. 2nd Ed. St. Louis, C. V. Mosby, 1970, pp. 153–154.
Johnson, D. R., and Burns, R. P.: Blepharoconjunctivitis associated with cancer chemotherapy. Trans. Pac. Coast Oto-Ophthalmol. Soc. 46:43, 1965.
Lischka, G.: Auffallend rasche Wirkung des Methotrexats bei Psoriasis eines 82 jahrigen Patienten mit gleichzeitigen Nebenwirkungen am Auge. Hautarzt. 19:473, 1968.
Physicians' Desk Reference. 28th Ed. Oradell, N. J., Medical Economics Co., 1974, p. 858.

* * * * * * * * * * * * *

Generic Name: Mithramycin

Proprietary Name: Mithracin

Primary Use: This cytostatic antibiotic is used primarily in the treatment of testicular neoplasms.

Ocular Side Effects

A. Systemic Administration
1. Subconjunctival or retinal hemorrhages
2. Periorbital pallor
3. Ocular teratogenic effects (?)

Clinical Significance: The main adverse reaction to mithramycin is severe thrombocytopenia which causes a bleeding diathesis which may also affect the eye. A striking periorbital pallor may occur in patients taking this drug. No reports of other drugs causing this unusual reaction have been made.

References

AMA Drug Evaluations. 2nd Ed., Acton, Mass., Publishing Sciences Group, 1973, pp. 854–856.
Blacow, N. W. (Ed.): Martindale: The Extra Pharmacopoeia. 26th Ed., London, Pharmaceutical Press, 1972, pp. 1215–1216.
Physicians' Desk Reference. 28th Ed., Oradell, N. J., Medical Economics Co., 1974, p. 1136.

* * * * * * * * * * * *

Generic Name: Mitotane

Proprietary Name: Lysodren

Primary Use: This adrenal cytotoxic agent is used in the treatment of inoperable adrenocortical carcinoma.

Ocular Side Effects

A. Systemic Administration
1. Decreased vision
2. Diplopia
3. Lens opacities
4. Retinal pigmentary changes
5. Papilledema
6. Retinal hemorrhages
7. Ocular teratogenic effects (?)

Clinical Significance: While systemic side effects due to mitotane occur commonly, adverse ocular reactions occur infrequently. Significant ocular side effects do occur, but seldom require discontinued drug use because of the seriousness of the underlying disease.

References

AMA Drug Evaluations. 2nd Ed., Acton, Mass., Publishing Sciences Group, 1973, p. 850.
Apt, L., and Gaffney, W. L.: Congenital eye abnormalities from drugs during pregnancy. In Leopold, I. H. (Ed.): Symposium on Ocular Therapy. St. Louis, C. V. Mosby, Vol. VII, 1974, pp. 1–22.
Goodman, L. S., and Gilman, A. (Eds.): The Pharmacological Basis of Therapeutics. 4th Ed., New York, Macmillan, 1970, p. 1383.
Physicians' Desk Reference. 28th Ed., Oradell, N. J., Medical Economics Co., 1974, p. 663.

* * * * * * * * * * * *

Generic Name: Procarbazine

Proprietary Name: Matulane, Natulan

Primary Use: This methylhydrazine derivative is used in the management of generalized Hodgkin's disease.

Ocular Side Effects

 A. Systemic Administration
  1. Subconjunctival or retinal hemorrhages secondary to drug-induced anemia
  2. Eyelids or conjunctiva
   a. Erythema
   b. Hyperpigmentation
   c. Photosensitivity
   d. Purpura
   e. Exfoliative dermatitis
   f. Lyell's syndrome
  3. Nystagmus
  4. Photophobia
  5. Diplopia
  6. Decreased accommodation
  7. Papilledema
  8. Loss of eyelashes or eyebrows (?)
  9. Ocular teratogenic effects (?)

Clinical Significance: Numerous adverse ocular reactions have been caused by procarbazine with the most frequent secondary to drug-induced hematologic disorders. Most ocular side effects are transitory and reversible with discontinued drug use, and seldom are of major clinical significance.

Interactions with Other Drugs

 A. Synergistic Activity
  1. Analgesics
  2. Antihistamines
  3. Barbiturates
  4. Phenothiazines
 B. Contraindications
  1. Local anesthetics
  2. Sympathomimetics
  3. Tricyclic antidepressants

References

AMA Drug Evaluations. 2nd Ed., Acton, Mass., Publishing Sciences Group, 1973, pp. 850–851.

Apt, L. and Gaffney, W. L.: Congenital eye abnormalities from drugs during pregnancy. In Leopold, I. H. (Ed.): Symposium of Ocular Therapy. St. Louis, C. V. Mosby Co., Vol. VII, 1974, pp. 1–22.

Goodman, L. S., and Gilman, A. (Eds.): The Pharmacological Basis of Therapeutics. 4th Ed. New York, Macmillan, 1970, pp. 1382–1383.

Meyler, L., and Herxheimer, A.: Side Effects of Drugs. Amsterdam, Excerpta Medica, 1972, pp. 599, 627–628.

Physicians' Desk Reference. 28th Ed. Oradell, N. J., Medical Economics Co., 1974, p. 1228.

* * * * * * * * * * * *

Generic Name: Thiotepa

Proprietary Name: Thio-Tepa (G.B.)

Primary Use: *Systemic:* This ethylenimine derivative is used in the management of carcinomas of the breast and ovary, lymphomas, Hodgkin's disease, and various sarcomas. *Ophthalmic:* This topical agent is used to inhibit pterygium recurrence and possibly to prevent corneal neovascularization after chemical injuries.

Ocular Side Effects

A. Systemic Administration
1. Subconjunctival or retinal hemorrhages secondary to drug-induced anemia
2. Loss of eyelashes or eyebrows
3. Acute fibrinous uveitis (?)
4. Ocular teratogenic effects (?)
B. Local Ophthalmic Use or Exposure
1. Irritation
2. Eyelids or conjunctiva
a Allergic reactions
b. Depigmentation
3. Delayed corneal wound healing
4. Keratitis
5. Corneal edema
6. Occlusion of lacrimal punctum
7. Corneal ulceration (?)
8. Ocular teratogenic effects (?)

Clinical Significance: Ocular side effects due to topical thiotepa application are rare. While ocular irritation and allergic reactions are the most common, depigmentation of the eyelids may be the most disturbing ocular reaction. Eyelid depigmentation has been reported to occur 6 years after topical ocular use of thiotepa and in some instances it has been permanent. This depigmentation due to thiotepa is probably enhanced by excessive exposure to sunlight. Corneal ulcerations have been attributed to thiotepa when it was used in alkaline injuries; however, this is difficult to substantiate due to the coexisting alkaline damage.

References

Asregadoo, E. R.: Surgery, thio-tepa, and corticosteroid in the treatment of pterygium. Am. J. Ophthalmol. 74:960, 1972.

Berkow, J. W., Gills, J. P., and Wise, J. B.: Depigmentation of eyelids after topically administered thiotepa. Arch. Ophthalmol. 82:415, 1969.

Burns, R. P., and Beighle, R.: Effects of triethylenethiophosphoramide on the carrageenin granuloma of the guinea pig cornea. Invest. Ophthalmol. 1:666, 1962.

Cassady, J. R.: The inhibition of pterygium recurrence by Thiotepa. Am. J. Ophthalmol. 61:886, 1966.

Grant, W. M.: Toxicology of the Eye. 2nd Ed., Springfield, Charles C Thomas, 1974, pp. 1010–1012.

Hornblass, A., et al.: A delayed side effect of topical thiotepa. Ann. Ophthalmol. 6:1155, 1974.
Howitt, D., and Karp, E. J.: Side-effect of topical thio-tepa. Am. J. Ophthalmol. 68:473, 1969.

* * * * * * * * * * * *

Generic Name: Urethan

Proprietary Name: Urethan

Primary Use: This carbamic acid ester is used in the management of multiple myeloma and leukemia.

Ocular Side Effects

A. Systemic Administration
    1. Subconjunctival or retinal hemorrhages secondary to drug-induced anemia
    2. Decreased vision
    3. Nystagmus
    4. Pupils
        a. Mydriasis
        b. Absence of reaction to light
    5. Ocular teratogenic effects (?)

Clinical Significance: Adverse ocular reactions due to urethan are rare and seldom of major significance. Nystagmus and pupillary changes have only been seen in extreme toxic states and are probably central in origin. While corneal crystals, iritis, ciliary body cysts, and corneal foreign body sensations have been attributed to urethan, these are more likely due to multiple myeloma and not the drug.

References

Aronson, S. B., and Shaw, R.: Corneal crystals in multiple myeloma. Arch. Ophthalmol. 61:541, 1959.
Ashton, N.: Cystic changes and urethane (Correspondence). Arch. Ophthalmol. 78:416, 1967.
Blacow, N. W. (Ed.): Martindale: The Extra Pharmacopoeia. 26th Ed., London, Pharmaceutical Press, 1972, pp. 1227–1228.
Grant, W. M.: Toxicology of the Eye. 2nd Ed., Springfield, Charles C Thomas, 1974, pp. 1074–1076.
Handley, G. J., and Arney, G. K.: Plasma cell myeloma and associated amino acid disorder: Case with crystalline deposition in the cornea and lens. Arch. Intern. Med. 120:353, 1967.

* * * * * * * * * * * *

Generic Name: 1. Vinblastine; 2. Vincristine

Proprietary Name: 1. Velban, Belbe (G.B.); 2. Oncovin

Primary Use: These vinca alkaloids are often used in conjunction with other antineoplastic agents. Vinblastine is primarily used in inoperable malignant neoplasms of the breast, the female genital tract, the lung, the testis, and the gastrointestinal tract. Vincristine is primarily used in Hodgkin's disease, lymphosarcoma, reticulum cell sarcoma, rhabdomyosarcoma, neuroblastoma, and Wilms' tumor.

Ocular Side Effects

A. Systemic Administration
   1. Ptosis
   2. Paresis or paralysis of extraocular muscles
   3. Diplopia
   4. Subconjunctival or retinal hemorrhages secondary to drug-induced anemia
   5. Ocular signs of gout (?)
   6. Loss of eyelashes or eyebrows (?)
   7. Ocular teratogenic effects (?)
B. Inadvertent Ocular Exposure — Vinblastine
   1. Irritation
      a. Lacrimation
      b. Hyperemia
      c. Photophobia
      d. Edema
   2. Keratitis
   3. Decreased vision
   4. Superficial gray corneal opacities
   5. Astigmatism

Clinical Significance: Vincristine more commonly causes extraocular muscle paresis and ptosis than vinblastine. These ocular side effects are dose-related and most patients obtain full recovery after these agents are discontinued. The onset of extraocular muscle paresis or paralysis may be seen as early as 2 weeks after commencing therapy. The ocular signs of gout which may occur include conjunctival hyperemia, uveitis, scleritis, and corneal deposits or ulcerations. An accidental splashing of vinblastine on a patient's eye caused corneal clouding, with vision reduced to seeing hand movements. Vision returned to near normal after a number of weeks with astigmatic correcting lens.

References

Albert, D. M., Wong, V. G., and Henderson, E. S.: Ocular complications of vincristine therapy. Arch. Ophthalmol. 78:709, 1967.
Bradley, W. G., et al.: The neuromyopathy of vincristine in man. Clinical, electrophysiological and pathological studies. J. Neurol. Sci. 10:107, 1970.
Grant, W. M.: Toxicology of the Eye. 2nd Ed., Springfield, Charles C Thomas, 1974, pp. 1083–1084.
Mosci, L.: Astigmatismo contro regola in un caso di causticazione corneale da vincaleucoblastina. Ann. Ottal. 93:94, 1967.
Physicians' Desk Reference. 28th Ed., Oradell, N. J., Medical Economics Co., 1974, pp. 926, 940.

* * * * * * * * * * * *

XII. Heavy Metal Antagonists and Miscellaneous Agents

Class: Agents Used to Treat Alcoholism

Generic Name: Disulfiram

Proprietary Name: Antabuse, Esperal (Fr.)

Primary Use: This thiuram derivative is used as an aid in the management of chronic alcoholism.

Ocular Side Effects

A. Systemic Administration
1. Decreased vision
2. Retrobulbar or optic neuritis
3. Scotomas — central or centrocecal
4. Problems with color vision — dyschromatopsia
5. Eyelids or conjunctiva
   a. Allergic reactions
   b. Urticaria
6. Visual hallucinations
7. Paresis of extraocular muscles
8. Anisocoria
9. Blindness

Clinical Significance: Adverse ocular side effects due to disulfiram are uncommon. Retrobulbar neuritis has been well documented by numerous authors, since each time the drug was restarted the optic neuritis, often bilateral, would recur. In most cases the vision lost during optic neuritis returned after the drug therapy was discontinued. Other ocular side effects are reversible and seldom of importance.

Interactions with Other Drugs

A. Effect of Disulfiram on Activity of Other Drugs
1. Barbiturates ↑
2. Sedatives and hypnotics ↑
3. Alcohol ↓

References

Blacow, N. W. (Ed.): Martindale: The Extra Pharmacopoeia. 26th Ed., London, Pharmaceutical Press, 1972, pp. 630–632.

Debrousse, J. Y.: L'examen systematique du fond d'oeil dans le traitement de l'alcoolisme par le disulfure de tetra-ethyl-thiourane. Sem. Hop. Paris 26:4132, 1950.

Grant, W. M.: Toxicology of the Eye. 2nd Ed. Springfield, Ill., Charles C Thomas, 1974, pp. 420–421.

Humblet, M.: Nevrite retrobulbaire chronique par Antabuse. Bull. Soc. Belge Ophtalmol. 104:297, 1953.

Perdriel, G., and Chevaleraud, J.: A propos d'un nouveau cas de nevrite optique due au disulfirame. Bull. Soc. Ophtalmol. Fr. 66:159, 1966.

Walsh, F. B., and Hoyt, W. F.: Clinical Neuro-Ophthalmology. 3rd Ed. Baltimore, Williams & Wilkins, Vol. III, 1969, p. 2597.

* * * * * * * * * * * *

Class: Chelating Agents

Generic Name: Deferoxamine

Proprietary Name: *Systemic:* Desferal, Desferrioxamine (G.B.), Desferyl *Ophthalmic:* Desferrioxamine (G.B.)

Primary Use: *Systemic:* This chelating agent is used in the treatment of iron-storage diseases and acute iron poisoning. *Ophthalmic:* This topical agent is used in the treatment of ocular siderosis and hematogenous pigmentation of the cornea.

Ocular Side Effects

A. Systemic Administration
   1. Eyelids or conjunctiva
      a. Allergic reactions
      b. Erythema
      c. Urticaria
   2. Decreased vision
   3. Cataracts
   4. Subconjunctival or retinal hemorrhages secondary to drug-induced anemia (?)
B. Local Ophthalmic Use or Exposure
   1. Eyelids or conjunctiva
      a. Allergic reactions
      b. Hyperemia

Clinical Significance: Adverse ocular side effects due to deferoxamine are rare and seldom significant. Cataracts have been observed in 3 patients who received this drug over prolonged periods in the treatment of chronic iron-storage diseases.

References

Ciba Pharmaceutical Company. Official literature on new drugs: Deferoxamine mesylate (desferal mesylate). A specific iron-chelating agent for treating acute iron intoxication. Clin. Pharmacol. Ther. *10*:595, 1969.

Davidson, S. I.: Report of ocular adverse reactions. Trans. Ophthalmol. Soc. U. K. *93*:495, 1973.

Goodman, L. S., and Gilman, A. (Eds.): The Pharmacological Basis of Therapeutics. 4th Ed., New York, Macmillan, 1970, pp. 954–955.

Grant, W. M.: Toxicology of the Eye. 2nd Ed., Springfield, Charles C Thomas, 1974, pp. 351–352.

Jacobs, J., Greene, H., and Gendel, B. R.: Acute iron intoxication. N. Engl. J. Med. *273*:1124, 1965.

Physicians' Desk Reference. 28th Ed., Oradell, N. J., Medical Economics Co., 1974, p. 673.

Valvo, A.: Desferrioxamine B in ophthalmology. Am. J. Ophthalmol. *63*:98, 1967.

* * * * * * * * * * * * *

Generic Name: Dimercaprol

Proprietary Name: BAL (British Anti-Lewisite)

Primary Use: This chelating agent is effective in the treatment of arsenic, gold, or mercury poisonings.

Ocular Side Effects

   A. Systemic Administration
      1. Nonspecific ocular irritation
         a. Lacrimation
         b. Edema
         c. Burning sensation
      2. Eyelids or conjunctiva
         a. Allergic reactions
         b. Conjunctivitis – nonspecific
         c. Blepharospasm
   B. Inadvertent Ocular Exposure
      1. Irritation
         a. Lacrimation
         b. Photophobia
         c. Burning sensation
      2. Blepharospasm

Clinical Significance: Approximately 50 percent of patients receiving intramuscular injections of dimercaprol experience a burning sensation around their eyes within 15 to 20 minutes. This persists for 1 to 2 hours and is completely reversible. Other ocular manifestations to systemic dimercaprol are also of little consequence, transitory, and reversible. Direct ocular contact with this drug causes significant local irritation which lasts for a few hours but without apparent ocular damage.

References

Blacow, N. W. (Ed.): Martindale: The Extra Pharmacopoeia. 26th Ed., London, Pharmaceutical Press, 1972, pp. 401–402.

Dimercaprol. Council on pharmacy and chemistry. "Bal" (British anti-lewisite) in the treatment of arsenic and mercury poisoning. JAMA 131:824, 1946.

Grant, W. M.: Toxicology of the Eye. 2nd Ed., Springfield, Charles C Thomas, 1974, pp. 398–399.

Peters, R. A., Stocken, L. A., and Thompson, R. H. S.: British anti-lewisite (BAL). Nature 156:616, 1945.

Scherling, S. S., and Blondis, R. R.: The effect of chemical warfare agents on the human eye. Milit. Surg. 96:70, 1945.

* * * * * * * * * * * *

Generic Name: Penicillamine

Proprietary Name: Cuprenil (Pol.), Cuprimine, Distamine (G.B.), D-Penamine (Austral.)

Primary Use: This amino acid derivative of penicillin is a potent chelating agent effective in the management of Wilson's disease, cystinuria, and copper, iron, lead, or mercury poisonings.

Ocular Side Effects

A. Systemic Administration
  1. Visual changes
     a. Myopia
     b. Hypermetropia
  2. Retinal hemorrhages
  3. Nonspecific ocular irritation
     a. Lacrimation
     b. Hyperemia
     c. Photophobia
     d. Edema
  4. Optic neuritis
  5. Papilledema
  6. Problems with color vision – dyschromatopsia
  7. Subconjunctival or retinal hemorrhages secondary to drug-induced anemia
  8. Cataracts (?)

Clinical Significance: Adverse ocular reactions to the three isomers of penicillamine (D, DL, and L) are rare. Probably most side effects are due to penicillamine-pyridoxine antagonism. This is most common with the DL or L isomers, and only rarely with the D form. Unfortunately, most of the literature does not differentiate which isomer was prescribed, although now only the D form is used. To date, myopia, optic neuritis, and papilledema have not been reported with the D isomer form of penicillamine.

Interactions with Other Drugs
  A. Cross Sensitivity
     1. Penicillins

References

Bigger, J. F.: Retinal hemorrhages during penicillamine therapy of cystinuria. Am. J. Ophthalmol. 66:954, 1968.

Blacow, N. W. (Ed.): Martindale: The Extra Pharmacopoeia. 26th Ed., London, Pharmaceutical Press, 1972, pp. 406–410.

Goodman, L. S., and Gilman, A. (Eds.): The Pharmacological Basis of Therapeutics. 4th Ed., New York, Macmillan, 1970, pp. 953–954.

McDonald, J. E., and Henneman, P. H.: Stone dissolution in vivo and control of cystinuria with D-penicillamine. N. Engl. J. Med. 273:578, 1965.

Scheinberg, I. H.: D-penicillamine with particular relation to Wilson's disease. J. Chronic Dis. 17:293, 1964.

* * * * * * * * * * * *

Class: Dermatologic Agents

Generic Name: Chrysarobin

Proprietary Name: Chrysarobin

Primary Use: This keratolytic agent is effective in the treatment of psoriasis and parasitic skin infections.

Ocular Side Effects
  A. Systemic Absorption from Topical Application to the Skin
     1. Nonspecific ocular irritation
     2. Eyelids or conjunctiva
        a. Hyperemia
        b. Brown-violet discoloration
     3. Keratoconjunctivitis
     4. Punctate keratitis
     5. Gray corneal opacities
  B. Inadvertent Ocular Exposure
     1. Irritation
        a. Lacrimation
        b. Hyperemia
        c. Photophobia

    2. Eyelids or conjunctiva
       a. Allergic reactions
       b. Conjunctivitis — nonspecific
       c. Edema
       d. Brown-violet discoloration
    3. Keratitis

Clinical Significance: Systemic absorption of chrysarobin through the skin has caused aggravating ocular symptoms. Irritation may be extensive and often takes the form of a keratoconjunctivitis which, in rare instances, may last for weeks. Chrysarobin is highly irritating as well if it comes into direct contact with the eye; however, rarely is permanent damage done. In general, ocular irritation secondary to direct ocular contact or systemic absorption usually subsides 8 to 10 days from the time of last exposure.

References

AMA Drug Evaluations. 2nd Ed., Acton. Mass., Publishing Sciences Group, 1973, p. 665.
Blacow, N. W. (Ed.): Martindale: The Extra Pharmacopoeia. 26th Ed., London, Pharmaceutical Press, 1972, pp. 560–561.
Duke-Elder, S.: Systems of Ophthalmology. St. Louis, C. V. Mosby, Vol. XIV, Part 2, 1972, p. 1189.
Grant, W. M.: Toxicology of the Eye. 2nd Ed., Springfield, Charles C Thomas, 1974, pp. 152, 291.
Willetts, G. S.: Ocular side-effects of drugs. Br. J. Ophthalmol. 53:252, 1969.

* * * * * * * * * * * *

Class: Immunosuppressants

Generic Name: Azathioprine

Proprietary Name: Imuran, Imurel (Aust., Fr.)

Primary Use: This imidazolyl derivative of mercaptopurine is used as an adjunct to help prevent rejection in homograft transplantation and to treat various possible autoimmune diseases.

Ocular Side Effects

A. Systemic Administration
    1. Decreased resistance to infection
    2. Delayed corneal wound healing
    3. Retinal pigmentary changes

    4. Subconjunctival or retinal hemorrhages secondary to drug-induced
        anemia
    5. Loss of eyelashes or eyebrows (?)
    6. Ocular teratogenic effects (?)

Clinical Significance: Ocular side effects due to azathioprine are uncommon
and, except for possible teratogenic effects, are reversible upon drug
withdrawal.

References

AMA Drug Evaluations. 2nd Ed., Acton, Mass., Publishing Sciences Group, 1973, pp.
    302–303, 900.
Blacow, N. W. (Ed.): Martindale: The Extra Pharmacopoeia. 26th Ed., London, Pharma-
    ceutical Press, 1972, pp. 1183–1187.
Ellis, P. P., and Smith, D. L.: Handbook of Ocular Pharmacology and Therapeutics. 4th Ed.,
    St. Louis, C. V. Mosby, 1973, pp. 171, 173.
Havener, W. H.: Ocular Pharmacology. 2nd Ed., St. Louis, C. V. Mosby, 1970, p. 153.
Physicians' Desk Reference. 28th Ed., Oradell, N. J., Medical Economics Co., 1974, p. 651.

* * * * * * * * * * * * *

Class: Solvents

Generic Name: Dimethyl Sulfoxide, DMSO

Proprietary Name: Dolicur (Germ.), Infiltrina (Germ.)

Primary Use: This is an exceptional solvent with controversial medical
therapeutic indications. It is possibly effective in the treatment of musculoskeletal pain, as a solvent for antivirals (IDU) or anticancer drugs, and as an
anti-inflammatory agent.

Ocular Side Effects

  A. Systemic or Topical Administration
      1. Potentiates the adverse effects of any drug it is combined with
  B. Local Ophthalmic Use or Exposure
      1. Irritation
          a. Burning sensation
      2. Eyelids or conjunctiva
          a. Erythema
          b. Photosensitivity

Clinical Significance: DMSO may enhance the ocular side effects of other drugs
by increasing the speed and volume of systemic absorption. No cases of any
lens changes in man have been reported due to systemic or local ocular

exposure. Topical ocular DMSO in high concentrations commonly causes ocular irritation.

References

Blacow, N. W. (Ed.): Martindale: The Extra Pharmacopoeia. 26th Ed., London, Pharmaceutical Press, 1972, pp. 1729–1730.

Gordon, D. M.: Dimethyl sulfoxide in ophthalmology, with special reference to possible toxic effects. Ann. N. Y. Acad. Sci. *141*:392, 1967.

Gordon, D. M., and Kleberger, K. E.: The effect of dimethylsulfoxide (DMSO) on animal and human eyes. Arch. Ophthalmol. *79*:423, 1968.

Hanna, C., Fraunfelder, F. T., and Meyer, S. M.: Effects of dimethylsulfoxide on ocular inflammation. In press. Ann. Ophthalmol.

Hull, F. W., Wood, D. C., and Brobyn, R. D.: Eye effects of DMSO. Report of negative results. Northwest. Med. *68*:39, 1969.

Kleberger, K. E.: An ophthalmological evaluation of DMSO. Ann. N. Y. Acad. Sci. *141*:381, 1967.

* * * * * * * * * * * * *

Class: Vaccines

Generic Name: Measles Virus Vaccine (Live, Attenuated)

Proprietary Name: Attenuvax, Lirugen, Mevilin-L (G.B.), M-Vac, Pfizer-Vax Measles L, Rubeovax

Primary Use: Measles virus vaccine is used for the active immunization against measles.

Ocular Side Effects

A. Systemic Administration
1. Strabismus
2. Conjunctivitis – nonspecific
3. Decreased vision
4. Subconjunctival or retinal hemorrhages secondary to drug-induced anemia

Clinical Significance: – Adverse ocular reactions due to measles virus vaccine are rare and transitory. Strabismus was primarily seen with the first available vaccines; however, this is an exceptionally rare ocular side effect with current preparations.

Interactions with Other Drugs

A. Effect of Other Drugs on Activity of Measles Virus Vaccine
1. Corticosteroids ↓

References

American Hospital Formulary Service. Washington, D. C., American Society of Hospital Pharmacists, Vol. II, *80*:12, 1969.

Blacow, N. W. (Ed.): Martindale: The Extra Pharmacopoeia. 26th Ed., London, Pharmaceutical Press, 1972, pp. 1917–1918.

Davidson, S. I.: Reports of ocular adverse reactions. Trans. Ophthalmol. Soc. U. K. *93*:495, 1973.

Kirkham, T. H., and MacLellan, A. V.: Strabismus following measles vaccination. Br. Orthop. J. *27*:108, 1970.

* * * * * * * * * * * *

XIII. Drugs Used Primarily in Ophthalmology

Class: Antibacterial Agents

Generic Name: 1. Colloidal Silver; 2. Mild Silver Protein; 3. Silver Nitrate; 4. Silver Protein

Proprietary Name: 1. Colloidal Silver; 2. Argyrol, Mild Protargin, Silvol; 3. Silver Nitrate; 4. Silver Protein

Primary Use: These topical ocular antibacterial agents are effective in the treatment of conjunctivitis and in the prophylaxis of ophthalmia neonatorum.

Ocular Side Effects

A. Local Ophthalmic Use or Exposure
    1. Silver deposits
        a. Cornea
        b. Conjunctiva
        c. Eyelids
        d. Lens
        e. Lacrimal sac
    2. Irritation
        a. Hyperemia
        b. Photophobia
        c. Ocular pain
        d. Edema
    3. Eyelids or conjunctiva
        a. Allergic reactions
        b. Conjunctivitis — nonspecific
        c. Edema
        d. Symblepharon
    4. Scarring or opacities of any ocular structure (silver nitrate — when exposed to caustic concentrations)
    5. Decreased vision
    6. Problems with color vision — objects have yellow tinge

Clinical Significance: The overall use of silver-containing medication has been decreasing; however, in some countries it is still commonly prescribed. Ocular side effects other than with silver nitrate in caustic concentrations seldom cause serious adverse reactions. Conjunctivitis is probably the most common side effect, but rarely requires discontinuation of the medication. Topical ocular silver application for even a few months may cause conjunctival silver deposition. Long-term dosage may cause corneal, lens, eyelid, or lacrimal sac silver deposition. Silver deposits in the cornea or lens rarely interfere with vision. Ocular and periocular silver deposits over many years are absorbed, if the drug is discontinued.

References

Bartlett, R. E.: Generalized argyrosis with lens involvement. Am. J. Ophthalmol. *38*:402, 1954.
Friedman, B., and Rotth, A.: Argyrosis corneae. Am. J. Ophthalmol. *13*:1050, 1930.
Goldstein, J. H.: Effects of drugs on cornea, conjunctiva, and lids. Int. Ophthalmol. Clin. *11*(2):13, 1971.
Grayson, M., and Pieroni, D.: Severe silver nitrate injury to the eye. Am. J. Ophthalmol. *70*:227, 1970.
Hanna, C., Fraunfelder, F. T., and Sanchez, J.: Ultrastructural study of argyrosis of the cornea and conjunctiva. Arch. Ophthalmol. *92*:18, 1974.
Rosen, E.: Argyrolentis. Am. J. Ophthalmol. *33*:797, 1950.

* * * * * * * * * * * *

Class: Antiviral Agents

Generic Name: 1. Adenine Arabinoside; 2. Idoxuridine; 3. Trifluorothymidine

Proprietary Name: 1. Ara-A, Vidarabine; 2. Dendrid, Herplex, IDU, Kerecid (G.B.), Stoxil; 3. F_3T

Primary Use: These topical ocular antiviral agents are used in the treatment of herpes simplex keratitis.

Ocular Side Effects

A. Local Ophthalmic Use or Exposure
   1. Irritation
      a. Lacrimation
      b. Hyperemia
      c. Photophobia
      d. Ocular pain
      e. Edema
   2. Corneal clouding
   3. Punctate keratitis
   4. Eyelids or conjunctiva
      a. Allergic reactions
      b. Conjunctivitis — follicular
      c. Eyelid thickening
   5. Narrowing or occlusion of lacrimal punctum

     6. Ptosis
     7. Corneal erosions
     8. Delayed corneal wound healing (?)

Clinical Significance: Adverse ocular reactions to these agents are often missed and frequently assumed to be worsening of the clinical disease. Ocular side effects seem to occur most frequently in eyes with decreased tear production. The occasional appearance of corneal clouding, stippling, and small punctate defects in the corneal epithelium is not uncommon. Not all signs and symptoms are reversible after discontinuing use of these drugs since in some cases ptosis and occlusion of the lacrimal punctum have been permanent. Simultaneous administration of boric acid may increase ocular irritation.

Interactions with Other Drugs

  A. Contraindications
     1. Boric acid

References

AMA Drug Evaluations. 2nd Ed., Acton, Mass., Publishing Sciences Group, 1973, p. 712.

Laibson, P. R.: Current therapy of herpes simplex virus infection of the cornea. Int. Ophthalmol. Clin. *13*(4):39, 1973.

McGill, J., et al.: Reassessment of idoxuridine therapy of herpetic keratitis. Trans. Ophthalmol. Soc. U. K. *94*:542, 1974.

McGill, J., Fraunfelder, F. T., and Jones, B. R.: Current and proposed management of ocular herpes simplex. Surv. Ophthalmol. *20*:358, 1976.

Physicians' Desk Reference. 28th Ed., Oradell, N. J., Medical Economics Co., 1974, p. 1382.

* * * * * * * * * * * *

Generic Name: Cytarabine

Proprietary Name: Ara-C, Cytosar

Primary Use: *Systemic:* This antimetabolite is effective in the management of acute granulocytic leukemia, polycythemia vera, and malignant neoplasms. *Ophthalmic:* This topical pyrimidine nucleoside is used in the treatment of herpes simplex keratitis.

Ocular Side Effects

  A. Systemic Administration
     1. Eyelids or conjunctiva
       a. Allergic reactions
       b. Conjunctivitis — nonspecific
       c. Hyperpigmentation
       d. Purpura
     2. Subconjunctival or retinal hemorrhages secondary to drug-induced anemia
     3. Keratitis
     4. Loss of eyelashes or eyebrows (?)
     5. Ocular teratogenic effects (?)

B. Local Ophthalmic Use or Exposure
    1. Ocular pain
    2. Iritis
    3. Corneal opacities
    4. Corneal ulceration

Clinical Significance: Ocular side effects due to systemic cytarabine are uncommon and seldom of major clinical significance. Other than the drug's possible teratogenic effects, all adverse ocular reactions are transitory and reversible with discontinued drug use. Because topical cytarabine causes significant corneal toxicity, it has been replaced by equally effective and less toxic antiviral agents.

References

Apt, L., and Gaffney, W. L.: Congenital eye abnormalities from drugs during pregnancy. In Leopold, I. H. (Ed.): Symposium on Ocular Therapy. St. Louis, C. V. Mosby, Vol. VII, 1974, pp. 1–22.
Blacow, N. W. (Ed.): Martindale: The Extra Pharmacopoeia. 26th Ed., London, Pharmaceutical Press, 1972, pp. 1197–1199.
Elliott, G. A. and Schut, A. L.: Studies with cytarabine HCl (CA) in normal eyes of man, monkey and rabbit. Am. J. Ophthalmol. 60:1074, 1965.
Grant, W. M.: Toxicology of the Eye. 2nd Ed., Springfield, Ill., Charles C Thomas, 1974, pp. 346–347.
Havener, W. H.: Ocular Pharmacology. 2nd Ed., St. Louis, C. V. Mosby, 1970, pp. 164–165.
Kaufman, H. E., et al.: Corneal toxicity of cytosine arabinoside. Arch. Ophthalmol. 72:535, 1964.

* * * * * * * * * * * *

Class: Carbonic Anhydrase Inhibitors

Generic Name: 1. Acetazolamide; 2. Dichlorphenamide; 3. Ethoxzolamide; 4. Methazolamide

Proprietary Name: 1. Acetazide (G.B.), Diamox, Diuramid (Pol.), Glaucomide (Austral.), Hydrazol; 2. Daranide, Oratrol; 3. Cardrase, Ethamide; 4. Neptazane

Primary Use: These enzyme inhibitors are effective in the treatment of all types of glaucomas. Acetazolamide is also effective in edema due to congestive heart failure, drug-induced edema, and centrencephalic epilepsies.

Ocular Side Effects

A. Systemic Administration
    1. Decreased intraocular pressure
    2. Decreased vision

3. Myopia
4. Decreased accommodation
5. Forward displacement of lens
6. Eyelids or conjunctiva
    a. Allergic reactions
    b. Urticaria
    c. Purpura
    d. Lyell's syndrome
7. Retinal or macular edema
8. Iritis
9. Ocular signs of gout
10. Globus hystericus
11. Subconjunctival or retinal hemorrhages secondary to drug-induced anemia
12. Problems with color vision (methazolamide)
    a. Dyschromatopsia
    b. Objects have yellow tinge

Clinical Significance: Ocular side effects due to carbonic anhydrase inhibitors are usually transient and insignificant. Myopia is a common adverse ocular reaction; but since most patients are already receiving miotics, these drugs are incriminated. Cases of gout have been induced by carbonic anhydrase inhibitors since they elevate serum uric acid. The ocular signs of gout include conjunctival hyperemia, uveitis, scleritis, and corneal deposits or ulcerations.

Interactions with Other Drugs

A. Effect of Carbonic Anhydrase Inhibitors on Activity of Other Drugs
    1. Diuretics ↑
    2. Erythromycin ↑
    3. Phenothiazines ↑
    4. Tricyclic antidepressants ↑
    5. Urea ↑
    6. Sympathomimetics ↑↓
    7. Salicylates ↓
B. Effect of Other Drugs on Activity of Carbonic Anhydrase Inhibitors
    1. Adrenergic blockers ↑
    2. Diuretics ↑
    3. Monoamine oxidase inhibitors ↑
    4. Sympathomimetics ↑
    5. Tricyclic antidepressants ↑
    6. Urea ↑

References

Back, M.: Transient myopia after use of acetazoleamide (Diamox). Arch. Ophthalmol. 55:546, 1956.
Beasley, F. J.: Transient myopia and retinal edema during ethoxzolamide (Cardrase) therapy. Arch. Ophthalmol. 68:490, 1962.
Galin, M. A., Baras, I., and Zweifach, P.: Diamox-induced myopia. Am. J. Ophthalmol. 54:237, 1962.

Halpern, A. E., and Kulvin, M. M.: Transient myopia during treatment with carbonic anhydrase inhibitors. Am. J. Ophthalmol. 48:534, 1959.
Physicians' Desk Reference for Ophthalmology. 3rd Ed., Oradell, N. J., Medical Economics Co., 1974/75, pp. 208, 222–224, 241.

* * * * * * * * * * * *

Class: Decongestants

Generic Name: Naphazoline

Proprietary Name: *Nasal:* Naphazoline *Ophthalmic:* Albalon, Clear Eyes, Privine, Vasocon

Primary Use: This topical sympathomimetic amine is effective in the symptomatic relief of both nasal and ophthalmic congestion of allergic or inflammatory origin.

Ocular Side Effects

A. Local Ophthalmic Use or Exposure
  1. Conjunctival vasoconstriction
  2. Irritation
    a. Lacrimation
    b. Reactive hyperemia
  3. Mydriasis — may precipitate narrow-angle glaucoma
  4. Decreased vision
  5. Punctate keratitis
  6. Eyelids or conjunctiva
    a. Allergic reactions
    b. Conjunctivitis — nonspecific
  7. Increased pigment granules in anterior chamber

Clinical Significance: No ocular side effects due to naphazoline are seen except with topical ocular application. Adverse ocular reactions are seldom significant except with frequent or long-term usage. The conjunctival vasculature may fail to respond to the vasoconstrictive properties of naphazoline if it is used excessively or for prolonged periods.

Interactions with Other Drugs

A. Effect of Naphazoline on Activity of Other Drugs
  1. Tricyclic antidepressants ↑
  2. Analgesics ↓
  3. Anticholinesterases ↓
B. Effect of Other Drugs on Activity of Naphazoline
  1. Alcohol ↑

   2. Anticholinergics ↑
   3. Antihistamines ↑
   4. Tricyclic antidepressants ↑
   5. Phenothiazines ↑↓
   6. Anticholinesterases ↓
 C. Contraindications
   1. Monoamine oxidase inhibitors

References

AMA Drug Evaluations. 2nd Ed., Acton, Mass., Publishing Sciences Group, 1973, pp. 471, 726–727.

Goodman, L. S., and Gilman, A. (Eds.): The Pharmacological Basis of Therapeutics. 4th Ed., New York, Macmillan, 1970, pp. 512–520.

Grant, W. M.: Toxicology of the Eye. 2nd Ed., Springfield, Charles C Thomas, 1974, p. 733.

Komi, T., et al.: Inhibitory effect of sodium chondroitin sulfate on epithelial keratitis induced by naphazoline. Am. J. Ophthalmol. 58:892, 1964.

Physicians' Desk Reference for Ophthalmology. 3rd Ed., Oradell, N. J., Medical Economics Co., 1974/75, pp. 201, 206, 234.

* * * * * * * * * * * *

Generic Name: Tetrahydrozoline

Proprietary Name: *Nasal:* Tyzine *Ophthalmic:* Murine 2, Visine

Primary Use: This topical sympathomimetic amine is effective in the symptomatic relief of both nasal and ophthalmic congestion of allergic or inflammatory origin.

Ocular Side Effects

 A. Local Ophthalmic Use or Exposure
   1. Conjunctival vasoconstriction
   2. Irritation
     a. Lacrimation
     b. Reactive hyperemia
   3. Mydriasis — may precipitate narrow-angle glaucoma
   4. Decreased intraocular pressure
   5. Decreased vision
   6. Orbital or periorbital pain
   7. Eyelids or conjunctiva
     a. Allergic reactions
     b. Conjunctivitis — nonspecific
   8. Increased pigment granules in anterior chamber (?)

Clinical Significance: No ocular side effects due to tetrahydrozoline are seen except with topical ocular application. In the drug concentrations available in commercial ophthalmic preparations, ocular side effects are quite rare and usually of little consequence. All adverse ocular reactions are reversible with discontinuation of the use of the drug.

Interactions with Other Drugs

A. Contraindications
  1. Monoamine oxidase inhibitors

References

AMA Drug Evaluations. 2nd Ed., Acton, Mass., Publishing Sciences Group, 1973, pp. 473, 726–727.
American Hospital Formulary Service. Washington, D. C., American Society of Hospital Pharmacists, Vol. II, 52:32, 1961.
Physicians' Desk Reference. 28th Ed., Oradell, N. J., Medical Economics Co., 1974, p. 875.
Physicians' Desk Reference for Ophthalmology. 3rd Ed., Oradell, N. J., Medical Economics Co., 1974/75, pp. 201, 224.

* * * * * * * * * * * *

Class: Miotics

Generic Name: Acetylcholine

Proprietary Name: Miochol

Primary Use: This intraocular quaternary ammonium parasympathomimetic agent is used to produce prompt, short-term miosis.

Ocular Side Effects

A. Local Ophthalmic Use or Exposure — Subconjunctival or Intracameral Injection
  1. Miosis
  2. Decreased intraocular pressure
  3. Conjunctival hyperemia
  4. Accommodative spasm
  5. Iris atrophy
  6. Blepharoclonus
  7. Lacrimation
  8. Retinal hemorrhages
  9. Paradoxical mydriasis
  10. Decreased anterior chamber depth

Clinical Significance: Very few ocular side effects due to acetylcholine are seen. While miosis is the primary ophthalmic effect, on rare occasions mydriasis may occur. Ocular side effects are rarely of clinical significance. If acetylcholine is given intraocularly, it may cause lacrimation.

Interactions with Other Drugs

  A. Effect of Other Drugs on Activity of Acetylcholine
   1. Anticholinergics ↓
   2. Sympathomimetics ↓

References

Barraquer, J. I.: Acetylcholine as a miotic agent for use in surgery. Am. J. Ophthalmol.
 57:406, 1964.
Catford, G. V., and Millis, E.: Clinical experience in the intraocular use of acetylcholine. Br.
 J. Ophthalmol. 51:183, 1967.
Harley, R. D., and Mishler, J. E.: Acetylcholine in cataract surgery. Br. J. Ophthalmol.
 50:429, 1966.
Rizzuti, A. B.: Acetylcholine in surgery of the lens, iris and cornea. Am. J. Ophthalmol.
 63:484, 1967.
Rongey, K. A., and Weisman, H.: Hypotension following intraocular acetylcholine.
 Anesthesiology 36:412, 1972.

* * * * * * * * * * * * *

Generic Name: 1. Demecarium; 2. Echothiophate; 3. Isoflurophate

Proprietary Name: 1. Humorsol, Tosmilen (G.B.); 2. Echothiopate (G.B.), Phospholine; 3. Dyflos (Austral.), Floropryl

Primary Use: These topical anticholinesterases are used in the management of open-angle glaucoma, conditions in which movement or constriction of the pupil is desired, and in accommodative esotropia. Demecarium is also used in the early management of ocular myasthenia gravis, and isoflurophate, in periocular louse infestations.

Ocular Side Effects

  A. Local Ophthalmic Use or Exposure
   1. Miosis
   2. Decreased vision
   3. Accommodative spasm
   4. Irritation
    a. Lacrimation
    b. Hyperemia
    c. Photophobia
    d. Ocular pain
    e. Edema
    f. Burning sensation
   5. Cataracts
    a. Anterior or posterior subcapsular
    b. Hydrational changes (?)
    c. Nuclear changes (?)
   6. Eyelids or conjunctiva
    a. Allergic reactions
    b. Conjunctivitis — follicular

        c. Conjunctival thickening
    7. Blepharoclonus
    8. Myopia
    9. Iris or ciliary body cysts — especially in children
  10. Intraocular pressure
        a. Increased — initial
        b. Decreased
  11. Iritis
        a. Occasionally fine K.P. (keratitic precipitates)
        b. Activation of latent iritis or uveitis
        c. Formation of anterior or posterior synechiae
  12. Decreased scleral rigidity
  13. Occlusion of lacrimal canaliculi
  14. Decreased anterior chamber depth
  15. Hyphema — during surgery
  16. Vitreous hemorrhages
  17. Decreased size of filtering bleb
  18. Corneal deposits (echothiophate)
  19. Retinal detachment (?)
  20. Atypical band keratopathy (?) (isoflurophate)

Clinical Significance: Ocular side effects are most common with isoflurophate followed by echothiophate and demecarium. Visual complaints with or without accommodative spasm are the most frequent adverse ocular reactions. Drug-induced lens changes are well documented and are primarily seen in the older age group. In shallow anterior chamber angles, these agents are contraindicated since in up to 10 percent of cases they may precipitate narrow-angle glaucoma. This is probably due to peripheral vascular congestion of the iris, which may further aggravate an already compromised angle. Also, these parasympathomimetic agents allow the iris lens diaphragm to come forward and, under certain circumstances, to induce a relative pupillary block. While irritative conjunctival changes are common with long-term usage, allergic reactions are rare. Some retinal surgeons are convinced that these agents cause retinal detachments by exerting traction on the peripheral retina. Cases of irreversible miosis due to long-term therapy have been reported. An atypical band-shaped keratopathy has been said to be due to long-term miotic therapy; however, others suggest this is due to long-term elevation of intraocular pressure and is not drug-induced.

Interactions with Other Drugs

  A. Effect of Anticholinesterases on Activity of Other Drugs
      1. Succinylcholine ↑

References

Grant, W. M.: Toxicology of the Eye. 2nd Ed., Springfield, Charles C Thomas, 1974, pp. 398, 441–442, 706–718.
Havener, W. H.: Ocular Pharmacology. 2nd Ed., St. Louis, C. V. Mosby, 1970, pp. 227–245.
Klendshoj, N. C., and Olmsted, E. P.: Observation of dangerous side effect of phospholine iodide in glaucoma therapy. Am. J. Ophthalmol. 56:247, 1963.

Shaffer, R. N., and Hetherington, J.: Anticholinesterase drugs and cataracts. Am. J.
  Ophthalmol. 62:613, 1966.
Westsmith, R. A., and Abernethy, R. E.: Detachment of retina with use of diisopropyl
  fluorophosphate (Fluropryl) in treatment of glaucoma. Arch. Ophthalmol. 52:779, 1954.

* * * * * * * * * * * * *

Generic Name: 1. Neostigmine; 2. Physostigmine

Proprietary Name: 1. Prostigmin; 2. Physostigmine

Primary Use: These topical parasympathomimetic agents are used in the
management of narrow- and open-angle glaucoma. Neostigmine is also used in
the management of ptosis caused by myasthenia gravis.

Ocular Side Effects

A. Local Ophthalmic Use or Exposure
    1. Miosis
    2. Decreased intraocular pressure
    3. Irritation
        a. Hyperemia
        b. Ocular pain
        c. Photophobia
    4. Blepharoclonus
    5. Accommodative spasm
    6. Decreased vision
    7. Eyelids or conjunctiva
        a. Allergic reactions
        b. Conjunctivitis — follicular
        c. Blepharoconjunctivitis
        d. Depigmentation
    8. Myopia
    9. Iritis
    10. Iris cysts
    11. Decreased anterior chamber depth
    12. Vitreous hemorrhages
    13. Cataracts
    14. Occlusion of lacrimal punctum (physostigmine)
    15. Retinal detachment (?)
    16. Atypical band keratopathy (?) (physostigmine)

Clinical Significance: Ocular side effects due to these anticholinesterases are
usually reversible with discontinued drug usage. These agents should be used
with caution since peripheral vascular congestion of the iris may precipitate
narrow-angle glaucoma. Long-term usage with these drugs is seldom possible,
since allergic or irritative conjunctivitis occurs frequently. An atypical band
keratopathy has been said to be due to long-term miotic therapy; however,
others suggest it is due to long-term elevation of intraocular pressure and is not
drug-induced. Physostigmine is sensitive to heat and light and becomes

discolored. Discolored solutions are irritating and clinically ineffective.

Interactions with Other Drugs

  A. Effect of Anticholinesterases on Activity of Other Drugs
      1. Succinylcholine ↑
      2. Local anesthetics ↓
  B. Effect of Other Drugs on Activity of Anticholinesterases
      1. Local anesthetics ↓

References

Cumming, G., Harding, L. K., and Prowse, K.: Treatment and recovery after massive overdose of physostigmine. Lancet 2:147, 1968.

Ellis, P. P., and Smith, D. L.: Handbook of Ocular Therapeutics and Pharmacology. 4th Ed., St. Louis, C. V. Mosby, 1973, pp. 205, 209–210.

Grant, W. M.: Toxicology of the Eye. 2nd Ed. Springfield, Ill., Charles C Thomas, 1974, pp. 706–718, 831–832.

Jacklin, H. N.: Depigmentation of the eyelids in eserine allergy. Am. J. Ophthalmol. 59:89, 1965.

Leopold, I. H. (Ed.): Glaucoma Drug Therapy: Monograph I Parasympathetic Agents. Irvine, Calif., Allergan Pharmaceuticals, 1975, pp. 19–21.

* * * * * * * * * * * *

Generic Name: Pilocarpine

Proprietary Name: Adsorbocarpine, Almocarpine, Isopto Carpine, Miocarpine SMP (G.B.), Mi-Pilo, Ocusert Pilo-20/40, Oculoguttae Pilocarpine (Scand.), Pilocar, Pilocel, Pilomiotin, Pilopt (Austral.), P.V. Carpine

Primary Use: This topical ocular parasympathomimetic agent is used in the management of glaucoma and in conditions in which constriction of the pupil is desired.

Ocular Side Effects

  A. Local Ophthalmic Use or Exposure
      1. Miosis
      2. Decreased vision
      3. Accommodative spasm
      4. Intraocular pressure
         a. Increased — initial
         b. Decreased
      5. Decreased anterior chamber depth
      6. Eyelids or conjunctiva
         a. Allergic reactions
         b. Hyperemia
         c. Conjunctivitis — follicular
      7. Irritation
         a. Lacrimation
         b. Hyperemia
         c. Ocular pain

8. Blepharoclonus
9. Iris cysts
10. Increased axial lens diameter
11. Decreased scleral rigidity
12. Cataracts
13. Atypical band keratopathy (?)

Clinical Significance: Probably the most frequent ocular side effect due to pilocarpine is decrease in vision secondary to miosis or accommodative spasms. Follicular conjunctivitis is common after long-term therapy, but it has minimal clinical significance. Iris cysts are quite rare, and drug-induced lens changes are still debatable. An atypical band-shaped keratopathy has been said to be due to long-term miotic therapy; however, others suggest it is due to long-term elevation of intraocular pressure and is not drug-induced.

Interactions with Other Drugs

A. Effect of Pilocarpine on Activity of Other Drugs
   1. Alcohol ↑
   2. Anticholinesterases ↑
   3. Urea ↑
   4. Anticholinergics ↓
B. Effect of Other Drugs on Activity of Pilocarpine
   1. Antihistamines ↑
   2. Anticholinesterases ↑
   3. Monoamine oxidase inhibitors ↑
   4. Phenothiazines ↑
   5. Tricyclic antidepressants ↑
   6. Urea ↑
   7. Adrenergic blockers ↓

References

Abraham, S. V.: Miotic iridocyclitis: Its role in the surgical treatment of glaucoma. Am. J. Ophthalmol. 48:634, 1959.
Abramson, D. H., et al.: Pilocarpine-induced lens changes. Arch. Ophthalmol. 92:464, 1974.
Forbes, M.: Influence of miotics on visual fields in glaucoma. Invest. Ophthalmol. 5:139, 1966.
Grant, W. M.: Toxicology of the Eye. 2nd Ed., Springfield, Charles C Thomas, 1974, pp. 706–718, 833–835.
Havener, W. H.: Ocular Pharmacology. 2nd Ed., St. Louis, C. V. Mosby, 1970, pp. 207–223.
Kennedy, R. E., Roca, P. D., and Landers, P. H.: Atypical band keratopathy in glaucomatous patients. Am. J. Ophthalmol. 72:917, 1971.
Levene, R. Z.: Uniocular miotic therapy. Trans. Am. Acad. Ophthalmol. Otolaryngol. 79:376, 1975.
Mills, P. V.: Atypical band-shaped keratopathy associated with chronic glaucoma or ocular hypertension. Trans. Ophthalmol. Soc. U. K. 94:450, 1974.
Physicians' Desk Reference for Ophthalmology. 3rd Ed. Oradell, N. J., Medical Economics Co., 1974/75, pp. 203, 211, 233.

* * * * * * * * * * * *

Class: Mydriatics and Cycloplegics

Generic Name: 1. Cyclopentolate; 2. Tropicamide

Proprietary Name: 1. Cyclogyl, Mydrilate (G.B.); 2. Mydriacyl

Primary Use: These topical ocular short-acting anticholinergic mydriatic and cycloplegic agents are used in refractions and fundus examination.

Ocular Side Effects

A. Local Ophthalmic Use or Exposure
1. Decreased vision
2. Mydriasis — may precipitate narrow-angle glaucoma
3. Irritation
   a. Hyperemia
   b. Photophobia
   c. Ocular pain
   d. Burning sensation
4. Decrease or paralysis of accommodation
5. Increased intraocular pressure
6. Eyelids or conjunctiva
   a. Allergic reactions
   b. Blepharoconjunctivitis
7. Visual hallucinations
8. Synechiae

Clinical Significance: Major ocular side effects due to these drugs are quite rare. Both cyclopentolate and tropicamide can elevate intraocular pressure in open-angle glaucoma and precipitate narrow-angle glaucoma. Visual hallucinations or psychotic reactions after topical applications are primarily seen with cyclopentolate.

Interactions with Other Drugs

A. Effect of Other Drugs on Activity of Anticholinergics
1. Antihistamines ↑
2. Phenothiazines ↑
3. Tricyclic antidepressants ↑

References

Grant, W. M.: Toxicology of the Eye. 2nd Ed., Springfield, Charles C Thomas, 1974, pp. 144–148, 344–345, 1067–1068.
Havener, W. H.: Ocular Pharmacology. 2nd Ed., St. Louis, C. V. Mosby, 1970, pp. 196–201.
Praeger, D. L., and Miller, S. N.: Toxic effects of cyclopentolate (Cyclogel). Am. J. Ophthalmol. 58:1060, 1964.
Simcoe, C. W.: Cyclopentolate (Cyclogyl) toxicity. Arch. Ophthalmol. 67:406, 1962.
Yamaji, R.: Study of pseudomyopia. Acta Soc. Ophthalmol. Jap. 72:2083, 1968.

* * * * * * * * * * * * *

Class: Ophthalmic Dyes ·

Generic Name: 1. Alcian Blue; 2. Fluorescein; 3. Rose Bengal; 4. Trypan Blue

Proprietary Name: *Systemic:* 2. Fluorescite, Funduscein *Ophthalmic:* 1. Alcian Blue; 2. Fluoreseptic, Fluorets (G.B.), Fluor-I-Strip-A.T., Ful-Glo; 3. Rose Bengal; 4. Trypan Blue

Primary Use: *Systemic:* Fluorescein is used to study the aqueous secretion of the ciliary body and to aid in the diagnosis of internal carotid artery insufficiency. *Ophthalmic:* These topical dyes are· used in various ocular diagnostic tests.

Ocular Side Effects
  A. Systemic Administration
      1. Stains ocular fluids and tissues yellow-green
      2. Eyelids or conjunctiva
          a. Allergic reactions
          b. Hyperemia
          c. Yellow-orange discoloration
          d. Angioneurotic edema
          e. Urticaria
  B. Local Ophthalmic Use or Exposure
      1. Stains mucus and connective tissue blue (alcian blue)
      2. Stains ocular fluids and tissues yellow-green (fluorescein)
      3. Stains degenerated epithelial cells and mucus red (rose bengal)
      4. Stains degenerated epithelial cells and mucus blue (trypan blue)
      5. Irritation
          a. Ocular pain
          b. Burning sensation
      6. Eyelids or conjunctiva
          a. Blue discoloration (alcian blue, trypan blue)
          b. Yellow-orange discoloration (fluorescein)
          c. Red discoloration (rose bengal)
      7. Problems with color vision (fluorescein)
          a. Objects have yellow tinge

Clinical Significance: Ocular side effects due to these ophthalmic dyes are rare and transient. Solutions of fluorescein can readily become contaminated with Pseudomonas because fluorescein inactivates the preservatives found in most ophthalmic solutions. Rose bengal, especially in concentrations above 1 percent, may cause significant ocular irritation after topical ocular instillation. If the corneal epithelium is not intact, the topical application of alcian blue may cause long-term or even permanent stromal deposits of the dye.

References

Grant, W. M.: Toxicology of the Eye. 2nd Ed. Springfield, Charles C Thomas, 1974, pp. 430–435, 495, 888, 1068–1069.
Havener, W. H.: Ocular Pharmacology. 2nd Ed. St. Louis, C. V. Mosby, 1970, pp. 323–332.
Norn, M. S.: Vital staining of cornea and conjunctiva. Acta Ophthalmol. (Suppl.) *113*:7, 1972.
Paterson, C. A.: Effects of drugs on the lens. Int. Ophthalmol. Clin. *11*(2):63, 1971.

* * * * * * * * * * * * *

Class: Ophthalmic Implants

Generic Name: Silicone

Proprietary Name: Silicone

Primary Use: Various silicone polymers of various viscosities or solids are used in ophthalmology as lubricants, implants, and volume expanders.

Ocular Side Effects

A. Local Ophthalmic Use or Exposure
   1. Burning sensation – topical application of liquid silicone
   2. Increase postoperative infections – silicone implants
   3. Granulomatous reactions – silicone implants
   4. Migration within the eye – intraocular liquid silicone
      a. Cataracts
      b. Endothelial damage with corneal edema or vascularization

Clinical Significance: Silicone solutions or solids rarely cause adverse ocular reactions; however, under certain circumstances significant side effects may occur. Like any foreign body buried within tissue, the implant, even if inert, will be encased by some scar tissue or even granulomatous tissue. Postoperative infection rates are also higher if an implant is included in the procedure. As with silicone liquids placed in other areas of the body, the solution within the eye may with time migrate to new locations. Since the usual site of injection is intravitreal, with time the solution may come in contact with the lens or enter the anterior chamber with the possibility of affecting the lens or cornea.

References

Armaly, M. F.: Ocular tolerance to silicones. Arch. Ophthalmol. *68*:390, 1962.
Cibis, P. A., et al.: The use of liquid silicone in retinal detachment surgery. Arch. Ophthalmol. *68*:590, 1962.
Havener, W. H.: Ocular Pharmacology. 2nd Ed., St. Louis, C. V. Mosby, 1970, p. 405.
Lee, P., et al.: Intravitreous injection of silicone. Ann. Ophthalmol. *1*:15, 1969.
Martola, E. L., and Dohlman, C. H.: Silicone oil in the anterior chamber of the eye. Acta Ophthalmol. *41*:75, 1963.

Morgan, J. F., and Hill, J. C.: Silicone fluid as a lubricant for artificial eyes. Am. J. Ophthalmol. *58*:767, 1964.

Rosengren, B.: Silicone injection into the vitreous in hopeless cases of retinal detachment. Acta Ophthalmol. *47*:757, 1969.

Schepens, C. L., et al.: Scleral buckling procedures. V. Synthetic sutures and silicone implants. Arch. Ophthalmol. *64*:868, 1960.

Spivey, B. E., Allen, L., and Burns, C. A.: The Iowa enucleation implant; a 10 year evaluation of technique and results. Am. J. Ophthalmol. *67*:171, 1969.

* * * * * * * * * * * *

Class: Ophthalmic Preservatives

Generic Name: Benzalkonium

Proprietary Name: Empiquat BAC (G.B.), Marinol (G.B.), Pheneen, Roccal (G.B.), Silquat B10/B50 (G.B.), Vantoc CL (G.B.), Zephiran

Primary Use: This topical ocular quaternary ammonium agent is used as a preservative in ophthalmic solutions and as a germicidal cleaning solution for contact lenses.

Ocular Side Effects

A. Local Ophthalmic Use or Exposure
1. Irritation
    a. Lacrimation
    b. Hyperemia
    c. Photophobia
    d. Edema
2. Punctate keratitis
3. Gray corneal epithelial haze
4. Pseudomembrane formation
5. Decreased corneal epithelial microvilli
6. Delayed corneal wound healing (?)

Clinical Significance: Adverse ocular reactions to benzalkonium are not uncommon, even at exceedingly low concentrations. Concentrations as low as 0.01 percent may cause cell damage by emulsification of the cell wall lipids. Almost all ocular side effects are reversible after use of the drug is discontinued, and most of the damage is fairly superficial. Benzalkonium may also destroy the corneal epithelial microvilli, and thereby possibly prevent adherence of the mucoid layer of the tear film to the cornea. This drug also allows for an increased penetration of some drugs through the corneal epithelium, and is added to some commercial ophthalmic preparations for this reason.

References

Goodman, L. S., and Gilman, A. (Eds.): The Pharmacological Basis of Therapeutics. 4th Ed., New York, Macmillan, 1970, pp. 1051–1052.

Lemp, M. A.: Artificial tear solutions. Int. Ophthalmol. Clin. *13*(1):221, 1973.

Lemp, M. A., and Holly, F. J.: Ophthalmic polymers as ocular wetting agents. Ann. Ophthalmol. *4*:15, 1972.

Leopold, I. H.: Local toxic effect of detergents on ocular structures. Arch. Ophthalmol. *34*:99, 1945.

Swan, K. C.: Reactivity of the ocular tissues to wetting agents. Am. J. Ophthalmol. *27*:1118, 1944.

* * * * * * * * * * * *

Generic Name: 1. Mercuric Oxide (Hydrargyric Oxide Flavum); 2. Nitromersol; 3. Phenylmercuric Acetate; 4. Phenylmercuric Nitrate (Phenylhydrargyric Nitrate); 5. Thimerosal

Proprietary Name: 1. Yellow Mercuric Oxide, Pagenstecher's Ointment (G.B.); 2. Nitromersol; 3. Controid (Austral.); 4. Clean-N-Soak, Vaxoid (Austral.), Visalens; 5. Merthiolate, Thiomersal (G.B.)

Primary Use: These topical ocular organomercurials are used as antiseptics, preservatives, and antibacterial or antifungal agents in ophthalmic solutions and ointments.

Ocular Side Effects

   A. Local Ophthalmic Use or Exposure
      1. Eyelids or conjunctiva
         a. Allergic reactions
         b. Erythema
         c. Blepharoconjunctivitis
      2. Bluish-gray mercury deposits
         a. Eyelids
         b. Conjunctiva
         c. Cornea (mercuric oxide)
         d. Lens (mercuric oxide and phenylmercuric acetate or nitrate)

Clinical Significance: Adverse ocular side effects due to these organomercurials are rare and seldom of significance. The most striking side effect is mercurial deposits in various ocular and periocular tissues. This is an apparently harmless side effect since it is asymptomatic, and no visual impairments due to it have been found. Conjunctival mercurial deposits are seen around blood vessels near the cornea, corneal deposits are in the peripheral Descemet's membrane, and lens deposits are mainly in the pupillary area. Mercurialentis has not been seen with thimerosal at concentrations of 0.005 percent, the concentration used as a preservative in some ophthalmic solutions. Unfortunately, in antifungal therapeutic concentrations, these mercurials are too toxic for ocular use.

References

Abrams, J. D.: Iatrogenic mercurialentis. Trans. Ophthalmol. Soc. U. K. *83*:263, 1963.
Abrams, J. D., and Majzoub, V.: Mercury content of the human lens. Br. J. Ophthalmol. *54*:59, 1970.
Blacow, N. W. (Ed.): Martindale: The Extra Pharmacopoeia. 26th Ed., London, Pharmaceutical Press, 1972, pp. 1058–1064.
Duke-Elder, S.: Systems of Ophthalmology. St. Louis, C. V. Mosby, Vol. XIV, Part 2, 1972, pp. 1095–1096.
Theodore, F. H.: Drug sensitivities and irritations of the conjunctiva. JAMA *151*:25, 1953.
Willetts, G. S.: Ocular side-effects of drugs. Br. J. Ophthalmol. *53*:252, 1969.

* * * * * * * * * * * *

Class: Proteolytic Enzymes

Generic Name: Alpha-Chymotrypsin

Proprietary Name: Alpha Chymar, Catarase, Chymar-Zon (G.B.), Quimotrase, Zolyse, Zonulysin (G.B.)

Primary Use: This intraocular proteolytic enzyme is effective in lysing zonular fibers in intracapsular lens extraction.

Ocular Side Effects

A. Local Ophthalmic Use or Exposure
1. Lyses zonular fibers
2. Forward displacement of lens
3. Increased intraocular pressure
4. Uveitis
5. Induce or aggravate scleritis
6. Corneal edema
7. Increased striate keratopathy (?)
8. Delayed corneal wound healing (?)
9. Retinal detachment (?)

Clinical Significance: Surprisingly few ocular side effects are seen with this potent enzyme when it is used in the concentrations recommended. The most common adverse ocular reaction is transient glaucoma, which usually appears 2 to 5 days after cataract surgery and spontaneously subsides within a week. This agent can affect the retina; however, clinically it would probably have to be injected directly into the vitreous to reach toxic retinal levels.

References

Havener, W. H.: Ocular Pharmacology. 2nd Ed., St. Louis, C. V. Mosby, 1970, pp. 27–45.
Kirsch, R. E.: Glaucoma following cataract extraction associated with use of alpha-chymotrypsin. Arch. Ophthalmol. *72*:612, 1964.

Maumenee, A. E.: Effects of alpha-chymotrypsin on the retina. Trans. Am. Acad. Ophthalmol. Otolaryngol. 64:33, 1960.
Rains, D. E., Rains, K. P., and Coker, H. G.: Enzymatic zonulolysis in cataract surgery: Historical review and present use. Ann. Ophthalmol. 6:511, 1974.
Troutman, R. C.: National survey on the facility of cataract extraction, operative and immediate postoperative complications. Trans. Am. Acad. Ophthalmol. Otolaryngol. 64:37, 1960.
Watson, P. G.: Treatment of scleritis and episcleritis. Trans. Ophthalmol. Soc. U. K. 94:76, 1974.

* * * * * * * * * * * *

Generic Name: Urokinase

Proprietary Name: Urokinase

Primary Use: This proteolytic enzyme is injected into the anterior chamber or vitreous to possibly aid in the removal of blood.

Ocular Side Effects

A.   Local Ophthalmic Use or Exposure
  1. Hypopyon
  2. Uveitis
  3. Intraocular pressure
      a. Increased
      b. Decreased
  4. Bleeding (?)

Clinical Significance: After intravitreal injections of urokinase, as high as a 50-percent incidence of sterile hypopyon has occurred. This is thought to be cellular debris in the anterior chamber which usually absorbs within 5 days. Uveitis usually is mild although severe cases have been seen.

References

Cleary, P. E., et al.: Intravitreal urokinase in the treatment of vitreous haemorrhage. Trans. Ophthalmol. Soc. U. K. 94:587, 1974.
Dugmore, W. N., and Raichand, M.: Intravitreal urokinase in the treatment of vitreous hemorrhage. Am. J. Ophthalmol. 75:779, 1973.
Forrester, J. V., and Williamson, J.: Lytic therapy in vitreous hemorrhage. Trans. Ophthalmol. Soc. U. K. 94:583, 1974.
Pierse, D.: The use of urokinase in the anterior chamber. Trans. Ophthalmol. Soc. U. K. 84:271, 1964.
Sellors, P. J. H., Kanski, J. J., and Watson, D. M.: Intravitreal urokinase in the management of vitreous haemorrhage. Trans. Ophthalmol. Soc. U. K. 94:591, 1974.

* * * * * * * * * * * *

Class: Topical Local Anesthetics

Generic Name: 1. Benoxinate; 2. Butacaine; 3. Cocaine; 4. Dibucaine; 5. Dyclonine; 6. Phenacaine; 7. Piperocaine; 8. Proparacaine; 9. Tetracaine

Proprietary Name: *Systemic:* 4. Cinchocaine (G.B.), Nupercaine, Nuporals; 7. Metycaine; 9. Amethocaine (G.B.), Pantocain (Germ.), Pontocaine *Ophthalmic:* 1. Dorsacaine, Novesine (G.B.); 2. Butyn; 3. Cocaine; 4. Nupercainal; 5. Dyclone; 6. Holocaine, Taricaine; 7. Metycaine; 8. Alcaine, Ophthaine, Ophthetic, Proxymetacaine (G.B.); 9. Amethocaine (G.B.), Pontocaine

Primary Use: *Systemic:* Dibucaine, piperocaine, and tetracaine are effective in infiltrative, nerve block, peridural, caudal, and spinal anesthesia. *Ophthalmic:* These topical local anesthetics are used in diagnostic and surgical procedures.

Ocular Side Effects

A. Systemic Administration
    1. Decreased vision
    2. Miosis
    3. Paralysis of extraocular muscles
    4. Diplopia
    5. Blepharoclonus
B. Local Ophthalmic Use or Exposure
    1. Corneal epithelium
        a. Punctate keratitis
        b. Gray, ground glass appearance
        c. Softening, erosions, and sloughing
        d. Filaments
        e. Ulceration
    2. Iritis
    3. Irritation
        a. Lacrimation
        b. Hyperemia
        c. Ocular pain
        d. Burning sensation
    4. Delayed corneal wound healing
    5. Eyelids or conjunctiva
        a. Allergic reactions
        b. Blepharoconjunctivitis
    6. Decreased stability of corneal tear film
    7. Subconjunctival hemorrhages
    8. Corneal edema
    9. Decreased blink reflex
    10. Hypopyon
    11. Inhibits bacterial growth

12. Inhibits fluorescence of fluorescein
13. Blindness
14. Conjunctival vasoconstriction (cocaine)
15. Mydriasis — may precipitate narrow-angle glaucoma (cocaine)
16. Paralysis of accommodation (cocaine)
17. Visual hallucinations — especially Lilliputian (cocaine)
18. Exophthalmos (cocaine)
19. Ptosis (?) (cocaine)

Clinical Significance: Few significant ocular side effects are seen with these agents if they are given topically for short periods of time; however, prolonged use may cause severe and permanent corneal damage and visual loss. Transient superficial corneal irregularities and edema may interfere with biomicroscopy or fundus examinations even after a single application. Recent data suggest that topical local anesthetics adversely affect superficial corneal epithelial microvilli. This may be the reason the stability of the tear film is adversely affected by these agents. Currently, proparacaine is probably the most commonly used topical local anesthetic since it causes the least irritation. Tetracaine may cause ocular irritation long after its local anesthetic effect wears off. Proparacaine has been reported to be one of the three more common topical ocular drugs causing allergic dermatitis. The other two drugs are atropine and neomycin. While most of these agents decrease the fluorescence of fluroescein, benoxinate decreases it the least. One case of an inadvertent anterior chamber injection of tetracaine has been reported, wherein wrinkling of Descemet's membrane, semidilated nonreactive pupils, and bullous keratopathy which did not respond to therapy occurred.

Interactions with Other Drugs

A. Effect of Topical Local Anesthetics on Activity of Other Drugs
    1. Succinylcholine ↑
    2. Sympathomimetics ↑
    3. Adrenergic blockers ↓
    4. Sulfonamides ↓

References

Bellows, J. G.: Surface anesthesia in ophthalmology; comparison of some drugs used. Arch. Ophthalmol. *12*:824, 1934.

Eerden, A. A. J. J. v. d.: Changes in corneal epithelium due to local anesthetics. Ophthalmologica *143*:154, 1962.

Epstein, D. L., and Paton, D.: Keratitis from misuse of corneal anesthetics. N. Engl. J. Med. *279*:396, 1968.

Grant, W. M.: Toxicology of the Eye. 2nd Ed., Springfield, Charles C Thomas, 1974, pp. 136–141.

Havener, W. H.: Ocular Pharmacology. 2nd Ed., St. Louis, C. V. Mosby, 1970, pp. 46–85.

Knapp, H.: On cocaine and its use in ophthalmic and general surgery. Arch. Ophthalmol. *68*:31, 1962.

* * * * * * * * * * * *

Class: Topical Osmotic Agents

Generic Name: Sodium Chloride

Proprietary Name: Adsorbonac, Ocean Mist

Primary Use: This topical ocular hypertonic salt solution is used to reduce corneal edema.

Ocular Side Effects

A. Local Ophthalmic Use or Exposure – Topical Application
1. Irritation
   a. Hyperemia
   b. Ocular pain
   c. Burning sensation
2. Corneal dehydration
3. Subconjunctival hemorrhages
B. Local Ophthalmic Use or Exposure – Subconjunctival Injection
1. Conjunctival hyperemia
2. Increased intraocular pressure

Clinical Significance: Few significant adverse ocular reactions are seen with commercial topical sodium chloride solutions. The most frequent ocular side effects are irritation and discomfort, which are primarily related to the frequency of application. At suggested dosages all ocular side effects are reversible and transient.

References

Grant, W. M.: Toxicology of the Eye. 2nd Ed., Springfield, Charles C Thomas, 1974, p. 929.

Maurice, D. M.: Influence on corneal permeability of bathing with solutions of differing reaction and tonicity. Br. J. Ophthalmol. *39*:463, 1955.

Physicians' Desk Reference for Ophthalmology. 3rd Ed., Oradell, N. J., Medical Economics Co., 1974/75, p. 221.

Walsh, F. B., and Hoyt, W. F.: Clinical Neuro-Ophthalmology. 3rd Ed., Baltimore, Williams & Wilkins, Vol. III, 1969, p. 2710.

* * * * * * * * * * * *

Index of Side Effects

Lists of drugs causing the following side effects appear on page 266 and following pages.

Abnormal Conjugate Deviations
Abnormal Visual Sensations
Absence of Foveal Reflex
Absence of Pupillary Reaction to Light
Accommodative Spasm
Achromatopsia, Blue-Yellow Defect
Achromatopsia, Red-Green Defect
Anisocoria
Blepharitis
Blepharoclonus
Blepharoconjunctivitis
Blepharospasm
Blindness
Cataracts
Central Serous Retinopathy
Colored Haloes around Lights
Congenital Cataracts
Conjunctival Deposits
Conjunctival Hyperemia
Conjunctivitis — Follicular
Conjunctivitis — Nonspecific
Constriction of Visual Fields
Corneal Deposits
Corneal Edema
Corneal Opacities
Cortical Blindness
Decreased Accommodation
Decreased Anterior Chamber Depth
Decreased Convergence
Decreased Corneal Reflex
Decreased Dark Adaptation
Decreased Depth Perception
Decreased Intraocular Pressure
Decreased Lacrimation
Decreased Pupillary Reaction to Light
Decreased Resistance to Infection
Decreased Spontaneous Eye
  Movements
Decreased Tolerance to Contact Lenses
Decreased Vision
Delayed Corneal Wound Healing
Diplopia
Dyschromatopsia
Enlarged Blind Spot

Exophthalmos
Eyelid Deposits
Eyelids — Depigmentation
Eyelids — Erythema
Eyelids — Exfoliative Dermatitis
Eyelids — Urticaria
Eyelids or Conjunctiva — Allergic
  Reactions
Eyelids or Conjunctiva —
  Angioneurotic Edema
Eyelids or Conjunctiva — Discoloration
Eyelids or Conjunctiva — Edema
Eyelids or Conjunctiva — Erythema
  Multiforme
Eyelids or Conjunctiva — Hyper-
  pigmentation
Eyelids or Conjunctiva — Lupoid
  Syndrome
Eyelids or Conjunctiva — Lyell's
  Syndrome
Eyelids or Conjunctiva — Purpura
Eyelids or Conjunctiva — Stevens-
  Johnson Syndrome
Heightened Color Perception
Hemianopsia
Hippus
Horner's Syndrome
Hypermetropia
Hypopyon
Increased Intraocular Pressure
Iris or Ciliary Body Cysts
Iritis
Jerky Pursuit Movements
Keratitis
Keratoconjunctivitis
Lacrimation
Lens Deposits
Loss of Eyelashes or Eyebrows
Macular Edema
Macular or Paramacular Degeneration
Miosis
Myasthenic Neuromuscular Blocking
  Effect
Mydriasis

264

Dimethindene
Diphenhydramine
Diphenylpyraline
Emetine
Ether
Glutethimide
Imipramine
Insulin
Isocarboxazid
Isoniazid
LSD
Lysergide
Meprobamate
Mescaline
Methyprylon
Neomycin
Nialamide
Nitrous Oxide
Nortriptyline
Orphenadrine
Pentylenetetrazol
Phenelzine
Protriptyline
Psilocybin
Sodium Antimonylgluconate
Sodium Salicylate
Stibocaptate
Stibophen
Tranylcypromine
Trichloroethylene
Tripelennamine
Urethan

Accommodative Spasm
Acetylcholine
Carbachol
Demecarium
Digitalis
Echothiophate
Guanethidine
Isoflurophate
Methylene Blue
Morphine
Neostigmine
Opium
Physostigmine
Pilocarpine

Achromatopsia, Blue-Yellow Defect
Acetyldigitoxin
Amodiaquine
Chloroquine
Deslanoside
Digitalis
Digitoxin
Digoxin
Erythromycin
Ethambutol
Gitalin
Hydroxychloroquine
Lanatoside C
Ouabain
Paramethadione
Quinine
Streptomycin
Trimethadione

Achromatopsia, Red-Green Defect
Acetophenazine
Alcohol
Amodiaquine
Aspirin
Butaperazine
Carphenazine
Chloroquine
Chlorpromazine
Diethazine
Epinephrine
Ethambutol
Ethopropazine
Fluphenazine
Hydroxychloroquine
Isocarboxazid
Isoniazid
Mesoridazine
Methdilazine
Methotrimeprazine
Morphine (?)
Nialamide
Opium (?)
Paramethadione
Pargyline
Perazine
Pericyazine
Perphenazine
Phenelzine

267

268

Secobarbital
Talbutal
Tetracaine
Thiamylal
Thiopental
Vinbarbital

Blepharoconjunctivitis
Aurothioglucose
Aurothioglycanide
Benoxinate
Bromide
Butacaine
Cocaine
Cyclopentolate
Dibucaine
Dyclonine
Epinephrine
Gold Au^{198}
Gold Sodium Thiomalate
Insulin
Iodine Solution
Mercuric Oxide
Methotrexate
Neostigmine
Nitromersol
Phenacaine
Phenylmercuric Acetate
Phenylmercuric Nitrate
Physostigmine
Piperocaine
Proparacaine
Tetracaine
Thimerosal
Tropicamide

Blepharospasm
Amphetamine (?)
Dextroamphetamine (?)
Dimercaprol
Emetine
Hashish
Levodopa
Marihuana
Methamphetamine (?)
Pentylenetetrazol
Phenmetrazine (?)
Tetrahydrocannabinol
THC

Blindness
Acetaminophen
Acetanilid
Acetophenazine
Adrenal Cortex Injection
Alcohol
Aldosterone
Allobarbital
Amitriptyline (?)
Amobarbital
Amodiaquine
Antimony Lithium Thiomalate
Antimony Potassium Tartrate
Antimony Sodium Tartrate
Antimony Sodium Thioglycollate
Antipyrine
Aprobarbital
Aspirin
Aurothioglucose
Aurothioglycanide
Barbital
Benoxinate
Benzathine Penicillin G
Betamethasone
Bishydroxycoumarin
Bupivacaine (?)
Butacaine
Butabarbital
Butalbital
Butallylonal
Butaperazine
Butethal
Capreomycin
Carbinoxamine
Carbon Dioxide
Carisoprodol
Carphenazine
Chloral Hydrate (?)
Chloramphenicol
Chlorisondamine
Chloroform
Chloroprocaine (?)
Chloroquine
Chlorpromazine
Cocaine
Cortisone
Cyclobarbital
Cyclopentyl Allylbarbituric Acid
Desipramine (?)

269

Quinidine (?)
Quinine
Radioactive Iodides
Secobarbital
Sodium Antimonylgluconate
Sodium Salicylate
Stibocaptate
Stibophen
Streptomycin
Sulfacetamide (?)
Sulfachlorpyridazine (?)
Sulfadiazine (?)
Sulfadimethoxine (?)
Sulfamerazine (?)
Sulfameter (?)
Sulfamethizole (?)
Sulfamethoxazole (?)
Sulfamethoxypyridazine (?)
Sulfanilamide (?)
Sulfaphenazole (?)
Sulfisoxazole (?)
Talbutal
Tetracaine
Thiamylal
Thiethylperazine
Thiopental
Thiopropazate
Thioproperazine
Thioridazine
Tranylcypromine (?)
Triamcinolone
Trichloroethylene
Trifluoperazine
Triflupromazine
Trimeprazine
Tripelennamine
Tryparsamide
Vinbarbital

Cataracts
Adrenal Cortex Injection
Aldosterone
Allopurinol
Amodiaquine (?)
Aurothioglucose
Aurothioglycanide
Betamethasone
Busulfan
Carbamazepine (?)

Carbromal (?)
Chloroquine (?)
Chlorprothixene
Clomiphene (?)
Cobalt
Colchicine (?)
Colloidal Silver
Cortisone
Deferoxamine
Demecarium
Desoxycorticosterone
Dexamethasone
Diazoxide
Droperidol (?)
Echothiophate
Edrophonium
Ergot (?)
Ethotoin (?)
Fludrocortisone
Fluorometholone
Fluprednisolone
Gold Au^{198}
Gold Sodium Thiomalate
Haloperidol (?)
Hydrocortisone
Hydroxychloroquine (?)
Ibuprofen (?)
Isoflurophate
Medrysone
Mephenytoin (?)
Methylprednisolone
Mild Silver Protein
Mitotane
Neostigmine
Paramethasone
Penicillamine (?)
Phenmetrazine
Physostigmine
Pilocarpine
Piperazine (?)
Prednisolone
Prednisone
Silicone
Silver Nitrate
Silver Protein
Thiothixene
Triamcinolone
Trifluperidol (?)
Vitamin A (?)

271

272

Conjunctival Deposits
Acetophenazine
Aurothioglucose
Aurothioglycanide
Butaperazine
Carphenazine
Chlorpromazine
Colloidal Silver
Diethazine
Epinephrine
Ethopropazine
Ferrocholinate
Ferrous Fumarate
Ferrous Gluconate
Ferrous Succinate
Ferrous Sulfate
Fluphenazine
Gold Au^{198}
Gold Sodium Thiomalate
Iron Dextran
Iron Sorbitex
Mercuric Oxide
Mesoridazine
Methdilazine
Methotrimeprazine
Mild Silver Protein
Nitromersol
Perazine
Pericyazine
Perphenazine
Phenylmercuric Acetate
Phenylmercuric Nitrate
Piperacetazine
Polysaccharide-Iron Complex
Prochlorperazine
Promazine
Promethazine
Propiomazine
Quinacrine
Silver Nitrate
Silver Protein
Sulfacetamide
Sulfamethizole
Sulfisoxazole
Thiethylperazine
Thimerosal
Thiopropazate
Thioproperazine
Thioridazine

Trifluoperazine
Triflupromazine
Trimeprazine
Vitamin D
Vitamin D$_2$
Vitamin D$_3$

Conjunctival Hyperemia
Acetohexamide
Acetylcholine
Adrenal Cortex Injection
Aldosterone
Alseroxylon
Aurothioglucose
Aurothioglycanide
Betamethasone
Carbachol
Chloral Hydrate
Chlorpropamide
Chrysarobin
Clindamycin
Colchicine
Cortisone
Deferoxamine
Deserpidine
Desoxycorticosterone
Dexamethasone
Erythromycin
Fludrocortisone
Fluorescein
Fluprednisolone
Gold Au^{198}
Gold Sodium Thiomalate
Hydrocortisone
Iodide and Iodine Solutions and
  Compounds
Lincomycin
Methacholine
Methylprednisolone
Oxyphenbutazone
Paramethasone
Phenoxybenzamine
Phenylbutazone
Pilocarpine
Practolol
Prednisolone
Prednisone
Propranolol
Radioactive Iodides

273

Conjunctival Hyperemia (Cont'd)
Rauwolfia Serpentina
Rescinnamine
Reserpine
Sodium Chloride
Syrosingopine
Thiabendazole
Thyroid
Tolazamide
Tolazoline
Tolbutamide
Triamcinolone
Vancomycin

Conjunctivitis — Follicular
Adenine Arabinoside
Amphotericin B
Atropine
Carbachol
Demecarium
Echothiophate
Framycetin
Gentamicin
Homatropine
Hyaluronidase
Idoxuridine
Isoflurophate
Neomycin
Neostigmine
Physostigmine
Pilocarpine
Scopolamine
Sulfacetamide
Sulfamethizole
Sulfisoxazole
Trifluorothymidine

Conjunctivitis — Nonspecific
Acenocoumarin
Acetaminophen
Acetanilid
Acetohexamide
Ampicillin
Anisindione
Antipyrine
Aspirin
Bishydroxycoumarin
Busulfan
Carbamazepine

Carbenicillin
Carbimazole
Chlorambucil
Chlorpropamide
Chrysarobin
Cloxacillin
Colloidal Silver
Cyclophosphamide
Cytarabine
Dicloxacillin
Diethylcarbamazine
Dimercaprol
Diphenadione
Edrophonium
Emetine
Ephedrine
Ethotoin
Heparin
Hetacillin
Hydralazine
Iodide and Iodine Solutions and
    Compounds
Measles Virus Vaccine
Mechlorethamine
Melphalan
Meperidine
Mephenytoin
Methicillin
Methimazole
Methocarbamol
Methyldopa
Methylthiouracil
Mild Silver Protein
Morphine
Nafcillin
Naphazoline
Opium
Oxacillin
Oxprenolol
Oxyphenonium
Phenacetin
Phenindione
Phenprocoumon
Propranolol
Propylthiouracil
Radioactive Iodides
Silver Nitrate
Silver Protein
Sodium Salicylate

Streptomycin
Sulfacetamide
Sulfachlorpyridazine
Sulfadiazine
Sulfadimethoxine
Sulfamerazine
Sulfameter
Sulfamethizole
Sulfamethoxazole
Sulfamethoxypyridazine
Sulfanilamide
Sulfaphenazole
Sulfisoxazole
Tetrahydrozoline
Tolazamide
Tolbutamide
Triethylenemelamine
Uracil Mustard
Warfarin

Constriction of Visual Fields
Acetophenazine
Alcohol
Allobarbital
Amobarbital
Amodiaquine
Aprobarbital
Aspirin
Barbital
Bromisovalum
Butabarbital
Butalbital
Butallylonal
Butaperazine
Butethal
Carbon Dioxide
Carbromal
Carisoprodol
Carphenazine
Chloramphenicol
Chloroquine
Chlorpromazine
Clomiphene
Cobalt (?)
Cortisone
Cyclobarbital
Cyclopentyl Allylbarbituric Acid
Dexamethasone
Diethazine

Digitalis
Emetine
Ergot
Ethambutol
Ethchlorvynol
Ethopropazine
Fluorometholone
Fluphenazine
Heptabarbital
Hexamethonium
Hexethal
Hexobarbital
Hydrocortisone
Hydroxychloroquine
Indomethacin (?)
Iodide and Iodine Solutions and
    Compounds
Isoniazid
Medrysone
Mephobarbital
Meprobamate
Mesoridazine
Metharbital
Methdilazine
Methitural
Methohexital
Methotrimeprazine
Methylprednisolone
Morphine (?)
Opium (?)
Oxygen
Pentobarbital
Perazine
Pericyazine
Perphenazine
Phenobarbital
Piperacetazine
Prednisolone
Primidone
Probarbital
Prochlorperazine
Promazine
Promethazine
Propiomazine
Quinidine
Quinine
Radioactive Iodides
Secobarbital
Sodium Salicylate

275

276

Benoxinate
Benzathine Penicillin G
Butacaine
Butaperazine
Carphenazine
Chloramphenicol
Chloroquine
Chlorpromazine
Chlortetracycline
Cocaine
Colistin
Dibucaine
Diethazine
Dyclonine
Epinephrine
Erythromycin
Ethopropazine
Fluphenazine
Hydrabamine Phenoxymethyl
   Penicillin
Hydroxychloroquine
Mesoridazine
Methdilazine
Methicillin
Methotrimeprazine
Neomycin
Perazine
Pericyazine
Perphenazine
Phenacaine
Phenoxymethyl Penicillin
Phenylephrine
Piperacetazine
Piperocaine
Polymyxin B
Potassium Penicillin G
Potassium Penicillin V
Potassium Phenethicillin
Potassium Phenoxymethyl Penicillin
Procaine Penicillin G
Prochlorperazine
Promazine
Promethazine
Proparacaine
Propiomazine
Quinacrine
Silicone
Streptomycin
Tetracaine

Tetracycline
Thiethylperazine
Thiopropazate
Thioproperazine
Thioridazine
Thiotepa
Trifluoperazine
Triflupromazine
Trimeprazine

Corneal Opacities
Alcohol
Busulfan (?)
Chlorambucil (?)
Chloroform
Chrysarobin
Cloxacillin
Cyclophosphamide (?)
Cytarabine
Diiodohydroxyquin (?)
Emetine
Ether
Ethotoin (?)
Iodochlorhydroxyquin (?)
Mechlorethamine (?)
Melphalan (?)
Mephenytoin (?)
Oxyphenbutazone
Phenylbutazone
Practolol
Protriptyline
Silver Nitrate
Trichloroethylene
Triethylenemelamine (?)
Uracil Mustard (?)
Vinblastine

Cortical Blindness
Bendroflumethiazide (?)
Benzthiazide (?)
Chloroform (?)
Chlorothiazide (?)
Chlorthalidone (?)
Cyclothiazide (?)
Ether (?)
Hydrochlorothiazide (?)
Hydroflumethiazide (?)
Methyclothiazide (?)
Nitrous Oxide (?)

277

278

Streptomycin
Tetrahydrocannabinol
THC
Thiothixene
Trifluperidol
Trihexyphenidyl
Tripelennamine
Tropicamide

Decreased Anterior Chamber Depth
Acetazolamide
Acetylcholine
Alpha-Chymotrypsin
Demecarium
Dichlorphenamide
Echothiophate
Edrophonium
Ethoxzolamide
Isoflurophate
Methazolamide
Neostigmine
Physostigmine
Pilocarpine
Sulfacetamide
Sulfachlorpyridazine
Sulfadiazine
Sulfadimethoxine
Sulfamerazine
Sulfameter
Sulfamethizole
Sulfamethoxazole
Sulfamethoxypyridazine
Sulfanilamide
Sulfaphenazole
Sulfisoxazole

Decreased Convergence
Alcohol
Allobarbital
Amobarbital
Amphetamine
Aprobarbital
Barbital
Bromide
Bromisovalum
Butabarbital
Butalbital
Butallylonal -
Butethal

Carbon Dioxide
Chloral Hydrate
Cyclobarbital
Cyclopentyl Allylbarbituric Acid
Dextroamphetamine
Dimethyl Tubocurarine Iodide
Diphenylhydantoin
Heptabarbital
Hexethal
Hexobarbital
Mephobarbital
Methamphetamine
Metharbital
Methitural
Methohexital
Morphine
Opium
Pentobarbital
Phenmetrazine
Phenobarbital
Primidone
Probarbital
Secobarbital
Talbutal
Thiamylal
Thiopental
Tubocurarine
Vinbarbital

Decreased Corneal Reflex
Amitriptyline
Amodiaquine
Benoxinate
Bromide
Butacaine
Carbon Dioxide
Carisoprodol
Chlordiazepoxide
Chloroquine
Cocaine
Desipramine
Diazepam
Dibucaine
Dyclonine
Flurazepam
Glutethimide
Hydroxychloroquine
Imipramine
Meprobamate

279

  Methyprylon
  Nortriptyline
  Paraldehyde
  Phenacaine
  Piperocaine
  Proparacaine
  Protriptyline
  Tetracaine
  Trichloroethylene

Decreased Dark Adaptation
  Alcohol
  Amodiaquine (?)
  Carbon Dioxide
  Chloroquine (?)
  Hydroxychloroquine (?)
  LSD
  Lysergide
  Mescaline
  Psilocybin

Decreased Depth Perception
  Alcohol
  Chlordiazepoxide
  Diazepam
  Flurazepam
  Sulfacetamide
  Sulfachlorpyridazine
  Sulfadiazine
  Sulfadimethoxine
  Sulfamerazine
  Sulfameter
  Sulfamethizole
  Sulfamethoxazole
  Sulfamethoxypyridazine
  Sulfanilamide
  Sulfaphenazole
  Sulfisoxazole

Decreased Intraocular Pressure
  Acetazolamide
  Acetylcholine
  Acetyldigitoxin
  Alcohol
  Allobarbital
  Alseroxylon
  Amobarbital
  Amyl Nitrite

Aprobarbital
Aspirin
Barbital
Bendroflumethiazide
Benzthiazide
Butabarbital
Butalbital
Butallylonal
Butethal
Carbachol
Carisoprodol (?)
Chlordiazepoxide
Chlorisondamine
Chloroform
Chlorothiazide
Chlorthalidone
Cortisone
Cyclobarbital
Cyclopentyl Allylbarbituric Acid
Cyclothiazide
Demecarium
Deserpidine
Deslanoside
Dexamethasone
Diazepam
Dichlorphenamide
Digitoxin
Digoxin
Dimethyl Tubocurarine Iodide
Diphenylhydantoin (?)
Droperidol
Echothiophate
Ephedrine
Epinephrine
Ergonovine
Ergotamine
Erythrityl Tetranitrate
Ether
Ethoxzolamide
Fluorometholone
Flurazepam
Furosemide
Gitalin
Glycerin
Guanethidine
Haloperidol
Hashish
Heparin
Heptabarbital

Hexamethonium
Hexethal
Hexobarbital
Hydrochlorothiazide
Hydrocortisone
Hydroflumethiazide
Insulin
Isoflurophate
Isosorbide
Isosorbide Dinitrate
Lanatoside C
Mannitol
Mannitol Hexanitrate
Marihuana
Mecamylamine
Medrysone
Meperidine
Mephenesin
Mephobarbital
Meprobamate (?)
Methacholine
Metharbital
Methazolamide
Methitural
Methohexital
Methoxyflurane
Methyclothiazide
Methyldopa
Methylergonovine
Methylprednisolone
Methysergide
Morphine
Neostigmine
Nitroglycerin
Nitrous Oxide
Opium
Oral Contraceptives
Ouabain
Pargyline
Pentaerythritol Tetranitrate
Pentobarbital
Pentolinium
Phenobarbital
Phenoxybenzamine (?)
Physostigmine
Pilocarpine
Polythiazide
Practolol
Prednisolone

Primidone
Probarbital
Propranolol
Protriptyline
Rauwolfia Serpentina
Rescinnamine
Reserpine
Secobarbital
Sodium Salicylate
Spironolactone
Succinylcholine
Syrosingopine
Talbutal
Tetraethylammonium
Tetrahydrocannabinol
Tetrahydrozoline
THC
Thiamylal
Thiopental
Tolazoline
Trichlormethiazide
Trichloroethylene
Trifluperidol
Trimethaphan
Trimethidinium
Trolnitrate
Tubocurarine
Urea
Urokinase
Vinbarbital
Vitamin A

Decreased Lacrimation
Acetophenazine
Amitriptyline
Atropine
Belladonna
Butaperazine
Carphenazine
Chlorisondamine
Chlorpromazine
Desipramine
Diethazine
Ether
Ethopropazine
Fluphenazine
Hexamethonium
Homatropine
Imipramine

281

282

Vitamin D_3

Decreased Resistance to Infection
Adrenal Cortex Injection
Aldosterone
Azathioprine
Betamethasone
Cortisone
Desoxycorticosterone
Dexamethasone
Fludrocortisone
Fluorometholone
Fluprednisolone
Hydrocortisone
Medrysone
Methylprednisolone
Paramethasone
Prednisolone
Prednisone
Triamcinolone

Decreased Spontaneous Eye
Movements
Alseroxylon
Amitriptyline
Bromide
Carbamazepine
Chlordiazepoxide
Deserpidine
Desipramine
Diazepam
Flurazepam
Imipramine
Lithium Carbonate
Nortriptyline
Protriptyline
Rauwolfia Serpentina
Rescinnamine
Reserpine
Syrosingopine

Decreased Tolerance to Contact Lenses
Brompheniramine
Carbinoxamine
Chlorpheniramine
Cyclizine
Cyproheptadine
Dexbrompheniramine
Dexchlorpheniramine

Dimethindene
Diphenhydramine
Diphenylpyraline
Furosemide
Oral Contraceptives
Orphenadrine (?)
Tripelennamine

Decreased Vision
Acetaminophen
Acetanilid
Acetazolamide
Acetohexamide
Acetophenazine
Acetyldigitoxin
Acid Bismuth Sodium Tartrate (?)
Adiphenine
Adrenal Cortex Injection
Alcohol
Aldosterone
Alkavervir
Allobarbital
Allopurinol
Alseroxylon
Aluminum Nicotinate
Amantadine
Ambenonium
Aminosalicylic Acid (?)
Amiodarone
Amithiozone
Amitriptyline
Amobarbital
Amodiaquine
Amphetamine
Amphotericin B
Amyl Nitrite
Anisindione
Anisotropine
Antimony Lithium Thiomalate
Antimony Potassium Tartrate
Antimony Sodium Tartrate
Antimony Sodium Thioglycollate
Antipyrine
Aprobarbital
Aspirin
Atropine
Atropine Methylnitrate
Bacitracin
Barbital

283

Doxepin
Doxycycline
Droperidol
Echothiophate
Edrophonium
Emetine
Ephedrine
Epinephrine
Ergonovine
Ergot
Ergotamine
Erythrityl Tetranitrate
Ethacrynic Acid
Ethambutol
Ethchlorvynol
Ether
Ethionamide
Ethopropazine
Ethosuximide
Ethoxzolamide
Floxuridine
Fludrocortisone
Fluorometholone
Fluorouracil
Fluphenazine
Fluprednisolone
Flurazepam
Furosemide
Gentamicin
Gitalin
Glutethimide
Glycopyrrolate
Griseofulvin
Guanethidine
Haloperidol
Hashish
Heptabarbital
Hexamethonium
Hexethal
Hexobarbital
Hexocyclium
Homatropine
Hydralazine
Hydrochlorothiazide
Hydrocortisone
Hydroflumethiazide
Hydromorphone
Hydroxyamphetamine
Hydroxychloroquine

Ibuprofen
Imipramine
Indomethacin
Insulin
Iodide and Iodine Solutions and
    Compounds
Iodochlorhydroxyquin
Iron Dextran
Isocarboxazid
Isoflurophate
Isoniazid
Isopropamide
Isosorbide
Isosorbide Dinitrate
Kanamycin
Ketamine
Lanatoside C
Levallorphan
Levodopa
Lidocaine
Lithium Carbonate
Mannitol
Mannitol Hexanitrate
Marihuana
Measles Virus Vaccine
Mecamylamine
Mechlorethamine
Medrysone
Mefenamic Acid
Melphalan
Mepenzolate
Meperidine
Mephenesin
Mephobarbital
Mepivacaine
Meprobamate
Mesoridazine
Methacycline
Methamphetamine
Methantheline
Methaqualone
Metharbital
Methazolamide
Methdilazine
Methitural
Methixene
Methocarbamol
Methohexital
Methotrexate

Methotrimeprazine
Methsuximide
Methyclothiazide
Methyldopa
Methylene Blue
Methylergonovine
Methylprednisolone
Methyprylon
Methysergide
Mild Silver Protein
Minocycline
Mitotane
Morphine
Nalidixic Acid
Nalorphine
Naloxone
Naphazoline
Neostigmine
Niacinamide
Nialamide
Nicotinic Acid
Nicotinyl Alcohol
Nitrofurantoin
Nitroglycerin
Nitrous Oxide
Nortriptyline
Nystatin
Opium
Oral Contraceptives
Orphenadrine
Ouabain
Oxprenolol
Oxygen
Oxymorphone
Oxyphenbutazone
Oxyphencyclimine
Oxyphenonium
Oxytetracycline
Paraldehyde
Paramethasone
Pentaerythritol Tetranitrate
Pentazocine
Pentobarbital
Pentolinium
Perazine
Pericyazine
Perphenazine
Phenacetin

Phendimetrazine
Phenelzine
Phenformin
Phenindione
Phenmetrazine
Phenobarbital
Phensuximide
Phentermine
Phenylbutazone
Phenylephrine
Physostigmine
Pilocarpine
Pipenzolate
Piperacetazine
Piperazine
Piperidolate
Piperocaine
Poldine
Polymyxin B
Polythiazide
Practolol
Pralidoxime
Prednisolone
Prednisone
Prilocaine
Primidone
Probarbital
Procaine
Prochlorperazine
Procyclidine
Promazine
Promethazine
Propantheline
Propiomazine
Propoxycaine
Propoxyphene
Propranolol
Protoveratrines A and B
Protriptyline
Pyridostigmine
Quinacrine
Quinidine
Quinine
Radioactive Iodides
Rauwolfia Serpentina
Rescinnamine
Reserpine
Scopolamine
Secobarbital

Silver Nitrate
Silver Protein
Sodium Antimonylgluconate
Sodium Salicylate
Spironolactone
Stibocaptate
Stibophen
Streptomycin
Sulfacetamide
Sulfachlorpyridazine
Sulfadiazine
Sulfadimethoxine
Sulfamerazine
Sulfameter
Sulfamethizole
Sulfamethoxazole
Sulfamethoxypyridazine
Sulfanilamide
Sulfaphenazole
Sulfisoxazole
Syrosingopine
Talbutal
Tetracaine
Tetracycline
Tetraethylammonium
Tetrahydrocannabinol
Tetrahydrozoline
THC
Thiabendazole
Thiamylal
Thiethylperazine
Thiopental
Thiopropazate
Thioproperazine
Thioridazine
Thiothixene
Thyroid
Tolazamide
Tolbutamide
Tranylcypromine
Triamcinolone
Trichlormethiazide
Trichloroethylene
Tridihexethyl
Triethylenemelamine
Trifluoperazine
Trifluperidol
Triflupromazine
Trihexyphenidyl

Trimeprazine
Trimethaphan
Trimethidinium
Tripelennamine
Trolnitrate
Tropicamide
Tryparsamide
Uracil Mustard
Urethan
Veratrum
Vinbarbital
Vinblastine

Delayed Corneal Wound Healing
Adenine Arabinoside (?)
Adrenal Cortex Injection
Aldosterone
Alpha-Chymotrypsin (?)
Azathioprine
Benoxinate
Benzalkonium (?)
Betamethasone
Butacaine
Cocaine
Cortisone
Desoxycorticosterone
Dexamethasone
Dibucaine
Dyclonine
Fludrocortisone
Fluorometholone
Fluprednisolone
Hydrocortisone
Idoxuridine (?)
Iodine Solution
Medrysone
Methylprednisolone
Paramethasone
Phenacaine
Piperocaine
Prednisolone
Prednisone
Proparacaine
Sulfacetamide
Sulfamethizole
Sulfisoxazole
Tetracaine
Thiotepa
Triamcinolone

Delayed Corneal Wound Healing (Cont'd)

Trifluorothymidine (?)

Diplopia

Acetohexamide
Acetophenazine
Acetyldigitoxin
Adrenal Cortex Injection
Alcohol
Aldosterone
Allobarbital
Ambenonium
Amitriptyline
Amobarbital
Amodiaquine
Amphotericin B
Ampicillin (?)
Aprobarbital
Aspirin
Aurothioglucose
Aurothioglycanide
Bacitracin
Barbital
Benzathine Penicillin G
Betamethasone
Bromide
Bromisovalum
Brompheniramine
Bupivacaine
Butabarbital
Butalbital
Butallylonal
Butaperazine
Butethal
Carbamazepine
Carbenicillin (?)
Carbinoxamine
Carbon Dioxide
Carisoprodol
Carphenazine
Cephaloridine
Chlordiazepoxide
Chloroprocaine
Chloroquine
Chlorpheniramine
Chlorpromazine
Chlorpropamide
Chlorprothixene
Clomiphene
Cloxacillin (?)
Colchicine
Colistimethate
Colistin
Cortisone
Cyclizine
Cyclobarbital
Cyclopentyl Allylbarbituric Acid
Cyproheptadine
Desipramine
Deslanoside
Desoxycorticosterone
Dexamethasone
Dexbrompheniramine
Dexchlorpheniramine
Diazepam
Dibucaine
Dicloxacillin (?)
Diethazine
Diiodohydroxyquin
Digitalis
Digitoxin
Digoxin
Dimethindene
Dimethyl Tubocurarine Iodide
Diphenhydramine
Diphenylhydantoin
Diphenylpyraline
Edrophonium
Ergot (?)
Ethchlorvynol
Ethionamide
Ethopropazine
Ethosuximide
Ethotoin
Fludrocortisone
Fluphenazine
Fluprednisolone
Flurazepam
Gitalin
Glutethimide
Gold Au^{198}
Gold Sodium Thiomalate
Guanethidine
Hashish
Heptabarbital
Hetacillin (?)
Hexethal
Hexobarbital

Hydrabamine Phenoxymethyl
  Penicillin
Hydrocortisone
Hydroxychloroquine
Imipramine
Indomethacin
Insulin
Iodochlorhydroxyquin
Isoniazid
Ketamine
Lanatoside C
Levodopa
Lidocaine
Marihuana
Mephenesin
Mephenytoin
Mephobarbital
Mepivacaine
Meprobamate
Mesoridazine
Methaqualone
Metharbital
Methdilazine
Methicillin (?)
Methitural
Methocarbamol
Methohexital
Methotrimeprazine
Methsuximide
Methylene Blue
Methylpentynol
Methylprednisolone
Methyprylon
Mitotane
Morphine
Nafcillin (?)
Nalidixic Acid
Nitrofurantoin
Nortriptyline
Oral Contraceptives
Orphenadrine
Opium
Ouabain
Oxacillin (?)
Oxyphenbutazone
Paramethadione
Paramethasone
Pentazocine
Pentobarbital

Perazine
Pericyazine
Perphenazine
Phenformin
Phenobarbital
Phenoxymethyl Penicillin
Phensuximide
Phenylbutazone
Piperacetazine
Piperocaine
Polymyxin B
Potassium Penicillin G
Potassium Penicillin V
Potassium Phenethicillin
Potassium Phenoxymethyl Penicillin
Pralidoxime
Prednisolone
Prednisone
Prilocaine
Primidone
Probarbital
Procaine
Procaine Penicillin G
Procarbazine
Prochlorperazine
Promazine
Promethazine
Propiomazine
Propoxycaine
Propranolol
Protriptyline
Pyridostigmine
Quinidine
Secobarbital
Sodium Salicylate
Talbutal
Tetracaine
Tetrahydrocannabinol
THC
Thiamylal
Thiethylperazine
Thiopental
Thiopropazate
Thioproperazine
Thioridazine
Thiothixene
Tolazamide
Tolbutamide
Triamcinolone

Diplopia (Cont'd)
Trichloroethylene
Trifluoperazine
Triflupromazine
Trimeprazine
Trimethadione
Tripelennamine
Tubocurarine
Vinbarbital
Vinblastine
Vincristine
Vitamin A

Dyschromatopsia
Acetaminophen
Acetanilid
Acetophenazine
Acetyldigitoxin
Adrenal Cortex Injection
Alcohol
Aldosterone
Allobarbital
Alseroxylon
Amitriptyline (?)
Amobarbital
Amodiaquine
Amyl Nitrite
Aprobarbital
Aspirin
Atropine
Barbital
Belladonna
Betamethasone
Bromide
Butabarbital
Butalbital
Butallylonal
Butaperazine
Butethal
Carbon Dioxide
Carphenazine
Chloramphenicol
Chloroquine
Chlorpromazine
Chlortetracycline
Cortisone
Cyclobarbital
Cyclopentyl Allylbarbituric Acid

Deserpidine
Desipramine (?)
Deslanoside
Desoxycorticosterone
Dexamethasone
Diethazine
Digitalis
Digitoxin
Digoxin
Diiodohydroxyquin
Disulfiram
Epinephrine
Ergonovine
Ergotamine
Erythromycin
Ethambutol
Ethchlorvynol
Ethionamide
Ethopropazine
Ferrocholinate (?)
Ferrous Fumarate (?)
Ferrous Gluconate (?)
Ferrous Succinate (?)
Ferrous Sulfate (?)
Fludrocortisone
Fluorometholone
Fluphenazine
Fluprednisolone
Furosemide
Gitalin
Hashish
Heptabarbital
Hexethal
Hexobarbital
Homatropine
Hydrocortisone
Hydroxychloroquine
Imipramine (?)
Indomethacin
Iodide and Iodine Solutions and
  Compounds
Iodochlorhydroxyquin
Iron Dextran (?)
Iron Sorbitex (?)
Isocarboxazid
Isoniazid
Lanatoside C
LSD

Lysergide
Marihuana
Medrysone
Mefenamic Acid
Mephobarbital
Mescaline
Mesoridazine
Metharbital
Methazolamide
Methdilazine
Methitural
Methohexital
Methotrimeprazine
Methylergonovine
Methylprednisolone
Methysergide
Morphine (?)
Nalidixic Acid
Nialamide
Nitrofurantoin (?)
Nortriptyline (?)
Opium (?)
Oral Contraceptives
Ouabain
Oxyphenbutazone
Paramethadione
Paramethasone
Pargyline
Penicillamine
Pentobarbital
Pentylenetetrazol
Perazine
Pericyazine
Perphenazine
Phenacetin
Phenelzine
Phenobarbital
Phenylbutazone
Piperacetazine
Piperazine
Piperidolate
Polysaccharide-Iron Complex (?)
Prednisolone
Prednisone
Primidone
Probarbital
Prochlorperazine
Promazine
Promethazine

Propiomazine
Protriptyline (?)
Psilocybin
Quinacrine
Quinidine
Quinine
Radioactive Iodides
Rauwolfia Serpentina
Rescinnamine
Reserpine
Secobarbital
Sodium Salicylate
Streptomycin
Sulfacetamide
Sulfachlorpyridazine
Sulfadiazine
Sulfadimethoxine
Sulfamerazine
Sulfameter
Sulfamethizole
Sulfamethoxazole
Sulfamethoxypyridazine
Sulfanilamide
Sulfaphenazole
Sulfisoxazole
Syrosingopine
Talbutal
Tetrahydrocannabinol
THC
Thiabendazole
Thiamylal
Thiethylperazine
Thiopental
Thiopropazate
Thioproperazine
Thioridazine
Tranylcypromine
Triamcinolone
Trichloroethylene
Trifluoperazine
Triflupromazine
Trimeprazine
Trimethadione
Vinbarbital

Enlarged Blind Spot
  Adrenal Cortex Injection
  Aldosterone
  Betamethasone

Carbon Dioxide
Chlortetracycline
Cortisone
Demeclocycline
Desoxycorticosterone
Dexamethasone
Doxycycline
Ergot
Fludrocortisone
Fluorometholone
Fluprednisolone
Hydrocortisone
Indomethacin (?)
Medrysone
Methacycline
Methylprednisolone
Minocycline
Oxytetracycline
Paramethasone
Prednisolone
Prednisone
Quinacrine
Tetracycline
Triamcinolone
Trichloroethylene
Vitamin A

Exophthalmos
Adrenal Cortex Injection
Aldosterone
Betamethasone
Carbimazole
Cocaine
Cortisone
Desoxycorticosterone
Dexamethasone
Digitalis (?)
Fludrocortisone
Fluprednisolone
Hydrocortisone
Iodide and Iodine Solutions and
  Compounds
Methimazole
Methylprednisolone
Methylthiouracil
Oral Contraceptives
Paramethasone
Prednisolone

Prednisone
Propylthiouracil
Radioactive Iodides
Thyroid (?)
Triamcinolone
Vitamin A

Eyelid Deposits
Acetophenazine
Aurothioglucose
Aurothioglycanide
Butaperazine
Carphenazine
Chlorpromazine
Colloidal Silver
Diethazine
Ethopropazine
Ferrocholinate
Ferrous Fumarate
Ferrous Gluconate
Ferrous Succinate
Ferrous Sulfate
Fluphenazine
Gold Au^{198}
Gold Sodium Thiomalate
Iron Dextran
Iron Sorbitex
Mercuric Oxide
Mesoridazine
Methdilazine
Methotrimeprazine
Mild Silver Protein
Nitromersol
Perazine
Pericyazine
Perphenazine
Phenylmercuric Acetate
Phenylmercuric Nitrate
Piperacetazine
Polysaccharide-Iron Complex
Prochlorperazine
Promazine
Promethazine
Propiomazine
Silver Nitrate
Silver Protein
Thiethylperazine
Thimerosal
Thiopropazate

292

Thioproperazine
Thioridazine
Trifluoperazine
Triflupromazine
Trimeprazine

Eyelids — Depigmentation
Carbimazole
Methimazole
Methotrexate
Methylthiouracil
Neostigmine
Physostigmine
Propylthiouracil
Thiotepa

Eyelids — Erythema
Actinomycin C
Aminopterin
Aurothioglucose
Aurothioglycanide
Benzphetamine
Bleomycin
Bromide
Busulfan
Chlorambucil
Chlorphentermine
Chlortetracycline
Cyclophosphamide
Dactinomycin
Deferoxamine
Demeclocycline
Diazoxide
Diethylpropion
Dimethyl Sulfoxide
DMSO
Doxycycline
Dromostanolone
Ethionamide
Floxuridine
Fluorouracil
Fluoxymesterone
Gold Au^{198}
Gold Sodium Thiomalate
Hydralazine
Hydroxyurea
Ibuprofen
Iron Dextran

Mechlorethamine
Melphalan
Mercuric Oxide
Methacycline
Methotrexate
Minocycline
Nitromersol
Oxprenolol
Oxytetracycline
Phendimetrazine
Phentermine
Phenylmercuric Acetate
Phenylmercuric Nitrate
Pipobroman
Procarbazine
Propranolol
Testolactone
Testosterone
Tetracycline
Thimerosal
Triethylenemelamine
Uracil Mustard

Eyelids — Exfoliative Dermatitis
Acetohexamide
Acetophenazine
Acid Bismuth Sodium Tartrate
Adiphenine
Allobarbital
Allopurinol
Aminosalicylic Acid (?)
Amithiozone
Amobarbital
Amodiaquine
Ampicillin
Anisindione
Anisotropine
Aprobarbital
Atropine Methylnitrate
Aurothioglucose
Aurothioglycanide
Barbital
Bismuth Carbonate
Bismuth Oxychloride
Bismuth Salicylate
Bismuth Sodium Tartrate
Bismuth Sodium Thioglycollate
Bismuth Sodium Triglycollamate

293

Eyelids — Exfoliative Dermatitis(Cont'd)
Busulfan
Butabarbital
Butalbital
Butallylonal
Butaperazine
Butethal
Carbamazepine
Carbenicillin
Carbimazole
Carisoprodol
Carphenazine
Chlorambucil
Chloroquine
Chlorpromazine
Chlorpropamide
Chlorprothixene
Clindamycin
Cloxacillin
Codeine
Cyclobarbital
Cyclopentyl Allylbarbituric Acid
Cyclophosphamide
Dicloxacillin
Dicyclomine
Diethazine
Diphemanil
Diphenadione
Diphenylhydantoin
Droperidol
Erythrityl Tetranitrate
Erythromycin
Ethionamide
Ethopropazine
Ethosuximide
Ethotoin
Fluphenazine
Furosemide
Glutethimide
Glycopyrrolate
Gold Au^{198}
Gold Sodium Thiomalate
Griseofulvin
Haloperidol
Heptabarbital
Hetacillin
Hexethal
Hexobarbital
Hexocyclium
Hydroxychloroquine

Isoniazid
Isopropamide
Isosorbide Dinitrate
Lincomycin
Mannitol Hexanitrate
Mechlorethamine
Melphalan
Mepenzolate
Mephenytoin
Mephobarbital
Meprobamate
Mesoridazine
Methantheline
Metharbital
Methdilazine
Methicillin
Methimazole
Methitural
Methixene
Methohexital
Methotrimeprazine
Methsuximide
Methylphenidate
Methylthiouracil
Methyprylon
Nafcillin
Nitroglycerin
Oxacillin
Oxyphenbutazone
Oxyphencyclimine
Oxyphenonium
Paramethadione
Pentaerythritol Tetranitrate
Pentobarbital
Perazine
Pericyazine
Perphenazine
Phenindione
Phenobarbital
Phensuximide
Phenylbutazone
Pipenzolate
Piperacetazine
Piperidolate
Poldine
Primidone
Probarbital
Procarbazine
Prochlorperazine
Promazine

294

Promethazine
Propantheline
Propiomazine
Propoxyphene
Propylthiouracil
Quinacrine
Quinidine
Secobarbital
Sulfacetamide
Sulfachlorpyridazine
Sulfadiazine
Sulfadimethoxine
Sulfamerazine
Sulfameter
Sulfamethizole
Sulfamethoxazole
Sulfamethoxypyridazine
Sulfanilamide
Sulfaphenazole
Sulfisoxazole
Talbutal
Thiabendazole
Thiamylal
Thiethylperazine
Thiopental
Thiopropazate
Thioproperazine
Thioridazine
Thiothixene
Tolazamide
Tolbutamide
Tridihexethyl
Triethylenemelamine
Trifluoperazine
Trifluperidol
Triflupromazine
Trimeprazine
Trimethadione
Trolnitrate
Uracil Mustard
Vancomycin
Vinbarbital

Eyelids — Urticaria
Acenocoumarin
Acetaminophen
Acetanilid
Acetazolamide
Aluminum Nicotinate

Anisindione
Antimony Lithium Thiomalate
Antimony Potassium Tartrate
Antimony Sodium Tartrate
Antimony Sodium Thioglycollate
Antipyrine
Aspirin
Benzphetamine
Bishydroxycoumarin
Capreomycin
Carbamazepine
Carbimazole
Cefazolin
Cephalexin
Cephaloglycin
Cephaloridine
Cephalothin
Chlorphentermine
Clomiphene
Deferoxamine
Dichlorphenamide
Diethylpropion
Diphenadione
Disulfiram
Ethoxzolamide
Fluorescein
Heparin
Hydralazine
Hydromorphone
Ibuprofen
Iodine Solution
Methazolamide
Methimazole
Methotrexate
Methylphenidate
Methylthiouracil
Morphine
Nalidixic Acid
Niacinamide
Nicotinic Acid
Nicotinyl Alcohol
Opium
Oral Contraceptives
Oxymorphone
Oxyphenbutazone
Phenacetin
Phendimetrazine
Phenindione
Phenprocoumon

295

Phentermine
Phenylbutazone
Piperazine
Propylthiouracil
Sodium Antimonylgluconate
Sodium Salicylate
Stibocaptate
Stibophen
Warfarin

Eyelids or Conjunctiva — Allergic Reactions
Acenocoumarin
Acetaminophen
Acetanilid
Acetazolamide
Acetohexamide
Acetophenazine
Acetyldigitoxin
Actinomycin C
Adenine Arabinoside
Adiphenine
Allobarbital
Allopurinol
Aluminum Nicotinate
Aminopterin
Aminosalicylic Acid (?)
Amithiozone
Amobarbital
Amodiaquine
Amphotericin B
Ampicillin
Amyl Nitrite
Anisindione
Anisotropine
Antipyrine
Aprobarbital
Aspirin
Atropine
Atropine Methylnitrate
Aurothioglucose
Aurothioglycanide
Bacitracin
Barbital
Bendroflumethiazide
Benoxinate
Benzathine Penicillin G
Benzthiazide

Bishydroxycoumarin
Bleomycin
Bromide
Busulfan
Butacaine
Butabarbital
Butalbital
Butallylonal
Butaperazine
Butethal
Carbachol
Carbamazepine
Carbenicillin
Carbimazole
Carisoprodol
Carphenazine
Cefazolin
Cephalexin
Cephaloglycin
Cephaloridine
Cephalothin
Chloral Hydrate
Chlorambucil
Chloramphenicol
Chloroquine
Chlorothiazide
Chlorpromazine
Chlorpropamide
Chlorprothixene
Chlortetracycline
Chlorthalidone
Chrysarobin
Clindamycin
Clomiphene
Cloxacillin
Cocaine
Colistin
Colloidal Silver
Cortisone
Cyclobarbital
Cyclopentolate
Cyclopentyl Allylbarbituric Acid
Cyclophosphamide
Cycloserine
Cyclothiazide
Cytarabine
Dactinomycin
Deferoxamine
Demecarium

Deslanoside
Dexamethasone
Diazoxide
Dibucaine
Dichlorphenamide
Dicloxacillin
Dicyclomine
Diethazine
Digitalis
Digitoxin
Digoxin
Dimercaprol
Diphemanil
Diphenadione
Diphenylhydantoin
Disulfiram
Dromostanolone
Droperidol
Dyclonine
Echothiophate
Edrophonium
Emetine
Erythromycin
Ephedrine
Epinephrine
Ethionamide
Ethopropazine
Ethosuximide
Ethotoin
Ethoxzolamide
Fluorescein
Fluorometholone
Fluorouracil
Fluoxymesterone
Fluphenazine
Framycetin
Furosemide
Gentamicin
Gitalin
Glutethimide
Glycopyrrolate
Gold Au[198]
Gold Sodium Thiomalate
Griseofulvin
Haloperidol
Heparin
Heptabarbital
Hetacillin
Hexethal

Hexobarbital
Hexocyclium
Homatropine
Hyaluronidase
Hydrabamine Phenoxymethyl
  Penicillin
Hydralazine
Hydrochlorothiazide
Hydrocortisone
Hydroflumethiazide
Hydromorphone
Hydroxyamphetamine
Hydroxychloroquine
Idoxuridine
Insulin
Iodide and Iodine Solutions and
  Compounds
Isoflurophate
Isoniazid
Isopropamide
Kanamycin
Lanatoside C
Levodopa
Lincomycin
Mechlorethamine
Medrysone
Melphalan
Mepenzolate
Mephenytoin
Mephobarbital
Meprobamate
Mercuric Oxide
Mesoridazine
Methacholine
Methantheline
Metharbital
Methazolamide
Methdilazine
Methicillin
Methimazole
Methitural
Methixene
Methohexital
Methotrexate
Methotrimeprazine
Methsuximide
Methyclothiazide
Methyldopa
Methylprednisolone

297

Eyelids or Conjunctiva — Allergic Reactions (Cont'd)

Methylthiouracil
Methyprylon
Mild Silver Protein
Morphine
Nafcillin
Naphazoline
Neomycin
Neostigmine
Niacinamide
Nicotinic Acid
Nicotinyl Alcohol
Nitrofurantoin
Nitromersol
Nystatin
Opium
Oral Contraceptives
Ouabain
Oxacillin
Oxprenolol
Oxymorphone
Oxyphenbutazone
Oxyphencyclimine
Oxyphenonium
Paramethadione
Pentobarbital
Perazine
Pericyazine
Perphenazine
Phenacaine
Phenacetin
Phenindione
Phenobarbital
Phenoxymethyl Penicillin
Phenprocoumon
Phensuximide
Phenylbutazone
Phenylephrine
Phenylmercuric Acetate
Phenylmercuric Nitrate
Physostigmine
Pilocarpine
Pipenzolate
Piperacetazine
Piperazine
Piperidolate
Piperocaine
Pipobroman
Poldine
Polymyxin B
Polythiazide
Potassium Penicillin G
Potassium Penicillin V
Potassium Phenethicillin
Potassium Phenoxymethyl Penicillin
Prednisolone
Primidone
Probarbital
Procaine Penicillin G
Prochlorperazine
Promazine
Promethazine
Propantheline
Proparacaine
Propiomazine
Propranolol
Propylthiouracil
Quinidine
Quinine
Radioactive Iodides
Scopolamine
Secobarbital
Silver Nitrate
Silver Protein
Sodium Salicylate
Streptomycin
Succinylcholine
Sulfacetamide
Sulfachlorpyridazine
Sulfadiazine
Sulfadimethoxine
Sulfamerazine
Sulfameter
Sulfamethizole
Sulfamethoxazole
Sulfamethoxypyridazine
Sulfanilamide
Sulfaphenazole
Sulfisoxazole
Talbutal
Testolactone
Testosterone
Tetracaine
Tetracycline
Tetrahydrozoline
Thiabendazole
Thiamylal

Thiethylperazine
Thimerosal
Thiopental
Thiopropazate
Thioproperazine
Thioridazine
Thiotepa
Thiothixene
Tolazamide
Tolbutamide
Trichlormethiazide
Tridihexethyl
Triethylenemelamine
Trifluoperazine
Trifluorothymidine
Trifluperidol
Triflupromazine
Trimeprazine
Trimethadione
Tropicamide
Uracil Mustard
Vancomycin
Vinbarbital
Warfarin

Eyelids or Conjunctiva —
Angioneurotic Edema
Acetaminophen
Acetanilid
Acetophenazine
Acetyldigitoxin
Adrenal Cortex Injection
Aldosterone
Allobarbital
Aluminum Nicotinate
Amobarbital
Ampicillin
Aprobarbital
Aspirin
Bacitracin
Barbital
Benzathine Penicillin G
Betamethasone
Butabarbital
Butalbital
Butallylonal
Butaperazine
Butethal
Carbenicillin

Carphenazine
Capreomycin
Carisoprodol
Cefazolin
Cephalexin
Cephaloglycin
Cephaloridine
Cephalothin
Chloramphenicol
Chlorpromazine
Chlorprothixene
Chlortetracycline
Clindamycin
Cloxacillin
Cortisone
Cyclobarbital
Cyclopentyl Allylbarbituric Acid
Demeclocycline
Deslanoside
Desoxycorticosterone
Dexamethasone
Dicloxacillin
Diethazine
Digitalis
Digitoxin
Digoxin
Doxycycline
Droperidol
Erythromycin
Ethopropazine
Ethosuximide
Ethotoin
Fludrocortisone
Fluorescein
Fluphenazine
Fluprednisolone
Gitalin
Griseofulvin
Haloperidol
Heparin
Heptabarbital
Hetacillin
Hexethal
Hexobarbital
Hydrabamine Phenoxymethyl
  Penicillin
Hydrocortisone
Indomethacin
Insulin

299

Iodide and Iodine Solution and
  Compounds
Iron Dextran
Isoniazid
Lanatoside C
Lincomycin
Mephenytoin
Mephobarbital
Meprobamate
Mesoridazine
Methacycline
Metharbital
Methdilazine
Methicillin
Methitural
Methohexital
Methotrimeprazine
Methsuximide
Methylprednisolone
Minocycline
Nafcillin
Nalidixic Acid
Niacinamide
Nicotinic Acid
Nicotinyl Alcohol
Nitrofurantoin
Ouabain
Oxacillin
Oxytetracycline
Paramethadione
Paramethasone
Pentobarbital
Perazine
Pericyazine
Perphenazine
Phenacetin
Phenobarbital
Phenoxymethyl Penicillin
Phensuximide
Piperacetazine
Potassium Penicillin G
Potassium Penicillin V
Potassium Phenethicillin
Potassium Phenoxymethyl Penicillin
Prednisolone
Prednisone
Primidone

Probarbital
Procaine Penicillin G
Prochlorperazine
Promazine
Promethazine
Propiomazine
Quinidine
Quinine
Radioactive Iodides
Secobarbital
Sodium Salicylate
Streptomycin
Tetracycline
Talbutal
Thiabendazole
Thiamylal
Thiethylperazine
Thiopental
Thiopropazate
Thioproperazine
Thioridazine
Thiothixene
Triamcinolone
Trifluoperazine
Trifluperidol
Triflupromazine
Trimeprazine
Trimethadione
Vancomycin
Vinbarbital

Eyelids or Conjunctiva — Discoloration
Acid Bismuth Sodium Tartrate (?)
Alcian Blue
Antimony Lithium Thiomalate
Antimony Potassium Tartrate
Antimony Sodium Tartrate
Antimony Sodium Thioglycollate
Antipyrine
Bismuth Carbonate (?)
Bismuth Oxychloride (?)
Bismuth Salicylate (?)
Bismuth Sodium Tartrate (?)
Bismuth Sodium Thioglycollate (?)
Bismuth Sodium Triglycollamate (?)
Chrysarobin
Ferrocholinate
Ferrous Fumarate
Ferrous Gluconate

Ferrous Succinate
Ferrous Sulfate
Fluorescein
Iron Dextran
Iron Sorbitex
Methylene Blue
Polysaccharide-Iron Complex
Quinacrine
Rose Bengal
Sodium Antimonylgluconate
Stibocaptate
Stibophen
Trypan Blue
Vitamin A

Eyelids or Conjunctiva — Edema
Acetohexamide
Acetophenazine
Actinomycin C
Adrenal Cortex Injection
Aldosterone
Allobarbital
Aminopterin
Aminosalicylic Acid (?)
Amobarbital
Antimony Lithium Thiomalate
Antimony Potassium Tartrate
Antimony Sodium Tartrate
Antimony Sodium Thioglycollate
Antipyrine
Aprobarbital
Aspirin
Aurothioglucose
Aurothioglycanide
Barbital
Betamethasone
Bleomycin
Butabarbital
Butalbital
Butallylonal
Butaperazine
Butethal
Carphenazine
Chlorisondamine
Chloral Hydrate
Chlorpromazine
Chlorpropamide
Chrysarobin
Colloidal Silver

Cortisone
Cyclobarbital
Cyclopentyl Allylbarbituric Acid
Dactinomycin
Desoxycorticosterone
Dexamethasone
Diethazine
Dromostanolone
Emetine
Ergonovine
Ergotamine
Ethopropazine
Floxuridine
Fludrocortisone
Fluorouracil
Fluoxymesterone
Fluphenazine
Fluprednisolone
Gold Au^{198}
Gold Sodium Thiomalate
Griseofulvin
Heptabarbital
Hexamethonium
Hexethal
Hexobarbital
Hydralazine
Hydrocortisone
Ibuprofen
Iodide and Iodine Solutions and
  Compounds
Iron Dextran
Levodopa
Lithium Carbonate
Mecamylamine
Mephobarbital
Mesoridazine
Metharbital
Methdilazine
Methitural
Methohexital
Methotrimeprazine
Methyldopa
Methylergonovine
Methylpentynol
Methylprednisolone
Methysergide
Mild Silver Protein
Oral Contraceptives
Oxyphenbutazone

301

Paramethasone
Pentobarbital
Pentolinium
Perazine
Pericyazine
Perphenazine
Phenobarbital
Phenylbutazone
Piperacetazine
Piperazine
Pipobroman
Prednisolone
Prednisone
Primidone
Probarbital
Prochlorperazine
Promazine
Promethazine
Propiomazine
Quinacrine
Radioactive Iodides
Secobarbital
Silver Nitrate
Silver Protein
Sodium Antimonylgluconate
Sodium Salicylate
Stibocaptate
Stibophen
Streptomycin
Talbutal
Testolactone
Testosterone
Tetraethylammonium
Thiamylal
Thiethylperazine
Thiopental
Thiopropazate
Thioproperazine
Thioridazine
Tolazamide
Tolbutamide
Triamcinolone
Trifluoperazine
Triflupromazine
Trimeprazine
Trimethaphan
Trimethidinium

Vinbarbital

Eyelids or Conjunctiva — Erythema Multiforme

Acetaminophen
Acetanilid
Acetohexamide
Amithiozone
Amodiaquine
Bendroflumethiazide
Benzthiazide
Carbamazepine
Chloroquine
Chlorothiazide
Chlorpropamide
Chlortetracycline
Chlorthalidone
Cyclothiazide
Demeclocycline
Diphenylhydantoin
Doxycycline
Ethosuximide
Ethotoin
Furosemide
Hydrochlorothiazide
Hydroflumethiazide
Hydroxychloroquine
Mephenytoin
Methacycline
Methsuximide
Methyclothiazide
Methylphenidate
Minocycline
Oxytetracycline
Paramethadione
Phenacetin
Phensuximide
Polythiazide
Quinine
Tetracycline
Tolazamide
Tolbutamide
Trichlormethiazide
Trimethadione

Eyelids or Conjunctiva — Hyperpigmentation

Actinomycin C
Aluminum Nicotinate
Aminopterin

Bleomycin
Busulfan
Cyclophosphamide
Cytarabine
Dactinomycin
Dromostanolone
Floxuridine
Fluorouracil
Fluoxymesterone
Mercaptopurine
Methotrexate
Niacinamide
Nicotinic Acid
Nicotinyl Alcohol
Pipobroman
Practolol
Procarbazine
Quinacrine
Testolactone
Testosterone
Thioguanine
Uracil Mustard

Eyelids or Conjunctiva — Lupoid Syndrome
Carbamazepine
Carbimazole
Diphenylhydantoin
Ethosuximide
Griseofulvin
Hydralazine
Isoniazid
Methimazole
Methsuximide
Methylthiouracil
Paramethadione
Phensuximide
Practolol
Propylthiouracil
Streptomycin
Trimethadione

Eyelids or Conjunctiva — Lyell's Syndrome
Acetazolamide
Adrenal Cortex Injection
Aldosterone
Allobarbital
Amobarbital
Ampicillin

Antipyrine
Aprobarbital
Aurothioglucose
Aurothioglycanide
Barbital
Benzathine Penicillin G
Betamethasone
Busulfan
Butabarbital
Butalbital
Butallylonal
Butethal
Carbenicillin
Chlorambucil
Cloxacillin
Cortisone
Cyclobarbital
Cyclopentyl Allylbarbituric Acid
Cyclophosphamide
Desoxycorticosterone
Dexamethasone
Dichlorphenamide
Dicloxacillin
Diphenylhydantoin
Ethoxzolamide
Fludrocortisone
Fluprednisolone
Gold Au^{198}
Gold Sodium Thiomalate
Heptabarbital
Hetacillin
Hexethal
Hexobarbital
Hydrabamine Phenoxymethyl
  Penicillin
Hydrocortisone
Kanamycin
Mechlorethamine
Melphalan
Mephobarbital
Metharbital
Methazolamide
Methicillin
Methitural
Methohexital
Methotrexate
Methylprednisolone
Nafcillin
Nitrofurantoin

Carbromal
Carisoprodol
Carphenazine
Chloroquine
Chlorothiazide
Chlorpromazine
Chlorpropamide
Chlortetracycline
Chlorthalidone
Clindamycin
Cloxacillin
Cyclobarbital
Cyclopentyl Allylbarbituric Acid
Cyclothiazide
Demeclocycline
Dicloxacillin
Diethazine
Diphenylhydantoin
Doxycycline
Erythromycin
Ethopropazine
Ethosuximide
Ethotoin
Fluphenazine
Gold Au^{198}
Gold Sodium Thiomalate
Heptabarbital
Hetacillin
Hexethal
Hexobarbital
Hydrabamine Phenoxymethyl
  Penicillin
Hydrochlorothiazide
Hydroflumethiazide
Hydroxychloroquine
Lincomycin
Mephenytoin
Mephobarbital
Meprobamate
Mesoridazine
Methacycline
Metharbital
Methdilazine
Methicillin
Methitural
Methohexital
Methotrimeprazine
Methsuximide
Methyclothiazide

Methylphenidate
Minocycline
Nafcillin
Oxacillin
Oxyphenbutazone
Oxytetracycline
Paramethadione
Pentobarbital
Perazine
Pericyazine
Perphenazine
Phenacetin
Phenobarbital
Phenoxymethyl Penicillin
Phensuximide
Phenylbutazone
Piperacetazine
Polythiazide
Potassium Penicillin G
Potassium Penicillin V
Potassium Phenethicillin
Potassium Phenoxymethyl Penicillin
Primidone
Probarbital
Procaine Penicillin G
Prochlorperazine
Promazine
Promethazine
Propiomazine
Propranolol
Quinine
Secobarbital
Sulfacetamide
Sulfachlorpyridazine
Sulfadiazine
Sulfadimethoxine
Sulfamerazine
Sulfameter
Sulfamethizole
Sulfamethoxazole
Sulfamethoxypyridazine
Sulfanilamide
Sulfaphenazole
Sulfisoxazole
Talbutal
Tetracycline
Thiabendazole
Thiamylal
Thiethylperazine

Eyelids or Conjunctiva – Stevens-Johnson Syndrome (Cont'd)

Thiopental
Thiopropazate
Thioproperazine
Thioridazine
Tolazamide
Tolbutamide
Trichlormethiazide
Trifluoperazine
Triflupromazine
Trimeprazine
Trimethadione
Vancomycin
Vinbarbital

Heightened Color Perception

Ethionamide
Hashish
LSD
Lysergide
Marihuana
Mescaline
Oxygen
Psilocybin
Tetrahydrocannabinol
THC

Hemianopsia

Aspirin
Epinephrine
Ergonovine
Ethambutol
Hexamethonium
Ibuprofen (?)
Iodide and Iodine Solutions and Compounds
Isoniazid
Morphine (?)
Opium (?)
Oral Contraceptives
Paraldehyde (?)
Radioactive Iodides
Sodium Salicylate
Vitamin D (?)
Vitamin D_2 (?)
Vitamin D_3 (?)

Hippus

Allobarbital
Amobarbital
Aprobarbital
Barbital
Butabarbital
Butalbital
Butallylonal
Butethal
Cyclobarbital
Cyclopentyl Allylbarbituric Acid
Heptabarbital
Hexethal
Hexobarbital
Mephobarbital
Metharbital
Methitural
Methohexital
Pentobarbital
Pentylenetetrazol
Phenobarbital
Primidone
Probarbital
Secobarbital
Talbutal
Thiamylal
Thiopental
Vinbarbital

Horner's Syndrome

Acetophenazine
Alseroxylon
Butaperazine
Carphenazine
Chlorpromazine
Deserpidine
Diethazine
Ethopropazine
Fluphenazine
Guanethidine
Levodopa
Mesoridazine
Methdilazine
Methotrimeprazine
Oral Contraceptives
Perazine
Pericyazine
Perphenazine
Piperacetazine
Prochlorperazine
Promazine
Promethazine

Propiomazine
Rauwolfia Serpentina
Rescinnamine
Reserpine
Syrosingopine
Thiethylperazine
Thiopropazate
Thioproperazine
Thioridazine
Trifluoperazine
Triflupromazine
Trimeprazine

Hypermetropia
Ergot
Penicillamine
Sulfacetamide (?)
Sulfachlorpyridazine (?)
Sulfadiazine (?)
Sulfadimethoxine (?)
Sulfamerazine (?)
Sulfameter (?)
Sulfamethizole (?)
Sulfamethoxazole (?)
Sulfamethoxypyridazine (?)
Sulfanilamide (?)
Sulfaphenazole (?)
Sulfisoxazole (?)
Tolbutamide (?)

Hypopyon
Benoxinate
Butacaine
Cocaine
Colchicine (?)
Dibucaine
Dyclonine
Ferrocholinate
Ferrous Fumarate
Ferrous Gluconate
Ferrous Succinate
Ferrous Sulfate
Iodide and Iodine Solutions and
  Compounds
Iron Dextran
Iron Sorbitex
Phenacaine
Piperocaine
Polysaccharide-Iron Complex

Proparacaine
Radioactive Iodides
Tetracaine
Urokinase

Increased Intraocular Pressure
Adrenal Cortex Injection
Aldosterone
Alpha-Chymotrypsin
Aluminum Nicotinate (?)
Amyl Nitrite
Atropine
Betamethasone
Carbon Dioxide
Cortisone
Cyclopentolate
Demecarium
Desoxycorticosterone
Dexamethasone
Echothiophate
Epinephrine
Erythrityl Tetranitrate (?)
Fludrocortisone
Fluorometholone
Fluprednisolone
Homatropine
Hydrocortisone
Hydroxyamphetamine
Isoflurophate
Isosorbide Dinitrate (?)
Ketamine
Mannitol Hexanitrate (?)
Medrysone
Methylphenidate (?)
Methylprednisolone
Morphine (?)
Niacinamide (?)
Nicotinic Acid (?)
Nicotinyl Alcohol (?)
Nitroglycerin
Nitrous Oxide
Oxyphenonium
Paramethasone
Pentaerythritol Tetranitrate (?)
Phenylephrine
Pilocarpine
Prednisolone
Prednisone
Scopolamine

308

Probarbital
Prochlorperazine
Promazine
Promethazine
Propiomazine
Protriptyline
Rauwolfia Serpentina
Rescinnamine
Reserpine
Secobarbital
Syrosingopine
Talbutal
Thiamylal
Thiethylperazine
Thiopental
Thiopropazate
Thioproperazine
Thioridazine
Trifluoperazine
Triflupromazine
Trimeprazine
Vinbarbital

Keratitis
Acetophenazine
Adenine Arabinoside
Alcohol
Amphotericin B
Antipyrine
Aspirin
Aurothioglucose
Aurothioglycanide
Benoxinate
Benzalkonium
Butacaine
Butaperazine
Carbimazole
Carphenazine
Chlorambucil
Chloroform
Chlorpromazine
Chlorprothixene
Chrysarobin
Cocaine
Colchicine (?)
Cytarabine
Dibucaine
Diethazine
Dyclonine

Emetine
Epinephrine
Ether
Ethopropazine
Fluphenazine
Framycetin
Gold Au^{198}
Gold Sodium Thiomalate
Guanethidine
Idoxuridine
Iodide and Iodine Solutions and
    Compounds
Isoniazid
Mesoridazine
Methdilazine
Methimazole
Methotrexate (?)
Methotrimeprazine
Methylthiouracil
Naphazoline
Neomycin
Oral Contraceptives
Oxyphenbutazone
Perazine
Pericyazine
Perphenazine
Phenacaine
Phenylbutazone
Phenylephrine
Piperacetazine
Piperocaine
Prochlorperazine
Promazine
Promethazine
Proparacaine
Propiomazine
Propylthiouracil
Radioactive Iodides
Sodium Salicylate
Sulfacetamide
Sulfachlorpyridazine
Sulfadiazine
Sulfadimethoxine
Sulfamerazine
Sulfameter
Sulfamethizole
Sulfamethoxazole
Sulfamethoxypyridazine
Sulfanilamide

Keratitis (Cont'd)
Sulfaphenazole
Sulfisoxazole
Tetracaine
Thiethylperazine
Thiopropazate
Thioproperazine
Thioridazine
Thiotepa
Thiothixene
Trichloroethylene
Trifluoperazine
Trifluorothymidine
Triflupromazine
Trimeprazine
Vinblastine

Keratoconjunctivitis
Aspirin
Aurothioglucose (?)
Aurothioglycanide (?)
Chrysarobin
Gold Au^{198} (?)
Gold Sodium Thiomalate (?)
Morphine
Opium
Practolol
Sodium Salicylate

Lacrimation
Acetophenazine
Acetylcholine
Alcohol
Ambenonium
Bishydroxycoumarin
Butaperazine
Carphenazine
Chloral Hydrate
Chlorpromazine
Diazoxide
Diethazine
Edrophonium
Epinephrine
Ether
Ethopropazine
Fluphenazine
Heparin
Indomethacin (?)
Ketamine

Levallorphan
Mesoridazine
Methacholine
Methaqualone
Methdilazine
Methotrimeprazine
Morphine
Nalorphine
Naloxone
Opium
Pentazocine
Perazine
Pericyazine
Perphenazine
Piperacetazine
Prochlorperazine
Promazine
Promethazine
Propiomazine
Pyridostigmine
Thiethylperazine
Thiopropazate
Thioproperazine
Thioridazine
Trifluoperazine
Triflupromazine
Trimeprazine

Lens Deposits
Acetophenazine
Aurothioglucose
Aurothioglycanide
Butaperazine
Carphenazine
Chlorpromazine
Chlorprothixene
Colloidal Silver
Diazepam (?)
Diethazine
Ethopropazine
Fluphenazine
Gold Au^{198}
Gold Sodium Thiomalate
Mercuric Oxide
Mesoridazine
Methdilazine
Methotrimeprazine
Mild Silver Protein
Perazine

310

Pericyazine
Perphenazine
Phenylmercuric Acetate
Phenylmercuric Nitrate
Piperacetazine
Prochlorperazine
Promazine
Promethazine
Propiomazine
Silver Nitrate
Silver Protein
Thiethylperazine
Thiopropazate
Thioproperazine
Thioridazine
Thiothixene
Trifluoperazine
Triflupromazine
Trimeprazine

Loss of Eyelashes or Eyebrows
Acenocoumarin (?)
Acetohexamide (?)
Actinomycin C (?)
Alcohol (?)
Allopurinol (?)
Aminopterin (?)
Amitriptyline (?)
Amodiaquine (?)
Anisindione (?)
Azathioprine (?)
Benzphetamine (?)
Bishydroxycoumarin (?)
Bleomycin (?)
Busulfan (?)
Carbamazepine (?)
Carbimazole (?)
Chlorambucil (?)
Chloroquine (?)
Chlorphentermine (?)
Chlorpropamide (?)
Colchicine (?)
Cyclophosphamide (?)
Cytarabine (?)
Dactinomycin (?)
Desipramine (?)
Dextrothyroxine (?)
Diethylcarbamazine
Diethylpropion (?)

Diphenadione (?)
Dromostanolone (?)
Droperidol (?)
Epinephrine
Ergonovine (?)
Ergotamine (?)
Ethionamide (?)
Ethotoin (?)
Floxuridine (?)
Fluorouracil (?)
Fluoxymesterone (?)
Gentamicin
Glycopyrrolate (?)
Haloperidol (?)
Heparin (?)
Hydroxychloroquine (?)
Hydroxyurea (?)
Imipramine (?)
Indomethacin (?)
Levodopa (?)
Mechlorethamine (?)
Melphalan (?)
Mephenytoin (?)
Methimazole (?)
Methotrexate (?)
Methylergonovine (?)
Methylthiouracil (?)
Methysergide (?)
Nortriptyline (?)
Paramethadione (?)
Phendimetrazine (?)
Phenindione (?)
Phenprocoumon (?)
Phentermine (?)
Pipobroman (?)
Procarbazine (?)
Propylthiouracil (?)
Protriptyline (?)
Testolactone (?)
Testosterone (?)
Thiotepa
Tolazamide (?)
Tolbutamide (?)
Triethylenemelamine (?)
Trifluperidol (?)
Trimethadione (?)
Uracil Mustard (?)
Vinblastine (?)
Vincristine (?)

311

Loss of Eyelashes or Eyebrows (Cont'd)
Vitamin A
Warfarin (?)

Macular Edema
Acetazolamide
Aluminum Nicotinate
Dichlorphenamide
Diiodohydroxyquin
Epinephrine
Ethambutol
Ethoxzolamide
Griseofulvin
Hexamethonium
Indomethacin (?)
Iodide and Iodine Solutions and
  Compounds
Iodochlorhydroxyquin
Methazolamide
Niacinamide
Nicotinic Acid
Nicotinyl Alcohol
Phenylephrine (?)
Quinine
Radioactive Iodides

Macular or Paramacular Degeneration
Adrenal Cortex Injection (?)
Aldosterone (?)
Allopurinol (?)
Amodiaquine
Betamethasone (?)
Chloroquine
Cortisone (?)
Desoxycorticosterone (?)
Dexamethasone (?)
Diiodohydroxyquin
Fludrocortisone (?)
Fluprednisolone (?)
Griseofulvin
Hydrocortisone (?)
Hydroxychloroquine
Indomethacin (?)
Iodochlorhydroxyquin
Methylprednisolone (?)
Oral Contraceptives
Paramethasone (?)
Prednisolone (?)
Prednisone (?)

Quinine
Triamcinolone (?)

Miosis
Acetophenazine
Acetylcholine
Alcohol
Allobarbital
Ambenonium
Amobarbital
Aprobarbital
Barbital
Bromide
Bromisovalum
Bupivacaine
Butabarbital
Butalbital
Butallylonal
Butaperazine
Butethal
Carbachol
Carbromal
Carisoprodol
Carphenazine
Chloral Hydrate
Chloroform
Chloroprocaine
Chlorpromazine
Chlorprothixene
Codeine
Cyclobarbital
Cyclopentyl Allylbarbituric Acid
Demecarium
Dibucaine
Diethazine
Digitalis (?)
Droperidol
Echothiophate
Edrophonium
Ephedrine (?)
Ergot
Ergotamine
Ether
Ethopropazine
Fluphenazine
Haloperidol
Heptabarbital
Hexethal
Hexobarbital

312

Hydromorphone
Iodide and Iodine Solutions and
  Compounds (?)
Isocarboxazid
Isoflurophate
Levallorphan
Levodopa
Lidocaine
Meperidine
Mephobarbital
Mepivacaine
Meprobamate
Mesoridazine
Methacholine
Methaqualone (?)
Metharbital
Methdilazine
Methitural
Methohexital
Methotrimeprazine
Methyprylon
Morphine
Nalorphine
Naloxone
Neostigmine
Nialamide
Nitrous Oxide
Opium
Oxymorphone
Paraldehyde
Pentazocine
Pentobarbital
Perazine
Pericyazine
Perphenazine
Phenelzine
Phenobarbital
Phenoxybenzamine
Phenylephrine
Physostigmine
Pilocarpine
Piperacetazine
Piperazine
Piperocaine
Prilocaine
Primidone
Probarbital
Procaine
Prochlorperazine

Promazine
Promethazine
Propiomazine
Propoxycaine
Propoxyphene
Propranolol
Pyridostigmine
Radioactive Iodides (?)
Secobarbital
Talbutal
Tetracaine
Thiamylal
Thiethylperazine
Thiopental
Thiopropazate
Thioproperazine
Thioridazine
Thiothixene
Tolazoline
Tranylcypromine
Trifluoperazine
Trifluperidol
Triflupromazine
Trimeprazine
Vinbarbital
Vitamin A

*Myasthenic Neuromuscular Blocking
Effect*
  Bacitracin
  Chlortetracycline
  Colistimethate
  Colistin
  Demeclocycline
  Diphenylhydantoin
  Doxycycline
  Ethotoin (?)
  Kanamycin
  Mephenytoin (?)
  Methacycline
  Minocycline
  Neomycin
  Oxytetracycline
  Paramethadione (?)
  Polymyxin B
  Streptomycin
  Sulfacetamide
  Sulfachlorpyridazine
  Sulfadiazine

313

Myasthenic Neuromuscular Blocking Effect (Cont'd)

Sulfadimethoxine
Sulfamerazine
Sulfameter
Sulfamethizole
Sulfamethoxazole
Sulfamethoxypyridazine
Sulfanilamide
Sulfaphenazole
Sulfisoxazole
Tetracycline
Trimethadione (?)

Mydriasis

Acetaminophen
Acetanilid
Acetophenazine
Acetylcholine
Adiphenine
Adrenal Cortex Injection
Alcohol
Aldosterone
Alkavervir
Allobarbital
Alseroxylon
Amitriptyline
Amobarbital
Amphetamine
Amyl Nitrite
Anisotropine
Antimony Lithium Thiomalate
Antimony Potassium Tartrate
Antimony Sodium Tartrate
Antimony Sodium Thioglycollate
Aprobarbital
Aspirin
Atropine
Atropine Methylnitrate
Barbital
Belladonna
Benzathine Penicillin G
Benzphetamine
Benztropine
Betamethasone
Biperiden
Bromide
Bromisovalum
Brompheniramine
Butabarbital
Butalbital
Butallylonal
Butaperazine
Butethal
Caramiphen
Carbamazepine
Carbinoxamine
Carbon Dioxide
Carbromal
Carisoprodol
Carphenazine
Chloral Hydrate
Chloramphenicol
Chlorisondamine
Chloroform
Chlorpheniramine
Chlorphenoxamine
Chlorphentermine
Chlorpromazine
Chlorprothixene
Clomiphene
Cocaine
Colistimethate
Colistin
Cortisone
Cryptenamine
Cyclizine
Cyclobarbital
Cyclopentolate
Cyclopentyl Allylbarbituric Acid
Cycrimine
Cyproheptadine
Deserpidine
Desipramine
Desoxycorticosterone
Dexamethasone
Dexbrompheniramine
Dexchlorpheniramine
Dextroamphetamine
Diazepam (?)
Dicyclomine
Diethazine
Diethylpropion
Digitalis
Digoxin
Dimethindene
Diphemanil
Diphenhydramine

Diphenylhydantoin
Diphenylpyraline
Doxepin
Droperidol
Emetine
Ephedrine
Epinephrine
Ergot
Ether
Ethopropazine
Fludrocortisone
Fluorometholone
Fluphenazine
Fluprednisolone
Glutethimide
Glycopyrrolate
Guanethidine
Haloperidol
Hashish (?)
Heptabarbital
Hexamethonium
Hexethal
Hexobarbital
Hexocyclium
Homatropine
Hydrabamine Phenoxymethyl
  Penicillin
Hydrocortisone
Hydromorphone
Hydroxyamphetamine
Imipramine
Indomethacin (?)
Insulin
Iodide and Iodine Solutions and
  Compounds
Isocarboxazid
Isoniazid
Isopropamide
Levallorphan
Levarterenol
Levodopa
LSD
Lysergide
Marihuana (?)
Mecamylamine
Medrysone
Mepenzolate
Meperidine
Mephentermine

Mephobarbital
Meprobamate
Mescaline
Mesoridazine
Metaraminol
Methamphetamine
Methantheline
Methaqualone (?)
Metharbital
Methdilazine
Methitural
Methixene
Methohexital
Methotrimeprazine
Methoxamine
Methylene Blue
Methylpentynol
Methylphenidate
Methylprednisolone
Methyprylon
Morphine
Nalidixic Acid
Nalorphine
Naloxone
Naphazoline
Nialamide
Nitrous Oxide
Nortriptyline
Opium
Oral Contraceptives
Orphenadrine
Oxygen
Oxymorphone
Oxyphencyclimine
Oxyphenonium
Paraldehyde
Paramethasone
Pargyline
Pentobarbital
Pentolinium
Pentylenetetrazol
Perazine
Pericyazine
Perphenazine
Phenacetin
Phendimetrazine
Phenelzine
Phenmetrazine
Phenobarbital

315

Mydriasis (Cont'd)
  Phenoxymethyl Penicillin
  Phentermine
  Phenylephrine
  Pipenzolate
  Piperacetazine
  Piperidolate
  Poldine
  Potassium Penicillin G
  Potassium Penicillin V
  Potassium Phenethicillin
  Potassium Phenoxymethyl Penicillin
  Prednisolone
  Prednisone
  Primidone
  Probarbital
  Procaine Penicillin G
  Prochlorperazine
  Procyclidine
  Promazine
  Promethazine
  Propantheline
  Propiomazine
  Protoveratrines A and B
  Protriptyline
  Psilocybin
  Quinidine
  Quinine
  Radioactive Iodides
  Rauwolfia Serpentina
  Rescinnamine
  Reserpine
  Scopolamine
  Secobarbital
  Sodium Antimonylgluconate
  Sodium Salicylate
  Stibocaptate
  Stibophen
  Syrosingopine
  Talbutal
  Tetraethylammonium
  Tetrahydrocannabinol (?)
  Tetrahydrozoline
  THC (?)
  Thiamylal
  Thiethylperazine
  Thiopental
  Thiopropazate
  Thioproperazine

Thioridazine
Thiothixene
Tranylcypromine
Triamcinolone
Tridihexethyl
Trifluoperazine
Trifluperidol
Triflupromazine
Trihexyphenidyl
Trimeprazine
Trimethaphan
Trimethidinium
Tripelennamine
Tropicamide
Urethan
Veratrum
Vinbarbital

Myopia
  Acetazolamide
  Acetophenazine
  Adrenal Cortex Injection
  Aldosterone
  Aspirin
  Bendroflumethiazide
  Benzthiazide
  Betamethasone
  Butaperazine
  Carbachol
  Carphenazine
  Chlorothiazide
  Chlorpromazine
  Chlortetracycline
  Chlorthalidone
  Codeine
  Cortisone
  Cyclothiazide
  Demecarium
  Demeclocycline
  Desoxycorticosterone
  Dexamethasone
  Dichlorphenamide
  Diethazine
  Digitalis (?)
  Doxycycline
  Echothiophate
  Ethopropazine
  Ethosuximide
  Ethoxzolamide

316

Fludrocortisone
Fluphenazine
Fluprednisolone
Hyaluronidase
Hydrochlorothiazide
Hydrocortisone
Hydroflumethiazide
Isoflurophate
Mesoridazine
Methacholine
Methacycline
Methazolamide
Methdilazine
Methotrimeprazine
Methsuximide
Methyclothiazide
Methylprednisolone
Minocycline
Morphine
Neostigmine
Opium
Oral Contraceptives
Oxytetracycline
Paramethasone
Penicillamine
Perazine
Pericyazine
Perphenazine
Phenformin
Phensuximide
Physostigmine
Piperacetazine
Polythiazide
Prednisolone
Prednisone
Prochlorperazine
Promazine
Promethazine
Propiomazine
Sodium Salicylate
Spironolactone
Sulfacetamide
Sulfachlorpyridazine
Sulfadiazine
Sulfadimethoxine
Sulfamerazine
Sulfameter
Sulfamethizole
Sulfamethoxazole

Sulfamethoxypyridazine
Sulfanilamide
Sulfaphenazole
Sulfisoxazole
Tetracycline
Thiethylperazine
Thiopropazate
Thioproperazine
Thioridazine
Triamcinolone
Trichlormethiazide
Trifluoperazine
Triflupromazine
Trimeprazine

Narrowing or Occlusion of Lacrimal Canaliculi or Punctum
Adenine Arabinoside
Demecarium
Echothiophate
Idoxuridine
Isoflurophate
Physostigmine
Thiotepa
Trifluorothymidine

Night Blindness
Acetophenazine
Amodiaquine
Butaperazine
Carphenazine
Chloroquine
Chlorpromazine
Diethazine
Ethopropazine
Fluphenazine
Hydroxychloroquine
Indomethacin (?)
Mesoridazine
Methdilazine
Methotrimeprazine
Paramethadione
Perazine
Pericyazine
Perphenazine
Piperacetazine
Prochlorperazine
Promazine
Promethazine
Propiomazine

317

318

Methoxamine
Methylpentynol
Methylthiouracil
Methyprylon
Nitrofurantoin
Paramethadione
Pentazocine
Pentobarbital
Phenelzine
Phenobarbital
Piperazine
Primidone
Probarbital
Procarbazine
Quinine
Secobarbital
Sodium Salicylate
Streptomycin
Talbutal
Tetrahydrocannabinol
THC
Thiamylal
Thiopental
Trichloroethylene
Trimethadione
Tripelennamine
Tubocurarine
Urea (?)
Urethan
Vinbarbital
Vitamin A
Vitamin D
Vitamin D_2
Vitamin D_3

Objects Have Blue Tinge
Acetyldigitoxin
Alcohol
Amphetamine
Deslanoside
Digitalis
Digitoxin
Digoxin
Gitalin
Hydroxyamphetamine
Lanatoside C
Methylene Blue
Nalidixic Acid
Oral Contraceptives

Ouabain
Quinacrine

Objects Have Brown Tinge
Acetophenazine
Butaperazine
Carphenazine
Chlorpromazine
Diethazine
Ethopropazine
Fluphenazine
Mesoridazine
Methdilazine
Methotrimeprazine
Perazine
Pericyazine
Perphenazine
Piperacetazine
Prochlorperazine
Promazine
Promethazine
Propiomazine
Thiethylperazine
Thiopropazate
Thioproperazine
Thioridazine
Trifluoperazine
Triflupromazine
Trimeprazine

Objects Have Green Tinge
Acetyldigitoxin
Allobarbital
Amobarbital
Aprobarbital
Barbital
Butabarbital
Butalbital
Butallylonal
Butethal
Cyclobarbital
Cyclopentyl Allylbarbituric Acid
Deslanoside
Digitalis
Digitoxin
Digoxin
Epinephrine
Gitalin
Griseofulvin

Cyclobarbital
Cyclopentyl Allylbarbituric Acid
Cyclothiazide
Deserpidine
Deslanoside
Diethazine
Digitalis
Digitoxin
Digoxin
Ethopropazine
Fluorescein
Fluphenazine
Gitalin
Hashish
Heptabarbital
Hexethal
Hexobarbital
Hydrochlorothiazide
Hydroflumethiazide
Hydroxychloroquine
Lanatoside C
Marihuana
Mephobarbital
Mesoridazine
Methaqualone
Metharbital
Methazolamide
Methdilazine
Methitural
Methohexital
Methotrimeprazine
Methyclothiazide
Mild Silver Protein
Nalidixic Acid
Nitrofurantoin (?)
Ouabain
Pentobarbital
Pentylenetetrazol
Perazine
Pericyazine
Perphenazine
Phenacetin
Phenobarbital
Piperacetazine
Polythiazide
Primidone
Probarbital
Prochlorperazine
Promazine

Promethazine
Propiomazine
Quinacrine
Rauwolfia Serpentina
Rescinnamine
Reserpine
Secobarbital
Silver Nitrate
Silver Protein
Sodium Salicylate
Streptomycin
Sulfacetamide
Sulfachlorpyridazine
Sulfadiazine
Sulfadimethoxine
Sulfamerazine
Sulfameter
Sulfamethizole
Sulfamethoxazole
Sulfamethoxypyridazine
Sulfanilamide
Sulfaphenazole
Sulfisoxazole
Syrosingopine
Talbutal
Tetrahydrocannabinol
THC
Thiabendazole
Thiamylal
Thiethylperazine
Thiopental
Thiopropazate
Thioproperazine
Thioridazine
Trichlormethiazide
Trifluoperazine
Triflupromazine
Trimeprazine
Vinbarbital
Vitamin A

Ocular Exposure — Irritation
Adenine Arabinoside
Alcian Blue·
Alcohol
Amphotericin B
Ampicillin
Atropine
Aurothioglucose

Aurothioglycanide
Bacitracin
Benoxinate
Benzalkonium
Benzathine Penicillin G
Butacaine
Carbenicillin
Cefazolin
Cephalexin
Cephaloglycin
Cephaloridine
Cephalothin
Chloramphenicol
Chloroform
Chlortetracycline
Chrysarobin
Cloxacillin
Cocaine
Colistin
Colloidal Silver
Cortisone
Cyclopentolate
Cytarabine
Demecarium
Dexamethasone
Dibucaine
Dicloxacillin
Dimercaprol
Dimethyl Sulfoxide
DMSO
Dyclonine
Echothiophate
Emetine
Ephedrine
Epinephrine
Erythromycin
Ether
Ferrocholinate
Ferrous Fumarate
Ferrous Gluconate
Ferrous Succinate
Ferrous Sulfate
Fluorescein
Fluorometholone
Fluorouracil
Framycetin
Gentamicin
Glycerin

Gold Au^{198}
Gold Sodium Thiomalate
Guanethidine
Hetacillin
Homatropine
Hyaluronidase
Hydrabamine Phenoxymethyl
  Penicillin
Hydrocortisone
Hydroxyamphetamine
Idoxuridine
Iodine Solution
Iron Dextran
Iron Sorbitex
Isoflurophate
Kanamycin
Lincomycin
Medrysone
Methicillin
Methylene Blue
Methylprednisolone
Mild Silver Protein
Nafcillin
Naphazoline
Neomycin
Neostigmine
Nystatin
Oxacillin
Phenacaine
Phenoxymethyl Penicillin
Phenylephrine
Physostigmine
Pilocarpine
Piperocaine
Polymyxin B
Polysaccharide-Iron Complex
Potassium Penicillin G
Potassium Penicillin V
Potassium Phenethicillin
Potassium Phenoxymethyl Penicillin
Pralidoxime
Prednisolone
Procaine Penicillin G
Proparacaine
Propranolol
Quinacrine
Rose Bengal
Scopolamine
Silicone

322

Silver Nitrate
Silver Protein
Sodium Chloride
Streptomycin
Sulfacetamide
Sulfamethizole
Sulfisoxazole
Tetracaine
Tetracycline
Tetrahydrozoline
Thiotepa
Trichloroethylene
Trifluorothymidine
Tropicamide
Trypan Blue
Vinblastine

Ocular Teratogenic Effects
Acenocoumarin (?)
Acetophenazine (?)
Actinomycin C (?)
Aminopterin (?)
Amodiaquine (?)
Aspirin
Azathioprine (?)
Bishydroxycoumarin (?)
Bleomycin (?)
Busulfan (?)
Butaperazine (?)
Carphenazine (?)
Chlorambucil (?)
Chloroquine (?)
Chlorpromazine (?)
Cyclizine (?)
Cyclophosphamide (?)
Cytarabine (?)
Dactinomycin (?)
Diethazine (?)
Diphenylhydantoin (?)
Dromostanolone (?)
Ethopropazine (?)
Floxuridine (?)
Fluorouracil (?)
Fluoxymesterone (?)
Fluphenazine (?)
Furosemide (?)
Hashish (?)
Hydroxychloroquine (?)
Hydroxyurea (?)

LSD (?)
Lysergide (?)
Marihuana (?)
Mechlorethamine (?)
Melphalan (?)
Mercaptopurine (?)
Mescaline (?)
Mesoridazine (?)
Methdilazine (?)
Methotrexate (?)
Methotrimeprazine (?)
Mithramycin (?)
Mitotane (?)
Perazine (?)
Pericyazine (?)
Perphenazine (?)
Phenprocoumon (?)
Piperacetazine (?)
Pipobroman (?)
Primidone (?)
Procarbazine (?)
Prochlorperazine (?)
Promazine (?)
Promethazine (?)
Propiomazine (?)
Psilocybin (?)
Quinacrine (?)
Quinine (?)
Radioactive Iodides
Sodium Salicylate
Testolactone (?)
Testosterone (?)
Tetrahydrocannabinol (?)
THC (?)
Thiethylperazine (?)
Thioguanine (?)
Thiopropazate (?)
Thioproperazine (?)
Thioridazine (?)
Thiotepa (?)
Triethylenemelamine (?)
Trifluoperazine (?)
Triflupromazine (?)
Trimeprazine (?)
Uracil Mustard (?)
Urethan (?)
Vinblastine (?)
Vincristine (?)
Vitamin D

Ferrous Sulfate (?)
Fluorometholone
Fluphenazine
Heptabarbital
Hexamethonium
Hexethal
Hexobarbital
Hydrocortisone
Hydroxychloroquine
Iodide and Iodine Solutions and
  Compounds
Iodochlorhydroxyquin
Iron Dextran (?)
Iron Sorbitex (?)
Isoniazid
Lidocaine (?)
Medrysone
Mephobarbital
Mepivacaine (?)
Mesoridazine
Metharbital
Methdilazine
Methitural
Methohexital
Methotrimeprazine
Methylene Blue
Methylprednisolone
Nitroglycerin (?)
Oral Contraceptives
Oxyphenbutazone
Pentobarbital
Perazine
Pericyazine
Perphenazine
Phenobarbital
Phenylbutazone
Piperacetazine
Polysaccharide-Iron Complex (?)
Prednisolone
Prilocaine (?)
Primidone
Probarbital
Procaine (?)
Prochlorperazine
Promazine
Promethazine
Propiomazine
Propoxycaine (?)
Quinine

Radioactive Iodides
Rauwolfia Serpentina (?)
Rescinnamine (?)
Reserpine (?)
Secobarbital
Sodium Antimonylgluconate
Sodium Salicylate
Stibocaptate
Stibophen
Streptomycin
Sulfacetamide (?)
Sulfachlorpyridazine (?)
Sulfadiazine (?)
Sulfadimethoxine (?)
Sulfamerazine (?)
Sulfameter (?)
Sulfamethizole (?)
Sulfamethoxazole (?)
Sulfamethoxypyridazine (?)
Sulfanilamide (?)
Sulfaphenazole (?)
Sulfisoxazole (?)
Syrosingopine (?)
Talbutal
Thiamylal
Thiethylperazine
Thiopental
Thiopropazate
Thioproperazine
Thioridazine
Thyroid (?)
Trichloroethylene
Trifluoperazine
Triflupromazine
Trimeprazine
Tryparsamide
Vinbarbital
Vitamin D
Vitamin D_2
Vitamin D_3

Oscillopsia
  Allobarbital
  Amobarbital
  Aprobarbital
  Barbital
  Butabarbital
  Butalbital
  Butallylonal

325

326

Propiomazine
Propoxycaine (?)
Quinine
Secobarbital
Sodium Antimonylgluconate
Sodium Salicylate
Stibocaptate
Stibophen
Sulfacetamide
Sulfachlorpyridazine
Sulfadiazine
Sulfadimethoxine
Sulfamerazine
Sulfameter
Sulfamethizole
Sulfamethoxazole
Sulfamethoxypyridazine
Sulfanilamide
Sulfaphenazole
Sulfisoxazole
Talbutal
Thiamylal
Thiethylperazine
Thiopental
Thiopropazate
Thioproperazine
Thioridazine
Tranylcypromine (?)
Trifluoperazine
Triflupromazine
Trimeprazine
Vinbarbital
Vitamin D
Vitamin D_2
Vitamin D_3

Papilledema Secondary to
Pseudotumor Cerebri
Adrenal Cortex Injection
Aldosterone
Betamethasone
Chlortetracycline
Cortisone
Demeclocycline
Desoxycorticosterone
Dexamethasone
Doxycycline
Fludrocortisone
Fluprednisolone

Gentamicin
Griseofulvin
Hydrocortisone
Methacycline
Methylprednisolone
Minocycline
Oral Contraceptives
Oxytetracycline
Paramethasone
Prednisolone
Prednisone
Tetracycline
Triamcinolone
Vitamin A

Paralysis of Accommodation
Acetophenazine
Adiphenine
Alcohol
Amitriptyline
Anisindione
Anisotropine
Atropine
Atropine Methylnitrate
Belladonna
Bendroflumethiazide
Benzthiazide
Benztropine
Biperiden
Butaperazine
Caramiphen
Carbinoxamine
Carbon Dioxide
Carphenazine
Chloramphenicol
Chlorisondamine
Chlorothiazide
Chlorphenoxamine
Chlorpromazine
Chlorthalidone
Cocaine
Cortisone
Cyclopentolate
Cyclothiazide
Cycrimine
Desipramine
Dexamethasone
Dicyclomine
Diethazine

327

328

Fludrocortisone
Fluprednisolone
Gold Au^{198}
Gold Sodium Thiomalate
Hydrocortisone
Hydroxychloroquine
Ibuprofen (?)
Imipramine
Iodide and Iodine Solutions and
  Compounds (?)
Lidocaine
Mepivacaine
Meprobamate
Methyldopa (?)
Methylprednisolone
Nitrofurantoin
Nortriptyline
Oral Contraceptives
Oxyphenbutazone
Paramethasone
Phenylbutazone
Piperazine
Piperocaine
Prednisolone
Prednisone
Prilocaine
Procaine
Propoxycaine
Protriptyline
Radioactive Iodides (?)
Sodium Salicylate
Succinylcholine
Tetracaine
Triamcinolone
Trichloroethylene
Tubocurarine
Vinblastine
Vincristine
Vitamin A

Paresis of Extraocular Muscles
  Acetohexamide
  Adrenal Cortex Injection
  Aldosterone
  Allobarbital
  Amitriptyline
  Amobarbital
  Amphotericin B
  Aprobarbital

Barbital
Betamethasone
Bupivacaine
Butabarbital
Butalbital
Butallylonal
Butethal
Chloroprocaine
Chlorpropamide
Colchicine
Cortisone
Cyclobarbital
Cyclopentyl Allylbarbituric Acid
Desipramine
Desoxycorticosterone
Dexamethasone
Digitalis
Digitoxin
Dimethyl Tubocurarine Iodide
Disulfiram
Ethambutol
Fludrocortisone
Fluprednisolone
Griseofulvin (?)
Heptabarbital
Hexethal
Hexobarbital
Hydrocortisone
Imipramine
Insulin
Isoniazid
Levodopa
Lidocaine
Mephenesin
Mephobarbital
Mepivacaine
Metharbital
Methitural
Methohexital
Methylene Blue
Methylprednisolone
Nalidixic Acid
Nortriptyline
Paramethasone
Pentobarbital
Phenobarbital
Prednisolone
Prednisone
Prilocaine

329

Paresis of Extraocular Muscles (Cont'd)
- Primidone
- Probarbital
- Procaine
- Propoxycaine
- Protriptyline
- Secobarbital
- Talbutal
- Thiamylal
- Thiopental
- Tolazamide
- Tolbutamide
- Triamcinolone
- Trichloroethylene
- Tubocurarine
- Vinbarbital
- Vinblastine
- Vincristine
- Vitamin A
- Vitamin D (?)
- Vitamin D_2 (?)
- Vitamin D_3 (?)

Periorbital Edema
- Carisoprodol
- Epinephrine
- Ethosuximide
- Fluorouracil
- Hexamethonium (?)
- Hydralazine
- Meprobamate
- Methsuximide
- Oral Contraceptives
- Phensuximide
- Sulfacetamide
- Sulfachlorpyridazine
- Sulfadiazine
- Sulfadimethoxine
- Sulfamerazine
- Sulfameter
- Sulfamethizole
- Sulfamethoxazole
- Sulfamethoxypyridazine
- Sulfanilamide
- Sulfaphenazole
- Sulfisoxazole

Photophobia
- Acetohexamide
- Acetophenazine
- Adiphenine
- Amodiaquine
- Anisotropine
- Atropine
- Atropine Methylnitrate
- Aurothioglucose
- Aurothioglycanide
- Belladonna
- Bromide
- Butaperazine
- Carbon Dioxide
- Carphenazine
- Chloroquine
- Chlorpromazine
- Chlorpropamide
- Chlortetracycline
- Clomiphene
- Demeclocycline
- Diazepam (?)
- Dicyclomine
- Diethazine
- Digitoxin
- Diphemanil
- Doxepin
- Doxycycline
- Edrophonium
- Ethambutol
- Ethionamide
- Ethopropazine
- Ethosuximide
- Ethotoin
- Fluphenazine
- Furosemide (?)
- Glycopyrrolate
- Gold Au^{198}
- Gold Sodium Thiomalate
- Hexocyclium
- Homatropine
- Hydroxychloroquine
- Isocarboxazid
- Isopropamide
- Levarterenol
- Mepenzolate
- Mephenytoin
- Mesoridazine
- Methacycline
- Methantheline
- Methdilazine

Methixene
Methotrimeprazine
Methsuximide
Minocycline
Nalidixic Acid
Nialamide
Oral Contraceptives
Oxyphencyclimine
Oxyphenonium
Oxytetracycline
Paramethadione
Perazine
Pericyazine
Perphenazine
Phenelzine
Phensuximide
Pipenzolate
Piperacetazine
Piperidolate
Poldine
Practolol
Procarbazine
Prochlorperazine
Promazine
Promethazine
Propantheline
Propiomazine
Quinidine
Quinine
Streptomycin
Tetracycline
Thiethylperazine
Thiopropazate
Thioproperazine
Thioridazine
Tolazamide
Tolbutamide
Tranylcypromine
Trichloroethylene
Tridihexethyl
Trifluoperazine
Triflupromazine
Trimeprazine
Trimethadione

Photosensitivity
Acetohexamide
Allobarbital
Amiodarone

Amitriptyline
Amobarbital
Amodiaquine
Aprobarbital
Aurothioglucose
Aurothioglycanide
Barbital
Bendroflumethiazide
Benzthiazide
Brompheniramine
Butabarbital
Butalbital
Butallylonal
Butethal
Carbamazepine
Carbinoxamine
Chlordiazepoxide
Chloroquine
Chlorothiazide
Chlorpropamide
Chlortetracycline
Chlorthalidone
Clindamycin
Cyclobarbital
Cyclopentyl Allylbarbituric Acid
Cycloserine
Cyclothiazide
Cyproheptadine
Demeclocycline
Desipramine
Diazepam
Dimethyl Sulfoxide
Diphenhydramine
Diphenylpyraline
DMSO
Doxepin
Doxycycline
Droperidol
Erythromycin
Floxuridine
Fluorouracil
Flurazepam
Gold Au^{198}
Gold Sodium Thiomalate
Griseofulvin
Haloperidol
Heptabarbital
Hexethal
Hexobarbital

331

Phenelzine
Phenobarbital
Phenoxybenzamine
Prednisolone
Prednisone
Primidone
Probarbital
Secobarbital
Succinylcholine
Talbutal
Tetraethylammonium
Thiamylal
Thiopental
Tolazoline
Tranylcypromine
Triamcinolone
Trichloroethylene
Trifluorothymidine
Tubocurarine
Vinbarbital
Vinblastine
Vincristine

Random Ocular Movements
Allobarbital
Amobarbital
Aprobarbital
Barbital
Butabarbital
Butalbital
Butallylonal
Butethal
Carisoprodol
Cyclobarbital
Cyclopentyl Allylbarbituric Acid
Heptabarbital
Hexethal
Hexobarbital
Ketamine
Mephobarbital
Meprobamate
Metharbital
Methitural
Methohexital
Pentobarbital
Phenobarbital
Primidone
Probarbital
Secobarbital

Talbutal
Thiamylal
Thiopental
Vinbarbital

Retinal Degeneration
Amodiaquine
Chloroquine
Cortisone
Dexamethasone
Ferrocholinate
Ferrous Fumarate
Ferrous Gluconate
Ferrous Succinate
Ferrous Sulfate
Fluorometholone
Hydrocortisone
Hydroxychloroquine
Indomethacin (?)
Iodide and Iodine Solutions and
    Compounds
Iron Dextran
Iron Sorbitex
Medrysone
Methylprednisolone
Polysaccharide-Iron Complex
Prednisolone
Radioactive Iodides

Retinal Edema
Acetazolamide
Acetophenazine
Adrenal Cortex Injection
Aldosterone
Amithiozone
Amodiaquine
Aspirin
Bendroflumethiazide
Benzthiazide
Betamethasone
Butaperazine
Carphenazine
Chloramphenicol
Chloroquine
Chlorothiazide
Chlorpromazine
Chlorthalidone
Cobalt (?)
Cortisone

333

Benzphetamine (?)
Butabarbital
Butalbital
Butallylonal
Butethal
Carbon Dioxide
Chloroquine
Chlorphentermine (?)
Clomiphene (?)
Cyclobarbital
Cyclopentyl Allylbarbituric Acid
Desipramine
Dextroamphetamine (?)
Diethylpropion (?)
Ergonovine
Ergot
Ergotamine
Ethambutol
Guanethidine (?)
Heptabarbital
Hexamethonium
Hexethal
Hexobarbital
Hydroxychloroquine
Imipramine
Iodide and Iodine Solutions and
  Compounds
Lidocaine (?)
Mephobarbital
Methamphetamine (?)
Metharbital
Methitural
Methohexital
Methylergonovine
Methysergide
Nitroglycerin
Nortriptyline
Oral Contraceptives
Oxygen
Pentobarbital
Phenacetin
Phendimetrazine (?)
Phenmetrazine (?)
Phenobarbital
Phentermine (?)
Primidone
Probarbital
Procaine (?)
Protriptyline

Quinine
Radioactive Iodides
Secobarbital
Streptomycin
Sulfacetamide
Sulfachlorpyridazine
Sulfadiazine
Sulfadimethoxine
Sulfamerazine
Sulfameter
Sulfamethizole
Sulfamethoxazole
Sulfamethoxypyridazine
Sulfanilamide
Sulfaphenazole
Sulfisoxazole
Talbutal
Thiamylal
Thiopental
Trichloroethylene
Vinbarbital

Retrobulbar or Optic Neuritis
Acetohexamide (?)
Acetyldigitoxin
Allobarbital
Aminosalicylic Acid (?)
Amitriptyline
Amobarbital
Aprobarbital
Barbital
Bromisovalum
Bupivacaine (?)
Butabarbital
Butalbital
Butallylonal
Butethal
Caramiphen (?)
Carbromal
Chloral Hydrate (?)
Chloramphenicol
Chloroprocaine (?)
Chlorpropamide (?)
Cyclobarbital
Cyclopentyl Allylbarbituric Acid
Cycloserine (?)
Desipramine
Deslanoside
Digitalis

335

Pericyazine
Perphenazine
Piperacetazine
Polysaccharide-Iron Complex
Prochlorperazine
Promazine
Promethazine
Propiomazine
Thiethylperazine
Thiopropazate
Thioproperazine
Thioridazine
Trifluoperazine
Triflupromazine
Trimeprazine
Vitamin D
Vitamin D_2
Vitamin D_3

Scotomas
Acetophenazine
Acetyldigitoxin
Adrenal Cortex Injection
Alcohol
Aldosterone
Allobarbital
Aluminum Nicotinate (?)
Amobarbital
Amodiaquine
Aminosalicylic Acid (?)
Aprobarbital
Aspirin
Barbital
Betamethasone
Bromide
Bromisovalum
Butabarbital
Butalbital
Butallylonal
Butaperazine
Butethal
Caramiphen (?)
Carbromal
Carphenazine
Chloramphenicol
Chloroquine
Chlorpromazine
Chlorpropamide (?)
Clomiphene

Cobalt (?)
Cortisone
Cyclobarbital
Cyclopentyl Allylbarbituric Acid
Deslanoside
Desoxycorticosterone
Dexamethasone
Diethazine
Digitalis
Digitoxin
Digoxin
Disulfiram
Emetine
Epinephrine
Ergot
Ethambutol
Ethchlorvynol
Ethopropazine
Fludrocortisone
Fluorometholone
Fluphenazine
Fluprednisolone
Gitalin
Heptabarbital
Hexethal
Hexobarbital
Hydrocortisone
Hydroxychloroquine
Ibuprofen
Indomethacin (?)
Iodide and Iodine Solutions and
    Compounds
Isoniazid
Lanatoside C
Lithium Carbonate
Medrysone
Mephobarbital
Mesoridazine
Metharbital
Methdilazine
Methitural
Methohexital
Methotrimeprazine
Methylprednisolone
Methysergide
Morphine (?)
Niacinamide (?)
Nicotinic Acid (?)
Nicotinyl Alcohol (?)

Fluorometholone
Fluorouracil
Fluprednisolone
Glycerin
Heparin
Hydrocortisone
Indomethacin (?)
Iodide and Iodine Solutions and
  Compounds (?)
Isosorbide
Lincomycin
Mannitol
Medrysone
Methylprednisolone
Mithramycin
Mitotane
Oxyphenbutazone
Paramethasone
Penicillamine
Phenacaine
Phenylbutazone
Piperocaine
Pralidoxime
Prednisolone
Prednisone
Proparacaine
Radioactive Iodides (?)
Rauwolfia Serpentina
Rescinnamine
Reserpine
Sodium Chloride
Sodium Salicylate
Sulfacetamide
Sulfachlorpyridazine
Sulfadiazine
Sulfadimethoxine
Sulfamerazine
Sulfameter
Sulfamethizole
Sulfamethoxazole
Sulfamethoxypyridazine
Sulfanilamide
Sulfaphenazole
Sulfisoxazole
Syrosingopine
Tetracaine
Triamcinolone
Trichloroethylene
Urea

Subconjunctival or Retinal
Hemorrhages Secondary to Drug-
induced Anemia
Acenocoumarin
Acetaminophen
Acetanilid
Acetazolamide
Acetohexamide
Acetophenazine
Actinomycin C
Allobarbital
Allopurinol
Aminopterin
Aminosalicylic Acid (?)
Amithiozone
Amitriptyline
Amobarbital
Amodiaquine
Amphotericin B
Ampicillin
Anisindione
Antimony Lithium Thiomalate
Antimony Potassium Tartrate
Antimony Sodium Tartrate
Antimony Sodium Thioglycollate
Antipyrine
Aprobarbital
Aurothioglucose
Aurothioglycanide
Azathioprine
Barbital
Bendroflumethiazide
Benzathine Penicillin G
Benzthiazide
Bishydroxycoumarin
Bleomycin
Brompheniramine
Busulfan
Butabarbital
Butalbital
Butallylonal
Butaperazine
Butethal
Carbamazepine
Carbenicillin
Carbimazole
Carbinoxamine
Carisoprodol
Carphenazine

339

Subjunctival or Retinal Hemorrhages Secondary to Drug-induced Anemia (Cont'd)

- Cefazolin
- Cephalexin
- Cephaloglycin
- Cephaloridine
- Cephalothin
- Chlorambucil
- Chloramphenicol
- Chlordiazepoxide
- Chloroquine
- Chlorothiazide
- Chlorpheniramine
- Chlorpromazine
- Chlorpropamide
- Chlorprothixene
- Chlortetracycline
- Chlorthalidone
- Clindamycin
- Cloxacillin
- Colchicine
- Cyclobarbital
- Cyclopentyl Allylbarbituric Acid
- Cyclophosphamide
- Cycloserine
- Cyclothiazide
- Cyproheptadine
- Cytarabine
- Dactinomycin
- Deferoxamine (?)
- Demeclocycline
- Desipramine
- Dexbrompheniramine
- Dexchlorpheniramine
- Diazepam
- Dichlorphenamide
- Dicloxacillin
- Diethazine
- Dimethindene
- Diphenadione
- Diphenhydramine
- Diphenylhydantoin
- Diphenylpyraline
- Doxycycline
- Dromostanolone
- Droperidol
- Erythromycin
- Ethacrynic Acid
- Ethopropazine
- Ethosuximide
- Ethotoin
- Ethoxzolamide
- Floxuridine
- Fluorouracil
- Fluoxymesterone
- Fluphenazine
- Flurazepam
- Furosemide
- Gentamicin
- Glutethimide
- Gold Au^{198}
- Gold Sodium Thiomalate
- Griseofulvin
- Guanethidine
- Haloperidol
- Heparin
- Heptabarbital
- Hetacillin
- Hexethal
- Hexobarbital
- Hydralazine
- Hydrabamine Phenoxymethyl Penicillin
- Hydrochlorothiazide
- Hydroflumethiazide
- Hydroxychloroquine
- Hydroxyurea
- Imipramine
- Indomethacin
- Isoniazid
- Levodopa
- Lincomycin
- Measles Virus Vaccine
- Mechlorethamine
- Mefenamic Acid
- Melphalan
- Mephenytoin
- Mephobarbital
- Meprobamate
- Mercaptopurine
- Mesoridazine
- Methacycline
- Methaqualone
- Metharbital
- Methazolamide

Methdilazine
Methicillin
Methimazole
Methitural
Methohexital
Methotrimeprazine
Methotrexate
Methsuximide
Methyclothiazide
Methyldopa
Methylene Blue
Methylphenidate
Methylthiouracil
Methyprylon
Minocycline
Nafcillin
Nalidixic Acid
Nitrofurantoin
Nitroglycerin
Nortriptyline
Oral Contraceptives
Orphenadrine
Oxacillin
Oxyphenbutazone
Oxytetracycline
Paramethadione
Penicillamine
Pentobarbital
Perazine
Pericyazine
Perphenazine
Phenacetin
Phenformin
Phenindione
Phenobarbital
Phenoxymethyl Penicillin
Phenprocoumon
Phensuximide
Phenylbutazone
Piperacetazine
Pipobroman
Polythiazide
Potassium Penicillin G
Potassium Penicillin V
Potassium Phenethicillin
Potassium Phenoxymethyl Penicillin
Primidone
Probarbital

Procaine Penicillin G
Procarbazine
Prochlorperazine
Promazine
Promethazine
Propiomazine
Propylthiouracil
Protriptyline
Quinacrine
Quinidine
Quinine
Secobarbital
Sodium Antimonylgluconate
Stibocaptate
Stibophen
Streptomycin
Talbutal
Testolactone
Testosterone
Tetracycline
Thiabendazole
Thiamylal
Thiethylperazine
Thioguanine
Thiopental
Thiopropazate
Thioproperazine
Thioridazine
Thiotepa
Thiothixene
Tolazamide
Tolbutamide
Trichlormethiazide
Triethylenemelamine
Trifluoperazine
Trifluperidol
Triflupromazine
Trimeprazine
Trimethadione
Tripelennamine
Uracil Mustard
Urethan
Vancomycin
Vinbarbital
Vinblastine
Vincristine
Vitamin A
Vitamin D

342

  Syrosingopine
  Tetrahydrocannabinol
  THC

Uveitis
  Alpha-Chymotrypsin
  Alseroxylon (?)
  Amodiaquine (?)
  Amphotericin B
  Bacitracin
  Benzathine Penicillin G
  Chloramphenicol
  Chloroquine (?)
  Chlortetracycline
  Colistin
  Cortisone
  Demecarium
  Deserpidine (?)
  Dexamethasone
  Diethylcarbamazine
  Echothiophate
  Erythromycin
  Fluorometholone
  Hydrabamine Phenoxymethyl
    Penicillin
  Hydrocortisone
  Hydroxychloroquine (?)
  Isoflurophate
  Medrysone
  Methicillin
  Methylprednisolone
  Neomycin
  Phenoxymethyl Penicillin
  Polymyxin B
  Potassium Penicillin G
  Potassium Penicillin V
  Potassium Phenethicillin
  Potassium Phenoxymethyl Penicillin
  Prednisolone
  Procaine Penicillin G
  Rauwolfia Serpentina (?)
  Rescinnamine (?)
  Reserpine (?)
  Streptomycin
  Syrosingopine (?)
  Tetracycline
  Thiotepa (?)

  Urokinase

Visual Agnosia
  Benzathine Penicillin G
  Hydrabamine Phenoxymethyl
    Penicillin
  Phenoxymethyl Penicillin
  Potassium Penicillin G
  Potassium Penicillin V
  Potassium Phenethicillin
  Potassium Phenoxymethyl Penicillin
  Procaine Penicillin G

Visual Hallucinations
  Acetophenazine
  Alcohol
  Allobarbital
  Amantadine
  Amitriptyline
  Amobarbital
  Amodiaquine
  Amphetamine
  Amyl Nitrite
  Aprobarbital
  Aspirin
  Atropine
  Barbital
  Belladonna
  Benzathine Penicillin G
  Benztropine
  Biperiden
  Bromide
  Butabarbital
  Butalbital
  Butallylonal
  Butaperazine
  Butethal
  Capreomycin (?)
  Carbamazepine
  Carbinoxamine
  Carbon Dioxide
  Carphenazine
  Cefazolin
  Cephalexin
  Cephaloglycin
  Cephaloridine
  Cephalothin
  Chloral Hydrate
  Chlordiazepoxide

Chloroquine
Chlorpheniramine
Chlorphenoxamine
Chlorpromazine
Chlortetracycline
Cocaine
Cyclizine
Cyclobarbital
Cyclopentolate
Cyclopentyl Allylbarbituric Acid
Cycloserine
Cycrimine
Cyproheptadine
Demeclocycline
Desipramine
Dextroamphetamine
Diazepam
Diethazine
Digitalis
Digoxin
Diphenhydramine
Diphenylhydantoin
Diphenylpyraline
Disulfiram
Doxycycline
Droperidol
Ephedrine
Ethchlorvynol
Ethopropazine
Flurazepam
Fluphenazine
Furosemide
Glutethimide
Glycerin
Griseofulvin
Haloperidol
Hashish
Heptabarbital
Hexethal
Hexobarbital
Homatropine
Hydrabamine Phenoxymethyl
  Penicillin
Hydroxychloroquine
Hydroxyurea
Imipramine
Indomethacin
Iodide and Iodine Solutions and
  Compounds

Isoniazid (?)
Isosorbide
Ketamine
Levallorphan
Levodopa
LSD
Lysergide
Mannitol
Marihuana
Mephobarbital
Mescaline
Mesoridazine
Methacycline
Methamphetamine
Metharbital
Methdilazine
Methitural
Methohexital
Methotrimeprazine
Methylpentynol
Methyprylon
Minocycline
Nalorphine
Naloxone
Nialamide
Nitroglycerin (?)
Nortriptyline
Oxprenolol
Oxyphenbutazone
Oxytetracycline
Paraldehyde
Pargyline
Pentazocine
Pentobarbital
Pentylenetetrazol
Perazine
Pericyazine
Perphenazine
Phenmetrazine
Phenobarbital
Phenoxymethyl Penicillin
Phenylbutazone
Piperacetazine
Piperazine
Potassium Penicillin G
Potassium Penicillin V
Potassium Phenethicillin
Potassium Phenoxymethyl Penicillin
Primidone
Probarbital

344

Procaine Penicillin G
Prochlorperazine
Procyclidine
Promazine
Promethazine
Propiomazine
Propranolol
Protriptyline
Psilocybin
Quinine
Radioactive Iodides
Scopolamine
Secobarbital
Sodium Salicylate
Sulfacetamide
Sulfachlorpyridazine
Sulfadiazine
Sulfadimethoxine
Sulfamerazine
Sulfameter
Sulfamethizole
Sulfamethoxazole
Sulfamethoxypyridazine
Sulfanilamide

Sulfaphenazole
Sulfisoxazole
Talbutal
Tetracycline
Tetrahydrocannabinol
THC
Thiamylal
Thiethylperazine
Thiopental
Thiopropazate
Thioproperazine
Thioridazine
Trichloroethylene
Trifluoperazine
Trifluperidol
Triflupromazine
Trihexyphenidyl
Trimeprazine
Tripelennamine
Tropicamide
Urea
Vinbarbital
Vitamin D
Vitamin D_2
Vitamin D_3

Index

347

65965